A Cast of Caregivers

Celebrity Stories to Help You Prepare to Care

Celebrity Stories to Help You Prepare to Care

A Cast of Caregivers

Sherri Snelling

BALBOA
PRESS
A DIVISION OF HAY HOUSE

Copyright © 2013 Sherri Snelling

Cover Artwork Design: Jennifer Jacquez
Cover Spotlight Image: Tuulijamala/Dreamstime
Interior Spotlight Image: Geopappas/Dreamstime

All rights reserved. No part of this book may be used or reproduced by any means, graphic, electronic, or mechanical, including photocopying, recording, taping or by any information storage retrieval system without the written permission of the publisher except in the case of brief quotations embodied in critical articles and reviews.

All brand or other names are trademarks, service marks or registered trademarks of their respective parties.

ISBN: 978-1-4525-5913-1 (sc)
ISBN: 978-1-4525-5914-8 (e)

Library of Congress Control Number: 2012918754

Balboa Press books may be ordered through booksellers or by contacting:

Balboa Press
A Division of Hay House
1663 Liberty Drive
Bloomington, IN 47403
www.balboapress.com
1-(877) 407-4847

Because of the dynamic nature of the Internet, any web addresses or links contained in this book may have changed since publication and may no longer be valid. The views expressed in this work are solely those of the author and do not necessarily reflect the views of the publisher, and the publisher hereby disclaims any responsibility for them.

The author of this book does not dispense medical advice or prescribe the use of any technique as a form of treatment for physical, emotional, or medical problems without the advice of a physician, either directly or indirectly. The intent of the author is only to offer information of a general nature to help you in your quest for emotional and spiritual well-being. In the event you use any of the information in this book for yourself, which is your constitutional right, the author and the publisher assume no responsibility for your actions.

Printed in the United States of America

Balboa Press rev. date: 11/29/2012

To my parents who cared for my grandparents,

my family who taught me how to care and love,

my friends who help me be fearless

and

my awe and appreciation for the

65 million Americans caring for a loved one today

For attractive lips, speak words of kindness.
For lovely eyes, seek out the good in people.
For a slim figure, share your food with the hungry.
For beautiful hair, let a child run his/her fingers through it
once a day.
For poise, walk with the knowledge that you never walk alone.
People, even more than things, have to be restored, renewed, revived, reclaimed, and redeemed; never throw out anyone.
Remember, if you ever need a helping hand,
you will find one at the end of each of your arms.
As you grow older, you will discover that you have two hands; one for helping yourself, and the other for helping others.

– Audrey Hepburn

Preface

When you become a caregiver, the spotlight in your life shifts. Your focus is now on your loved one – whether the person needing care is your parent, your spouse, your sibling, your friend or a child with special needs. I wrote this book to put the spotlight back on you – the caregiver. Your needs, your health, your happiness – are as important as those of the person for whom you are caring. You are the real star – for without you there is nothing but an empty stage. We are a nation of caregivers – 65 million Americans caring for loved ones who are ill, disabled, dying or aging. We are a cast of caregivers.

For the last few years I have been thinking about writing a book about caregiving. There were already a lot of good books on the shelves – mostly about a caregiver's personal journey, educational tomes and the *how-to* books. What could I add?

I knew I wanted to write something different. Mostly I wanted to write a book people would actually read. Knowing caregivers have precious little time to sit down with a book I wanted to make it a quick read with short and digestible chapters. I wanted to wrap all the science, information and expertise into something readable and relatable. And I wanted it to be helpful and hopeful.

Think of this book like mini appetizers, a buffet or snacks rather than a 7-course dinner – you can pick and choose what you want rather than sitting through the whole meal. You can read just one chapter and be informed and empowered.

And like anything that has to do with food, this book is for you but it is also to be shared. You may read this book for yourself or you may give it to a friend, spouse, sister, brother, mom or dad who may be caregiving or needs to realize the journey you will face together.

I noodled around with what I thought were great ideas and themes for the book but as my blogs started to get published by numerous online sites I came to a realization. The articles that got the most attention were my stories about celebrities who were caregivers. That was my *a ha* moment.

I have always had a love for movies, TV, music, sports and news. As a young girl I had asthma and allergies. Unfortunately, this kept me inside a lot since the pollens prevented me from playing softball or running track. While I eventually took to indoor sports such as gymnastics, my early childhood afternoons were spent inside dark movie theaters escaping into the magic of the latest Disney movie or watching TV with my little brother. So began my love affair with the movies and television.

We are a celebrity-driven culture. If we weren't, *People* magazine, *Entertainment Tonight* and the entire E! cable channel would not exist. And we are a society that largely pays more attention to pop culture than important facts. If you have ever watched the Jay Leno late night show you know this. He does a bit called *Jay Walking* where he asks questions of people on the street. An example: "What are the three main branches of government?" No one came up with the correct answer. Then he asked, "What are the names of the three elves in the Rice Krispies commercials?" Everyone got the correct answer (Snap, Crackle, Pop). I'm not saying we're a silly society – but pop culture is our touchstone in many ways. If you can't beat 'em, join 'em.

If I can get current and future caregivers to read this book because of the celebrity stories and entertainment references, I could wrap those stories in the helpful information I know caregivers need.

When I told my close friends and family about my idea, their first reaction was probably your reaction: celebrities don't have a lot of worries when it comes to caregiving. They have money and assistants and an entourage who will handle all those time-consuming, bank account-depleting activities regular caregivers face. In some instances, you are correct. Some of these celebrities have more financial resources than the average Joes and Jills to address their caregiving needs. But, they are still mothers, wives, daughters, husbands, sons, brothers and they experience the emotional roller coaster of caregiving just like we do – they just do it under the constant glare of intrusive paparazzi.

As I began to interview these celebrities I realized these stars are just like the rest of us. They feel guilt, they feel hopeless and they feel helpless. They struggle with making the right decisions for their loved one. They learn everything they can about the disease or disability changing their world and the one they love. And you'll read they aren't all sitting on goldmines to cover the costs of care today – financially speaking they are as ill-prepared as the rest of us for a caregiving future.

To hear the pain still fresh in Holly Robinson Peete's voice as she talked about her father with Parkinson's disease 10 years after losing him. To hear Joan Lunden, an intrepid journalist, admit she did not have a clue about where to start to find the care needed for her mom with dementia. To hear Alana Stewart quietly say she sometimes feels like she failed Farrah Fawcett in finding a cure for cancer. All of a sudden I realized caregiving is the great equalizer in our society. No matter who you are the caregiving path is not always easy and none of us know where to start. The caregiving emotional journey is a universal one and the statistics show most, if not all of us, will be taking it. In fact, many of the stars in the caregiving world – the experts in various areas I interviewed for the book – started their companies and nonprofit organizations or pursue their programs and services because they have been caregivers themselves.

I experienced caregiving in my late teens and early 20s as a supporting player to my mom who took care of my maternal grandparents. I was a senior in high school when my grandmother was felled by a devastating stroke and a college student when my grandfather went through a series of illnesses including cancer. I remember coming home on weekends and giving my mom a little respite after hearing about all the things she was doing to care for my beloved grandparents. She was often exhausted but also appreciative to give back to the parents who had given her so much.

In the case of my father, I watched him and my stepmom lovingly care for my ailing paternal grandmother who had the serenity of hospice care at home at the end of her life. Hospice teams are special angels in the health care world who help manage the loved one's pain and bring comfort to their daily existence while also giving emotional and spiritual support to the caregiver and other family.

While I was not the star of these caregiving scenes it prepared me for a role I know I will one day play. I was a caregiving understudy and have been learning and honing my craft ever since. Over the last decade I have focused on bringing more awareness and information to the nation's 65 million family caregivers. I have worked on several of the wonderful research projects conducted by the National Alliance for Caregiving as well as other projects through my career at one of the world's largest health and wellness companies.

Talking to caregivers all around the country has taught me a lot – mostly about what is needed to support this valuable yet overlooked and underappreciated cast of caregivers. Caregivers are the first responders in our health care crisis. As we experience the *age boom* happening in our society today – baby boomers and older generations who are living longer – caregivers will continue to take on an essential role.

The two biggest issues I saw with most caregivers were how to balance caring for themselves and how to start the caregiving conversations so they can prepare to care. This book is dedicated to helping you with both challenges.

In the end, one of the main messages of this book is to show you are not alone. Caregiving is a role which most of us will star or at least be a co-star. It is up to us whether we triumph or flop. When you become a caregiver, you have stepped into a spotlight. You will be a superstar and I applaud you.

Contents

Preface ix

Introduction xix

ACT I — STAR PERFORMANCES 1
Celebrity Caregiving Journeys, Lessons Learned and "Me Time" 3

Holly Robinson Peete 7
Superstar Sandwich Generation Caregiver 7

Joan Lunden 23
Coast to Coast Caregiving Coverage 23

Marg Helgenberger 41
Collecting Clues on Caregiving 41

Jill Eikenberry and Michael Tucker 55
Cooking Up a New Caregiving Recipe 55

Sylvia Mackey – "Mrs. 88" 71
A Football Wife Tackles Dementia and the NFL 71

Alan and David Osmond 85
Like Father, Like Son – In Perfect Harmony 85

Alana Stewart 103
Caring for an Angel 103

ACT II — THE ROLE OF A LIFETIME: CAREGIVER — 119

Casting Calls – Which Caregiver Role Will You Play? — 121

Trading Places — 127
Caring for a Parent — 127

The Parent Trap — 137
Sandwich Generation Juggling Act — 137

When Harry Met Sally — 143
Spousal and Partner Caregiving — 143

Bringing Up Baby — 149
Caring for Children with Special Needs — 149

The Sons Also Rise — 155
Men as Caregivers — 155

Brothers & Sisters — 161
Caring for a Young Adult — 161

Far and Away — 167
Long-Distance Caregiving — 167

Bravehearts — 173
Caregivers of Veterans — 173

The Joy Luck Club — 179
Caring for Multiple Loved Ones — 179

Lost Generation — 185
Children as Caregivers — 185

Angels in America — 191
Gay, Lesbian, Bisexual, Transgender Caregivers — 191

It's A Small World After All — 197
Multicultural Caregivers — 197

Away From Her — 203
Alzheimer's Caregivers — 203

Rehearsals – Which Caregiving Responsibilities Will You Face?   209

One Singular Sensation or A Chorus Line?   211
Solo act or team caregiving   211

Martin Scorsese or Woody Allen?   215
Family drama or comedy   215

The Three Faces of Eve   219
From hospital to home to hospice - care transitions   219

Raiders of the Lost Ark   225
Elder Law attorneys, Medicare, Medicaid   225

The Money Pit   233
Costs and savings of caregiving   233

Driving Miss Daisy   243
Senior driving safety, driving retirement and alternative transportation   243

Cocoon   253
Home safety modifications, home care services, respite care, senior living options   253

My Man Godfrey   279
Caregiving information, online matchmakers, telemedicine, advocates/navigators and professional geriatric care managers   279

Lost in Translation   295
Health care literacy and expert support   295

Drugstore Cowboy   303
Medication safety and adherence   303

Breakfast At Tiffanys   309
Nutrition and meals for your loved one and for you   309

Nine to Five   315
Working caregivers and employer support   315

The Jetsons   321
Aging and technology   321

Twister   337
Disaster planning when caregiving   337

Planes, Trains and Automobiles	**345**
Traveling with a loved one, caregiving vacations, hotels & services	345
Dr. Doolittle and The Sound of Music	**355**
Alternative therapies: pets and music	355

Curtain Call – How Will You Prepare for the End? — 363

Beyond the Bucket List	**365**
End-of-life wishes	365
Twilight	**369**
Hospice and palliative care	369
Sequels	**373**
Life after caregiving – coping with loss and paying it forward	373

Refreshments – How Will You Overcome Stress, Burn-out, Guilt and Depression? — 383

From Ghostbusters to Stressbusters	**387**
Learn to relax, reconnect	387
Backdraft and the Magnificent Seven – 7 Ways to Put Out the Flames of Burn-out	**399**
Sleep, sunshine, sustenance, sweating, soothing, sex, setting limits	399
Two for the Road – Get Off the Guilt Trip	**413**
Seek forgiveness, let go gracefully, find kindness	413
Misery – Dealing with Depression	**421**
Finding nature and words	421

Cue Cards – How Will You Find Happiness and Support? — 431

The Pursuit of Happyness	**433**
Humor, Hope, Having Fun	433
LOST and Found	**443**
Support Groups, Professionals, Personal Board of Directors, Friends	443

ACT III — COMING ATTRACTIONS 449

Dialogue Coach – How Do You Start the Conversation? 451
Becoming Meryl Streep 451

C-A-R-E Conversations^{SM} 453

Reality Show – How Do You Find Time for Yourself? 461
Me Time Monday^{SM} 461

That's a Wrap 467
You as Director of the Caregiving Show 467

Subtitles 471
Alphabetical List of Caregiving Acronyms, Jargon 471

Resources – You Are Not Alone 489

- Caregiving Advocacy and Service Organizations 489
- Caregiving Products and Technology 491
- Celebrity Web Sites 492
- Disease Organizations and Support Groups 492
- Driving 493
- Employers 494
- Financial - Costs of Caregiving 494
- Government Services 495
- Healthy Caregiver 496
- Home, Housing and Caregiving Hotels 496
- Legal 498
- Meals and Nutrition 498
- Membership Groups 498
- Specialized Caregiving Help 498
- Travel 499
- Veterans Caregiver 499
- Volunteer to Help Caregivers 499

End Credits 501

Acknowledgements 501
References and Notes 503
About the Author 511
Index 513

Introduction

Life is not so much about beginnings and endings as it is about going on and on and on. It is about muddling through the middle.

— *Anna Quindlen*

Every good screenplay – whether for a movie or TV series – has a similar story arc: a beginning, a middle and an end (kind of like life). One of my writing/film directing heroes is Nora Ephron, famous for *When Harry Met Sally, Sleepless in Seattle, Heartburn* and *You've Got Mail* among many other movies I'm sure you know. As I was writing this book, the sad news came Nora had passed away after a battle with leukemia. It makes me blue there will be no more Nora Ephron movies or books. But her wisdom and wit lives on. I read something she said to actress Rita Wilson about how to write a good article or book, "Tell them what you're going to tell them, tell them, then tell them what you told them." Thanks Nora.

What I am Going To Tell You

I'm going to start by telling you caregiving is complicated. Not just the act of caregiving but the entire universe you enter as a caregiver is complicated and a little chaotic. It can also consume you if you let it. There is no 1-800-CAREGIVER to help you (although some services and experts come close).

Since every caregiving situation is unique it is hard to predict the path your caregiving journey will take. This is why so many of us simply ignore planning for caregiving until it hits us on the head similar to how those anvils and cases of dynamite are always falling on Wile E. Coyote in the *Roadrunner* cartoons.

It would be easier if I could write about caregiving in a similar way Heidi Murkoff wrote about impending motherhood in *What to Expect When You're Expecting*. In fact, for many caregivers, I'm sure it would help to know your caregiving journey would only be nine months long. On average, caregivers spend 4.6 years caring for a loved one. The latest aging statistics point to the fact we will have more aging parents to care for than children over the next 20 years. Consider this book your *What to Expect When You're Caregiving* guide.

What is one of the most important messages of this book is this: *You are not alone*. You are part of a vast army of caregivers, celebrities are caregiving just like you, experts are there to guide you, speaking up and having conversations about caregiving will bring a circle of friends and others to support you. When you become a caregiver, there is hope. You can conquer caregiving. In fact, I am going to help you conquer caregiving in three easy steps:

1. Knowledge.

2. Communication.

3. Self-care.

What I'm Telling You

Knowledge is power. It allows us to take control, it empowers us. It can save us money and time. Knowledge is your friend in the caregiving world. This book will give you caregiving knowledge. You will learn all the ways you can become a caregiver – a role in life you probably won't miss playing.

This knowledge will better prepare you to care. You will learn about many of the things you may encounter as a caregiver and you will gather some expert information and resources to help you. You will read about celebrities and how they became caregivers. In their personal stories you may see similar emotions and challenges you face or have faced as a caregiver and you will realize you are not alone in this world of caregiving. You will learn tips and techniques about how to care for yourself as lovingly and intensely as you care for your loved one.

In many ways, caregiving is like the environmental movement: *Think Global. Act Local.* You will read about many national organizations that offer good information, tips and insights but the actual help you will need will be on a local basis.

Communication is the key to success. First of all, you need to learn the language of caregiving. It is mostly English but it's like speaking English with a Scottish dialect or accent. Don't get me wrong – I love the Scots – only three generations back through one of my grandparents and we're proud kilt wearers. However, if you come across a Scot who has a really thick accent, he's speaking English but you have to ask him to repeat what he said several times and even then you may still be confused.

This is what the language of health care is like. I have included a listing of acronyms and other jargon you will come across in the Subtitles chapter and you will learn other valuable language tips throughout the Rehearsals chapters. For instance, do you know what a GCM is and how valuable they will be to you as a caregiver? If you wanted to search for the latest technology to help you keep your loved one at home and safe, do you know what words to put into your Google search? Do you know what CAPS, CNA, DNR, ADL, PERS mean? You will learn…read on brave caregiver.

For instance, let's start with the word *caregiver*. To some, this means a professional – maybe a nurse or home health aide. To others, it means the unpaid family member caring for a loved one. This ambiguity has created confusion for all mankind. They've solved the riddle in the U.K. and Australia where family caregivers are known as *carers*. However, try saying that three times really fast. It trips on your tongue.

For our purposes, when I write the word *caregiver* – I am talking about the 65 million Americans who provide more than $450 billion worth of unpaid care to a loved one to keep the health care system afloat every year. This statistic is from AARP's 2011 survey called *Valuing the Invaluable - The Economic Value of Family Caregiving* in which they put a dollar amount on the unpaid care caregivers represent to society and came up with the whopping $450 billion. What does that mean exactly? AARP compared it this way: that is $89 billion more than the total spent by the U.S. government and state agencies for Medicaid in both health care and long-term care services and support; it is $42 billion more than the total sales of the country's largest company – Walmart – and $11 billion more than the total sales of the three largest auto makers – Toyota, Ford, Daimler – *combined;* and it would be equal to these caregivers handing each and every American citizen $1,500. If you are a caregiver, you deserve medals, parades and awards for the service you provide.

After you have learned the language, then you must practice your new linguistic skills. There are two ways to communicate but they both start with identifying yourself as a caregiver and understanding the valuable role you play in your loved one's care. The first part of this communication process is to stand up and be heard as a caregiver.

We are at the beginning of what I call The Caregiving Movement and you are part of it. Mary Furlong, PhD, author, professor and noted baby boomer trend expert identifies caregiving as one of the next big revolutions for our society.

"Since the 1960s, the baby boomers have ushered in social and cultural revolutions driven primarily by two things: health and life stage needs," says Furlong. "In the 1960s, the oldest boomers questioned authority and promoted the civil rights movement; in the 1970s it was the women's movement and equal rights; in the 1980s is was gay rights and a health and fitness craze; in the 1990s it became the era of connectivity through technology with the rise of the Internet, and the desire for nutritional supplements; in 2000 it was the environmental movement and a focus on wellness and alternative medicine. Our next revolution will include longevity, which is the business of living longer, and with it, the caregiver revolution."

Now that you realize you are part of this fierce and fabulous Caregiving Movement, it is time to also have the conversations with your loved ones. This is what I call the C-A-R-E Conversation[SM] and it is one of the hardest things you will face as a caregiver but it is essential to your mental health and your wallet that you do. The chapter on C-A-R-E Conversations will coach you through some simple concepts about starting these critical conversations with your loved one. As Americans, we are guaranteed Freedom of Speech under the First Amendment to the Constitution. Exercise your rights – as a caregiver, it's time to speak up.

Becoming a self-care expert is essential. The balancing act of caring for yourself while you are caring for a loved one is my mantra. It is essential. It is critical. If you ignore your own health and wellness needs you may become more ill than your loved one. Where does that leave us? We still have a loved one – your loved one – needing care and we now have you needing care as well. You can start to see the domino effect I am talking about.

When it comes to caregiving and caring for yourself, you will face mortal enemies: Stress, Burn-out, Depression and Guilt. What you will learn is how to take on these four big bad guys. You are Gary Cooper and it's *High Noon* time. Actually, it's more like a Fellini film or Cirque de Soleil. As a caregiver, you will need to learn to juggle, balance, work the high wire when having delicate conversations, you'll have to stretch and become more flexible and you might do some dancing. As a caregiver you will see it's time to join the circus.

Once you have the tools for caring for yourself you need a sure-fire plan to find the time for *me time*. Many caregivers know they should take better care of themselves but finding the time is like *Mission Impossible*. I have a plan you will read about that will ensure your mission is possible and it's called Me Time Monday[SM].

What I Have Told You

To recap: You will gain knowledge about caregiving, you will learn to speak the language of caregiving and health care and how to have the C-A-R-E Conversation, you will join the circus (learning how to care for yourself while caregiving) and learn how to find Me Time Monday. You may feel like you are on this caregiving journey alone. The following story may help you see how in your solitary as a caregiver you are always surrounded by love.

Caregiver Walkabout

There is a cultural tradition among Australian Aborigines that very closely resembles the journey caregivers take. It is called a *walkabout* and is a rite of passage for adolescent boys to become men. These young boys have no choice on whether they want to do this or not – it is a long-held tradition these people believe connects them to the land they love. They are sent out alone into the Outback, sometimes spending months in solitude. Many of the boys follow ancient *songlines* or *dreaming tracks* where they learn to find food and shelter – the same types of food and rock formations their ancestors found before them. During this quest, they develop deep self-awareness and when they return to their families they have a greater sense of who they are, their importance to their family and their heritage.

In many ways, caregivers are on a walkabout. You may feel you had no choice to become a caregiver. You may spend months or years feeling all alone in your journey. But along the way, you learn about food, shelter (and legal paperwork and insurance rules) in the care of your aging or ill loved one. When you return from your caregiving journey, hopefully you will feel a sense of connectedness to your past and your future. In this journey called life, you understand your purpose, your role. And while you may have felt alone in the *Caregiving Outback*, friends, experts and others were helping to guide you. They were in the stars and the whispers of the wind at night. When you open your eyes and realize you are or will be a caregiver, you will know you are not alone. Welcome to the cast of caregivers.

Act I

Star Performances

I've been through it all baby, I'm mother courage.
— Elizabeth Taylor

Star Performances

Celebrity Caregiving Journeys, Lessons Learned and "Me Time"

In the following pages you will read about some famous names and faces who have stepped into the same caregiving spotlight as you. Your first reaction may be, "But celebrities have all the money and resources in the world to ease the burdens of caregiving." While for some this may be true, the reality is that celebrities are still sons and daughters, wives and husbands, sisters and brothers, partners and friends. And the emotional caregiving journey is one they take with the rest of us. You will read about:

Holly Robinson Peete
SuperStar Sandwich Generation Caregiver

A father with Parkinson's disease, a son with autism – Holly has been a caregiver across the life spectrum. This actress, singer, talk show host, author and advocate did not accept defeat by these challenging back-to-back caregiving situations; instead she made her *mess* her *message*. Holly talks about the emotional tolls: the guilt of a long good-bye to a beloved parent, the impact of caring for a child with special needs on a marriage and nurturing her family to create a *new normal*.

Joan Lunden
Coast to Coast Caregiving Coverage

This iconic TV morning show host became a mom of twins (for the second time!) at age 54, manages a career and business enterprise and cares for a mother with dementia who lives clear across the country – all at the same time. Joan Lunden gives us the headlines on being better prepared, really understanding your loved one's needs and keeping the lines of communication strong so everyone thrives.

Marg Helgenberger
Collecting Clues on Caregiving

Before she was a film (*Erin Brockovich*) and TV star (*CSI*) she was a small town Nebraska girl with dreams of becoming an actress in the Big Apple. As this young starlet was finding her way, both of her parents were rocked by devastating illness – first her mom with breast cancer immediately followed by her father with aggressive multiple sclerosis. Marg talks about bridging the distance through these crises that brought her closer to family, home and her own heart.

Jill Eikenberry and Michael Tucker
Cooking Up a New Caregiving Recipe

They left *L.A. Law* for a little R&R in the Italian countryside. However, Jill and Mike became unexpected co-stars as caregivers of her mother with dementia. Moving mom from Los Angeles to New York City became the little slice of the Italy they longed for and created the family affair that has been at the heart of their careers and lives.

Sylvia Mackey "Mrs. 88"
Football Wife Tackles Dementia and the NFL

Her husband was considered one of the NFL's best tight ends earning credit for his Baltimore Colts' 1971 Super Bowl win and a place in the National Football League Hall of Fame. When knocked down by dementia, his resilient wife came up with a decade-long game plan to care for him. Along the way she also encouraged the NFL to support retired players and the families hit hard by brain-related illness resulting in the game-changing 88 Plan of health care benefits.

David and Alan Osmond
Like Father, Like Son – In Perfect Harmony

The say lighting never strikes twice but for the legendary entertainment Osmond clan it did just that. Not only is David following in his famous father's footsteps as a musician, singer/songwriter and entertainer, he is also living and thriving with multiple sclerosis which affects both father and son. Taking a look at caregiving from the perspective of the persons with the disease, these men talk about family, especially their wives at their sides, their faith and their power of positive thinking which they believe are the prescription needed to battle a chronic illness.

Alana Stewart
Caring for An Angel

Some friendships are special but the bond between Texans turned California girls, Alana Stewart and Farrah Fawcett, took them on a journey neither expected. Across oceans and emotions, Alana and Farrah prove that girl power can be healing power even in the face of the devastating *C-word*. And in the aftermath of loss, Alana talks about carrying on after caregiving and how there are still footprints in the sand.

Their stories are unique but you will recognize yourself in their emotional journeys. They share their caregiving stories, the lessons they learned along the way and how they find their "Me Time" with you.

Holly Robinson Peete

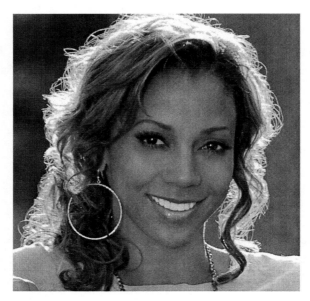

Photo: Courtesy of Holly Robinson Peete

Through humor, you can soften some of the worst blows that life delivers. And once you find laughter, no matter how painful your situation might be, you can survive it.

— Bill Cosby

Holly Robinson Peete

Superstar Sandwich Generation Caregiver

When it comes to superstars in this game we call *life* Holly Robinson Peete is a top draft pick. An actress, talk show host, singer, author, passionate advocate, wife and mother, Holly appears to have the perfect life. But even some of the most perfect pearls are formed through being tossed about in rough seas.

Holly's perfect life has faced two unforeseen and often devastating blows. While juggling a thriving acting career, marriage and motherhood, she was also caring long-distance for her father who suffered with Parkinson's disease (PD) and simultaneously learned one of her twins had autism.

What struck me the most when I spoke to Holly is how she uses humor to rule her household. On the day we talked, the kids were on their way to Starbucks but called several times with questions about mom's order that cracked Holly up. She joked to me, "Do you believe how crazy it is to just get a coffee around here?"

The Sandwich Generation of family caregivers – more than 24 million strong according to the National Alliance for Caregiving – is defined as someone who is sandwiched between generational care. You are caring for a child or children still at home while also providing assistance or full-time care to an older parent. In Holly's case, she is Super Sandwich Generation: dealing with a father with a progressive disease of the central nervous system, and raising twins, one who was healthy and active (her daughter Ryan), and the other (son R.J.), who was withdrawn and showing the symptoms of a special needs child.

For some people, this double hit would be enough to bring them down before the game even gets started. But Holly Robinson Peete learned to fight through to get to the goal line.

From *Sesame Street* to *21 Jump Street*

It was in the 1980s when Holly was at Sarah Lawrence College in Bronxville, New York, when her father started showing the early signs of what would be eventually diagnosed as Parkinson's disease. He was only 46 years old.

Her father, Matthew T. Robinson, Jr., was a producer and also played *Gordon* on the award-winning PBS-TV children's program *Sesame Street* in the 1960s and 70s. In the late '70s and '80s he went on to become one of the most prolific screenwriters for several TV series including the wildly popular, *The Cosby Show*. Just as her father thrived in TV, Holly wound up making her mark on the small screen as well.

In the 1980s and '90s, she decided to give acting a go, and was riding high on a career that saw her become a breakout TV star on *21 Jump Street* alongside a then unknown Johnny Depp, followed by her star turn on *Hangin' with Mr. Cooper*. During this time, since Holly's parents were divorced, it was up to Holly and her brother to support their father as his disease progressed.

It is estimated 1 million people are diagnosed with Parkinson's disease and each year there are 60,000 new cases in the U.S. This neurodegenerative brain disorder is characterized by a progressive destruction of cells in the central nervous system. The brain's inability to produce an adequate amount of dopamine causes nerve cells to fire incorrectly which then causes afflicted individuals to lose control of their normal body movements.

While later stages of the disease are devastating, early warning signs can be subtle and progress gradually. Not every PD patient has the same symptoms. Some experience poor balance and frequent falls, rigidity or muscle stiffness, tremors, and *Bradykinesia* which is the slowing down or loss of movement (shuffling steps, loss of one arm swing when walking, and difficulty or inability to turn the body). The most high profile people living with PD today are the actor Michael J. Fox and former world heavyweight boxing champion Muhammad Ali.

"My first reaction to my dad's diagnosis was what is Parkinson's?" says Holly. As a young college student, she raced to the library to find out everything she could about the disease. "I saw two words in the books I read: neurological and incurable. I felt helpless and in a dark place and it was hard. This was in a pre-Google period and there was no Michael J. Fox or Muhammad Ali who had raised awareness about Parkinson's." Holly struggled with whether or not she should quit college to take care of her father. "It was a very helpless time."

Double Dose of Devastation

While still providing care to her dad, Holly's career was taking off and so was her love life. She had fallen for Rodney Peete, who had been a superstar college football player at USC and one of the NFL's best quarterbacks with a 16-year career playing for the Philadelphia Eagles, Washington Redskins, Dallas Cowboys and Carolina Panthers. They were married in 1995, and two years later Holly was a sought-after actress, NFL wife and new mom to fraternal twins Rodney Jackson and Ryan Elizabeth.

It was at this exciting time for Holly, that life gave her two blows. Her father's illness was progressing to a point he needed around-the-clock care and Holly and her brother decided he needed to live in a special care facility. Since Holly lived in Los Angeles and her father was in New York, Holly became one of the 7-8 million long-distance caregivers.

"The day we moved my dad into the facility was singlehandedly the worst day of my life; to this day I still have regrets about the decision, but there really were not a lot of choices," says Holly with the pain still evident in her voice almost 10 years later. She had her twins, a husband who was on the road for six months out of the year and she was pregnant again. Moving her family to New York or moving her father in with her in LA really was not an option.

What was hard for Holly in those years was not being able to share the father-daughter moments with her dad. "I remember when 9/11 happened, and I wanted to talk to my dad about it, it was just so devastating but he wasn't really *here* anymore." In the end he was suffering from mild dementia, and any communication was difficult if not impossible. Holly couldn't bring him back into the world, and this emotional loss before the physical loss of her dad was really hard on her – she encountered a lot of dark moments. She says what is hardest for those caring for loved ones with brain-related illnesses is, "You break your butt to be there for them and help them and at the end of the day they don't even know who you are. You really have to dig deep to keep going."

Despite his decline, Holly still wishes she could have changed things. "To this day since my father passed away I still feel a tremendous amount of guilt," says Holly, her voice growing quieter. "That I wasn't there, that it didn't happen on my watch, the guilt, to be honest, never really goes away."

As Holly struggled with her dad's disease, she was noticing something did not seem right with her two-year-old son R.J. After watching some of his unexplainable behaviors continue, Holly took R.J. to be tested when he was three years old. The result was a devastating diagnosis: autism.

"I know it sounds like every cliché imaginable but when we were told about R.J., I felt like I was kicked in the gut, the carpet was pulled out from under me and my life just stopped right there in the doctor's office," says Holly. "I call that day the *never day* – we were told all the things my beautiful baby boy would *never* do. I felt 10 times more than helpless."

Holly recalls how the diagnosis of her son was very different from learning about her dad's disease. "Even though my dad was young when he was diagnosed with Parkinson's, it was totally different to be told that your three-year-old child will never really be anything."

What Holly and Rodney found as they struggled with their son's diagnosis and started to speak to other parents around the country is the best message is: Hope. "Every parent who gets a devastating diagnosis and is not given much hope by medical professionals should leave that office saying, 'I'm not going to let anyone tell me what my kid will or will not be.'" What you do have to do according to Holly is roll up your sleeves and become your child's best advocate. "You'll have a period of denial after you get the news. It's OK, you're human. Just move through denial quickly so that it does not steal time from you and your child when you can be discovering new interventions." Holly learned when it comes to autism, you have to move fast. Getting therapies underway, trying new diets, etc., are all critical in terms of time to intervene and improve your child's situation.

What Holly also learned from her journey is the healing power of time can be so essential to caregivers. "R.J. was diagnosed 11 years ago and in all fairness, a lot was not known about autism back then." Now with new books, talk shows, clinical studies, Internet information, as well as new drugs and alternative medicine techniques, knowledge is at our fingertips, and hope grows every day around new therapies and maybe even cures.

Mars vs. Venus

While Holly was recovering and regrouping over R.J.'s diagnosis, what happened next came out of left field. Her husband Rodney had been "my rock while I cared for my dad," always there to support his wife and the father-in-law who adored him. But suddenly with RJ's diagnosis, Rodney became withdrawn, frustrated and living in denial a lot longer than Holly did.

Since Rodney was on the road still playing in the NFL, Holly would send him books to read and magazine articles on autism, most of which she says he ignored. Because Rodney was in denial about R.J.'s condition, as is typical of fathers of special needs children, he distanced himself and was less involved in the daily struggle.

While it is estimated 85 percent of parents with special needs children divorce, Holly actually thinks the distance saved their marriage. "It gave me time to cope on my own without facing Rodney's different attitude and ideas about R.J.," says Holly. "Rodney originally thought R.J. just needed more discipline; I knew it wasn't about that at all."

In a study that looked at men and women caregivers of spouses and parents, Bowling Green State University researcher I-Fen Lin says, "Men take a block and tackle approach to caregiving. They're problem solvers and they'll look to finish a task and move on whereas women caregivers are more nurturing but also have higher expectations of themselves – they're more concerned with how their performance as a caregiver is judged, especially by the person they're caring for."

"This was the classic men are from Mars, women are from Venus scenario," says Holly. "Men and women just think and do things differently." Holly says Rodney struggled with being a world-class athlete and having a son who he could not toss the football around with. Holly says for a lot of men, "it impacts their manhood."

Holly encouraged Rodney to do two things. First, she thought Rodney would benefit from talking to other dads of sons with autism. While most men struggle with group therapy and see it as *touchy feely*, being able to hear other dads felt the same as Rodney really helped him. In addition, Holly encouraged her husband to write down his thoughts about being a father of a special needs child, which eventually became his book, *Not My Boy! A Father, A Son and One Family's Journey with Autism* chronicling his discovery about autism through his son R.J.'s eyes.

As she looks back on this period, Holly says if she could play Monday morning quarterback, "I would have been way more respectful of Rodney's denial, and I would not have looked at it like it was an affront to me and my child." Holly says spouses, especially women, need to be patient, since parents process things differently as men and women. They're each struggling with the emotional tools needed to deal with this challenge.

Although Holly admits she and her husband struggled with their marriage through this period, she credits Rodney with coming up with the winning game plan. "Rodney had that 'oh my god' moment when he realized he could lose his family, but he chose instead to enter into the fight and save us all." Holly said when she and Rodney got the same game plan going, everything changed.

"As I look back, I talk about Rodney's denial over R.J.'s autism, but I realize now that his denial over our son was the same denial I had with my dad – different people, different times – but still denial."

After 17 years of marriage, the night before Valentine's Day, February 13, 2012, Holly and Rodney renewed their marriage vows and their commitment to each other and their family with all four children as their attendants.

The Miracle Worker

After R.J.'s diagnosis while Rodney retreated, Holly got to work. She learned everything she could about autism in the same way she had educated herself about Parkinson's disease. Holly learned autism impairs a person's ability to communicate and socialize normally with others, and it often has a physical manifestation of repetitive behaviors. According to the Centers for Disease Control and Prevention (CDC), one in every 88 children has autism spectrum disorder (ASD), and symptoms can be subtle or significant. She also learned there is no cure for autism.

Given little hope by doctors for R.J.'s ability to assimilate into normal childhood, Holly refused this dismal outlook for her son and turned to alternative measures. She found a wonderful autism therapist who ran a preschool called SmartStart; she established a gluten-free diet for R.J. with very positive effects and she brought music into his life, which she found soothed her son.

"Music therapy became very powerful for my son," says Holly. In fact, R.J. has recorded his first music single and Holly believes it was a way for him to not feel *judged*, as he often did during sports or other activities. She says both music and animals have magical powers when it comes to autistic children and especially for R.J. Holly learned autistic children are very present – they know exactly what is going on around them; they just cannot verbally respond or express their emotions, and this is very frustrating for them. "I believe when you have a brain disorder or disease, music can make all the difference in the world." She also relates how music really soothed her father who along with his Parkinson's developed dementia in his last years.

She also maintained as normal a life as possible for her other children, which in addition to R.J.'s twin sister Ryan now included sons Robinson and Roman. One of the challenges for parents of special needs children is focusing so much on one child that the others don't get the same kind of attention. This can breed anger and resentment with those children who may feel overlooked or neglected. All children want to be the center of attention but when you have a sibling who pulls the focus all the time it can be difficult. Holly says since Ryan and R.J. are twins, the attention R.J. gets can sometimes make it even harder on Ryan. At one point, Ryan was feeling slighted. Holly feels sometimes she puts pressure on Ryan to be her brother's keeper and pushes her to help him fight his battles. "I have to remember she has her own popularity dramas and teenage angst," says Holly. "I have to stop myself and say she's 14 and trying to figure out who she is."

One of the ways Holly put Ryan on center stage was to co-author a book with her daughter about R.J.'s autism. "It was Ryan's idea," says Holly. "She looked for a children's book on autism and could not find one." At the same time, "She really wanted to have kids at school understand R.J. and what made him the way he is." The result was the book, *My Brother Charlie*, published by Scholastic. This project gave Ryan a hero's role in her brother's daily challenges and eventually won Holly and Ryan an NAACP Image Award. They are currently working on a follow-up book that addresses the teenage years of a girl with an autistic brother.

White Elephant in the Room

One of the biggest challenges facing the parents of special needs children is what will happen to their child after they are gone – it is the *big white elephant in the room*. Many children with disorders such as autism or genetic conditions such as Down syndrome are living longer and they are living at home. Easter Seals statistics show more than 80 percent of adults (ages 18-30) with autism still live at home. While this has helped these children have longevity and better quality of life, it also creates a huge fear for their folks.

"Ask any parent of a special needs kid and the number one fear is: What happens when I'm gone? Who's going to take care of him? How is he going to make it in this world?" Holly says all parents have some concern over their child's future, but a special needs parent has added woes. Her six-year-old son has been asking Holly a lot of questions about autism, and she had him read his sister's book. When Holly said to him, "So what have you learned about autism?" he replied, "Autism means you don't have friends." It is enough to break your heart, but Holly is grateful and confident her children will always be there for each other.

When you think about the future of your special needs child, you add to the basket of parental concern people's lack of empathy for special needs kids and adults, lack of understanding of disorders like autism, mean people, missed social cues that cause problems for your child and the list goes on. When contemplating this picture, the future can be frightening. "I still wake up in cold sweats about it," says Holly.

For the Peete family, the plan is Ryan and her younger brothers will always be there to take care of R.J. once Holly and Rodney are gone. "Some people say you put too much pressure on your other kids to ask that of them but it is understood when we're gone, you're all taking care of this guy." It's the team mentality and it works for the Peetes.

As R.J. has entered his teen years, he started traveling with Holly to do speaking engagements. The proud mom says, "He is lovely and sweet and articulate about his autism, and has crafted a great message about himself and what it is like to be a teenager going through this." Holly says R.J. realizes he is an advocate for autism and "he's working that." R.J. often asks his mom if he can go with her when he sees something on her calendar and he tells her, "Can I go with you? I have something to say to them." Laughing Holly says she thinks he's being a typical teen boy and may just want to get out of school, but his speaking has made a difference to other teens and she is really proud of him.

Holly's wish is as a society we come to understand more about autism and how these special needs people have special gifts and value they can give. The Center for Autism and Related Disorders (CARD) says 81 percent of adults ages 18-30 with autism are unemployed. In 10 years, ½ million autistic children will be adults with typical expectations for living into their 60s and 70s. The significant difference they face is a society that does not understand how to assimilate them and support them once their parents are gone. Right now, many autistic adults are homeless, and law enforcement and other officials struggle to understand the issues concerning autistic indigents.

In addition, because brain-related disorders still have a stigma in certain cultures, African American, Asian and Latino children are typically diagnosed 2-5 years later for autism than their Caucasian counterparts – a time period that can be critical for interventions. More knowledge about autism in general, but especially in minority communities, is Holly's dream, and she often speaks to church groups and nonprofit organizations about this topic.

"I hope we get to a place of empathy and eventually remove the stigma of autism," says Holly. It might take a little extra effort, but if you include them or hire them to do certain things, they can be valuable to society."

Holly told me one day she was in a bakery and noticed a special needs adult stocking the shelves in the back of the store. She took the time to find the manager and thank him for hiring that person. She told him, "I really appreciate that you hired that special person because that could be my son someday."

Finding Your Vault

As Holly was caring for her dad, her mom, despite having divorced Holly's father years ago, really stepped up to support Holly. "She also is a great grandma to all my kids, but she has a really deep connection with R.J." Holly says out of all the family and friends, her mom was the #1 cheerleader and so proactive in finding support for R.J. and for Holly. "She would bring over books or new research studies or spend time with R.J. – what she gave was unconditional love."

One of the hardest challenges in R.J.'s diagnosis was Holly watching friends fall away unable to cope with the issues of her autistic son. She told me of one incident when she and her children were at a friend's child's birthday party as R.J. began to cause a commotion by crying. While Holly tried to soothe him, her friend later told her she couldn't watch her child's birthday video because of R.J. crying in the background.

"I had a lot of friends who just really couldn't handle it; they kind of abandoned me emotionally," says Holly. "I was surprised how far removed they were. Now looking back I think they were fearful." Holly says having a special needs child becomes a great litmus test for who is truly in your corner.

What Holly found is she had to find a new language to explain to friends and family what autism is not just that her son has it.

"When I first told my friends about R.J., I would simply tell them he had autism; that was it," says Holly. Because there was not a lot of attention on autism even a decade ago when R.J. was diagnosed, this did little to help Holly's friends see into her world.

"One day, my son was repetitively twirling around in circles in the corner when a friend was at my house," says Holly. "She asked what he was doing." Instead of telling her friend, like she had told so many others, that R.J. has autism, she explained why he twirled.

"He needs that to stimulate himself – it calms him down." All of a sudden, the friend got it and was more interested in discussing this than what they had been talking about – she realized there is a reason for this behavior and while not normal to us, it is how R.J. copes. "It was like a light bulb went on for my friend."

When it comes to friendship, there is one person who has always been there for Holly. Her longtime friend Terri Ellis, who is part of the R&B group En Vogue.

"Terri does not judge, and our relationship is so pure – she was just there, she didn't know a lot of what autism is but she was there for me." Holly told me when she was on Oprah Winfrey's show she told Oprah, "Terri is *my personal vault*, meaning I know there is nothing I could say to her anyone else would ever hear from her lips. It's the most comforting feeling ever, and I don't have it with anybody else."

Team Peete Scores

One of the things Holly is grateful for is the special bond her husband and her father shared. Since her dad was a Philadelphia native, he could not have been more thrilled when his daughter married the star quarterback of the Philadelphia Eagles at that time. "My dad adored Rodney and Rodney adored him." When Holly was struggling with the decisions over her father's care, it was Rodney who suggested they do something to help others in the same situation.

"It was really Rodney who pointed out that we knew all these people and we owed it to ourselves, my dad and other people to start a nonprofit to help people. He was instrumental in saying we should use our sad situation for the good of others." The HollyRod Foundation was born in 1997.

Ever since, Holly and Rodney's passion play has been the HollyRod Foundation. Originally created to support families facing Parkinson's to honor her father, their mission was expanded to also help families living with autism.

The entire family works on fund-raising efforts and activities, as the foundation is the sole source of funding for the Compassionate Care Program for Parkinson's disease at the USC Keck School of Medicine. In addition, the foundation launched its *Give the Gift of Voice* program that provides augmentative communications devices, such as iPads with specially designed software, to help nonverbal children with autism communicate to family, peers and community.

Holly also competed on the third season of TV's *Celebrity Apprentice* in 2010 to vie for a position to work at Donald Trump's side. Showing her competitive drive, Holly raised the most money for any task in the show's history. She eventually was a semi-finalist on the show coming in second to that season's ultimate winner, singer Bret Michaels. She says about the experience, "The best part about being on that crazy show was my ability to have one of the challenges be about raising funds and awareness for the HollyRod Foundation and particularly for the kids with autism."

The Peetes are a great example of a family that has faced several challenges but have become stronger through those times by coming at life like a winning team.

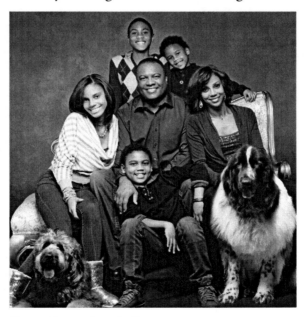

Photo: Christopher Voelker

Meet the Peetes

From Guilt to Gratitude

Holly says while she still has pangs of guilt of not being by her father's side when he passed, for the most part she has learned to work through her guilt over not being there more for her dad. She's done this by slowly not holding herself accountable anymore. But she has so much empathy for other caregivers who struggle with guilt over a loved one. "You know you shouldn't carry around guilt forever, but it's so hard to shake," she says. "It's important for people to understand that you have to move on with your life." Holly says the guilt of not doing enough, not being there 24/7, not making it better for your loved one is inevitable for all caregivers.

When it comes to her son, she says one of the blessings of caregiving is being there in the trenches every day and realizing as time goes on you are making a difference in your loved one's life. "One thing you tell yourself as a caregiver is, if you want something done right you do it yourself." But Holly says the burden of this attitude is you "chip away at your own physical and emotional stamina."

She recommends caregivers find a break for themselves, such as embracing a higher power and spiritual awareness. You have to have something that refreshes and replenishes your soul. And she says you have to constantly remind yourself of the good job you are doing as a caregiver. If you can do this, Holly feels the job of caregiving becomes easier.

How she finally overcame the guilt, both from caregiving for her dad and also helping her son, is by celebrating the impact of the HollyRod Foundation. The foundation has helped so many families just like hers who needed answers and support. She feels grateful her family has created a place where other families can find hope and help.

"At some point, you take your guilt and you move on, and I did that by paying it forward," says Holly. "Knowing my family can help others and maybe ease their caregiving journey is the best gift of all."

Spoken like a true superstar.

Holly's Lessons Learned

1. Lifelong Learning

Life is really about learning – we never stop being students. As Holly's story demonstrates, she began her caregiver journey as a young student and continues her caregiving education to this day with the ongoing challenges of R.J. and his autism. Now that R.J. is a teenager, Holly is coping with the typical teen dramas of her twins but also how to help R.J. develop into a young man who society will see as someone who can add value.

Holly's caregiving journey spanned two different information eras: one without the Internet or much available information and one where Google has given us even more information than we could have imagined. This is both a blessing and a burden. We now can arm ourselves with questions to ask physicians, specialists and others through our online research. However, what is difficult for caregivers is having the time to troll every Internet site that offers information about a loved one's disease and then knowing where to turn next and what information to trust.

One of the best places to start is with the online organization for the disease that your loved one has. In Holly's case this would have been the National Parkinson Foundation (founded 50 years ago) and Autism Speaks (which was founded four years after R.J. was diagnosed and where Holly is on the board). From there, you can continue to search for other resources such as Holly's organization, the HollyRod Foundation or the Michael J. Fox Foundation for Parkinson's Research, where innovative or local programs outside the typical nonprofit disease organizations may exist.

These online resources are very reliable and often have information vital to caregivers such as recent research, clinical trials, information about the disease and how to connect with others who are facing the same challenges as you. Information is power and the wonderful world of the digital age has given us this gift. See the Resource section of the book for contact information for many of these organizations.

2. Let Go of the Guilt

Guilt is a very basic human emotion, and in caregiving situations, guilt is very common. If you are feeling sad, regretful, powerless or even grieving about your loved one's situation – this is actually *good guilt* – embrace these emotions and don't let them swallow you up. Instead of feeling guilty about her dad, Holly and family celebrate him every January 1 – his birthday and the start of a new year. "We play the same old tunes he used to love, we dance, we laugh, we tell our kids who didn't know him stories about him, we watch old episodes of *Sesame Street* and *The Cosby Show*." In other words, rather than mourning their loss, they celebrate the life and the man.

3. Educate and Communicate

In Holly's story we see how little we all know about chronic illness until it strikes us or someone we love. Part of our role as caregivers is to help others understand the disease or disorder. Holly found once she started explaining R.J.'s autism to her friends who really cared rather than just simply telling them about his condition, people started to provide her with support rather than avoiding her.

4. Build Your Team

Any good captain knows you have to have a strong team if you want to win. If you are the captain of your caregiving team – find strong recruits and focus on their strengths. Every member of the Peete family has a role in caring for R.J. in some way. Ryan has a role in educating her younger friends about R.J.'s autism, Rodney runs their foundation which helps hundreds of other families and that helps Holly feel better about what their family has faced. Holly's other kids are also involved in helping with R.J. And Holly has her mom and other strong, real friendships that give her an emotional and physical break when she needs it.

Another part of Holly's team are the professionals she has learned from. Having trusted experts in your circle of care is essential to give you the peace of mind you have researched all the avenues available. These experts also give you confidence the choices you help make for your loved one are the best available.

How Holly Finds Her "Me Time"

Holly admits she has great help from both her husband and her mother to get a break and take care of herself. When she has the time, she indulges in an occasional spa day or even a quick massage. "Just to pamper yourself is so important." If she cannot find time to break away for a massage – a long, luxurious bath will do – anything that provides a warm embrace and soothes body and mind.

She also indulges in quiet time. "I try to find an afternoon just for a couple of hours when I can grab a book and go to the beach. Listening to the waves break on the sand, the relative quiet and solitude of the ocean refreshes me. It is very difficult to find these moments, but when I can I have long since given up feeling guilty about it." She says she learned if she shuts down, the whole "Robinson Peete operation shuts down."

She also has her *girl time* – spending a long lunch with a good friend like Terri lets her recharge her batteries.

But mostly Holly revels in being a mom. She loves being with her kids, teaching them to help each other and help others.

Joan Lunden

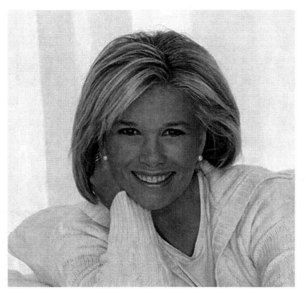

Photo: Courtesy of Joan Lunden

Life is a voyage that is homeward bound.

— Herman Melville

Joan Lunden

Coast to Coast Caregiving Coverage

For 17 years throughout the 1980s and 1990s, she woke us all with "Good Morning America" as co-host of ABC-TV's morning broadcast. But it was only a few years ago that Joan Lunden, the sunny, blonde, adventurous TV journalist got her own wake-up call.

She remembers it like it was yesterday. In her words, "it 100 percent shook me up."

I first met Joan when she hosted a caregiving special series on the RLTV cable channel, *Taking Care with Joan Lunden*. I was one of the featured experts that Joan interviewed on the show and we had a chance to talk about her caregiving situation with her mom. Her story was so poignant; I called her a year later to talk more about the details of her caregiving journey for several articles and this book.

It was back in 2006 that her brother Jeff, who had long suffered from type 2 diabetes, passed away. Joan had been caregiving for both her ailing brother as well as her then 87-year-old mother, Gladyce. While her brother suffered the ravages of diabetes – blurred vision, headaches, operations on his hands and feet – her mom suffered from signs of dementia and had several mini strokes over the years. For both their safety and Joan's peace of mind, she had purchased a condominium in the Sacramento, California area where Joan had grown up, and paid for them both to live there together.

Meanwhile, Joan lived across the country in her home base of Connecticut, where she was raising two sets of twins under the age of 10 with her second husband and playing empty nest mom to her three older daughters from her first marriage. In addition, she had not slowed down since leaving *Good Morning America* in 1997. She has traveled the country as a spokesperson on healthy living for Walgreens, authored several books and manages a growing business under the Joan Lunden Healthy Living brand.

Joan was both a Sandwich Generation caregiver – caring for children and a parent simultaneously and thus, sandwiched between caregiving duties – and a long-distance caregiver. Approximately 7-8 million caregivers care for a loved one long-distance – whether they are one hour away or across the country as in Joan's case. This makes caregiving more difficult – you are not there every day to see the small things that can be warning signs that something is changing and your loved one needs more care.

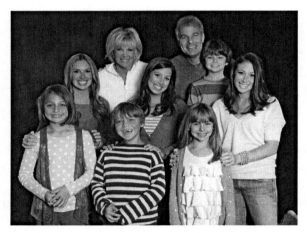

Photo: Angie Watson

Joan with her husband and children

Sunrise, Sunset

Joan's first caregiving role was actually not for her mom it was for her brother. She had been taking care of her brother since she was in her 30s, when she was reporting and then filling the anchor seat for ABC-TV's top-rated *Good Morning America*. Her brother was suffering from the impact of type 2 diabetes and Joan laments that he had not taken better care of his health.

According to the American Diabetes Association, type 2 diabetes is the most common form of the disease affecting millions of Americans. Having this form of diabetes means your body is not producing enough insulin or your cells are ignoring the insulin, a hormone that is necessary for the body to be able to use blood glucose (sugar) for energy. Insulin takes the glucose developed in the blood and transfers it to the cells. If the glucose builds up in the blood without migrating to the cells, complications of diabetes occur.

Health problems of diabetes can range from eye issues such as glaucoma or cataracts; numbness in the extremities; hypertension, which is high blood pressure that can lead to kidney and heart disease; hearing loss; higher risk for skin rashes and other dermatological issues; and increased mental health issues such as depression. And diabetics have a 2 to 4 times higher risk of stroke than non-diabetics. The American Diabetes Association says there are more than 25 million people – children and adults – living with either type 1 or type 2 diabetes, and an additional 79 million Americans who are pre-diabetic.

When her brother finally succumbed to all the health problems associated with his diabetes, it was not his death that rocked Joan's world. She mourned her brother's passing, but she also quickly came to a stunning realization: her mother's dementia was so much worse than even she knew. Joan had hired an in-home care agency that sent a personal care worker six hours a day to help her brother and mom take care of their household. This personal care worker helped with housekeeping, grocery shopping, transportation to doctor appointments, etc.

Joan says it is the typical long-distance caregiver scenario – everyone puts on a happy face when you get together, and you don't see the little cracks in the façade. Joan also believes that many caregivers don't want to see the cracks – you don't want to believe your parent is declining as much as she is so you ignore the red flags.

"I think it probably started well before I became aware of it," says Joan. "My mom was always comfortable around my brother and me, so when we got together her dementia seemed so minimal. I also did not realize that my brother's health was failing as rapidly as it was, because everybody puts on a good face when you live far away and you visit maybe half a dozen times a year. You leave thinking great they're doing really well."

"There is also the psychological part of this – you want them to be doing well," says Joan. That is what gets caregivers in trouble. Denial can be a huge barrier to planning ahead and getting the proper systems in place for the future care of your loved one.

Joan realized she had been overlooking her mother's real needs and issues. This is easy to do when an older loved one is relatively healthy and appears fine on the outside but is suffering from dementia that can cause sudden mood shifts, or other emotional problems especially frightfulness and forgetfulness. It is only through the activities of daily living that one sees how critical proper care becomes, and Joan did not have the benefit of seeing her mom on a daily basis. It quickly became apparent to Joan that her mom could not live alone in the condo she had shared with Joan's brother, even with the in-home help Joan was providing.

According to *The Shriver Report: A Woman's Nation Takes on Alzheimer's*, there are more than 10 million American women who are impacted by Alzheimer's or other dementias – either as the woman living with the disease or the woman caring for a loved one with the disease. Dementia can be sneaky. And the Alzheimer's Association tells us that 50 percent of those with dementia are not even diagnosed yet.

For a long-distance caregiver, it becomes even more difficult to know if something is wrong because you may only be visiting and you don't see the day-to-day issues that are impacting your loved one. The other difficulty is that dementia itself is not a specific disease, it is an overall term to describe a wide range of symptoms associated with a decline in memory and impact to other thinking skills. It can also reduce a person's ability to perform activities of daily living (ADLs). Alzheimer's disease is the most common form of dementia representing 60-80 percent of dementia cases. For Joan's mom, dementia was slowly sneaking up on her, which made it difficult for Joan to see it while caring for her mom from a distance.

"I think my brother's passing had a profound impact on my mom's dementia and her physicians all agreed," says Joan. Gladyce also had surgery a few years before, and there is the possibility that the anesthesia had a more pronounced effect on her dementia. In her 50s, Gladyce had two mini heart attacks, and later in her 70s she had a series of mini strokes that did not severely impair her but affected her balance and created some disconnects in her brain.

Joan says what is scary as a caregiver is to watch a loved one decline in health. "There would be times when my mom would blink her eyes and then stop talking for a minute then look at me and say, 'Where am I?'" Joan says this is not only disconcerting for a caregiver but it makes us more aware of our own mortality and vulnerabilities.

Eventually, Joan discovered that her mom had *sundowners* or *sundowning*, a typical symptom of those with dementia and Alzheimer's which causes the person to become irritated, irrational and sometimes violent during the time of day when the sun is setting. While researchers still do not know the cause of sundowning, they believe that Alzheimer's and dementia disturbs our inner clock and causes those afflicted to have increased behavioral changes that begin at dusk and continue throughout the night.

"Many Alzheimer's patients are confused, and they become tired navigating all their daily activities – just getting through the day is hard," says Beth Kallmyer, vice president of constituent services for the Alzheimer's Association. "What can help is ensuring they are engaged throughout the day, so they do want to sleep through the night. Also, keeping the lights on seems to help. People living with Alzheimer's can become afraid of shadows and this causes more confusion, which then causes the patient to be restless or agitated."

Joan's mother started showing signs of paranoia especially after Joan moved her mother into an assisted living facility. "Mom was afraid to go downstairs and visit with the other residents; they frightened her and yet she could not tell us why," says Joan. A lot of times this happened around the dinner hour at dusk.

"I think the biggest problem for caregivers of someone with dementia or Alzheimer's is that you still see them as the person they were but they just are not that person anymore," Joan says in a wistful voice. Getting to this reality is hard for caregivers who are dealing with denial over their parent's decline.

His Girl Friday

When Joan's brother passed away, it was left to Joan to decide if her mother could continue living independently with some personal care assistance from an outside agency or a professional. In addition, Joan needed to go through all the paperwork for her mother that her brother had been handling. Joan, her brother and her mother had been a threesome as Joan grew up since her father was tragically killed in a plane accident when Joan was only 14 years old.

What Joan found "was just stacks of everything – stacks of mail, stacks of newspapers, stacks of old bills, everything except the important documentation I needed to find. I had touched 20,000 pieces of paper and still could not put my hands on the paperwork I really needed."

I call this situation, about which I have heard from so many caregivers, the *adult scavenger hunt*. Joan called it her detective hour or more precisely her journalistic skills put to the test.

Like all the great heroines in Howard Hawks movies (who directed *His Girl Friday*), Joan was a smart, spunky woman who got down to doing what she does best – investigating. As a journalist you have to be inquisitive and look for clues to the real story. In Joan's case she had to search through mountains of paperwork and become an amateur genealogist to be able to help her mother.

"Mom did not know where her driver's license was, her passport, her social security card, etc." Joan could not access her mother's bank account without this form of ID. She knew she was not going to be able to help her mom until she could verify her mother's identity.

Joan found the counsel and guidance of an Elder Law attorney critical to her success. Joan was capable of doing the research, but she needed an expert to tell her what she was looking for. Elder Law attorneys are specialists at understanding Medicare and Medicaid and other services that support older Americans. In the same way you want a lawyer who specializes in divorce or criminal law, there is a specialty in the legal field where these Elder Law attorneys understand the nuances to medical privacy laws, senior and gerontological issues, senior housing, etc. You also want to ensure you engage an Elder Law attorney in the same state where your loved one currently resides because laws vary from state to state. (You can read more about Elder Law attorneys in the Raiders of the Lost Ark chapter).

The Elder Law attorney advised Joan to find her mother's birth and marriage certificates, since she knew her mother's maiden name. He said this would be enough information to then get copies of the identifying documents for her mom she needed. After securing copies of her mom's birth and marriage certificates, Joan and her mom went to the Social Security office. In order to get a duplicate Social Security card, two forms of official identification are required. Joan thought they were home free with the birth and marriage certificates. Not so fast.

"When we got to the Social Security office with our documentation, they asked my mom for her mother's maiden name (which was not on her birth certificate)," says Joan. "My mom could not remember her mother's maiden name, and I could not remember it either." Joan says the next few minutes were like a tragic game show – both women standing in the Social Security line playing 20 questions, with Joan trying to get her mom to remember the name. The Social Security representative said without the maiden name, there would be no new card and no continuation of the search for other important forms of identification and authorization such as a Medicare card, bank account access, etc. Eventually her mom did remember the name, and they left Social Security triumphant.

"It was one of my toughest journalistic endeavors to track all of these important documents down to get the ID cards that were essential," laments Joan. "I literally had to put her identity back together."

In addition, Gladyce had to authorize Joan as a co-signer on her bank account and grant her access to her health insurance and other critical information that has privacy protection. Thank goodness in Joan's case Gladyce was still lucid enough to authorize her daughter to help. In many caregiving situations the loved one can no longer provide that authorization and it becomes a costly and time-consuming burden for the caregiver to seek guardianship that gets this done.

You think you know your parents but then something like this happens and you realize maybe you do not know as much as you should. This is especially true when it comes to verifying records and making decisions on their behalf.

"The more I learned, the more I became determined to see if anyone I knew is prepared for this," says Joan. "I asked my attorney, my accountant, my hairdresser if they knew where their parents banked, if their parents had an Advance Directive, where the deed to their parents' house is or who the mortgage lender is, where is the title to their car is and what their grandmother's maiden name was – everyone said, 'I don't know.'"

In retrospect, Joan says, "I wish I had the family meeting before the crisis in care happened, but I am typical of most caregivers. The crisis happened and all of a sudden you have to become an instant expert at so many issues around elder care."

Home Sweet Home

One of the biggest issues facing Joan after her brother was gone was where her mom was going to live. For long-distance caregivers, this becomes an even more agonizing issue. Even if Joan felt her mom would have been OK at home with round-the-clock care, "The cost of care at home can be really prohibitive for a lot of people; it can really take you down," says Joan.

Nora Jean Levin, executive director of the nonprofit organization Caring From a Distance, advises, "A lot of caregivers find it difficult to orchestrate finding a more suitable living arrangement for their loved one when they only have a couple of days off work, drive or fly in, and try to get everything handled in 48-72 hours." Levin says many caregivers struggle with the dilemma of whether they should move their loved one closer to them or whether they should consider moving closer to their loved one.

The other difficulty according to Levin is the world of senior care is "a patchwork quilt with more holes than patches," and caregivers can be at a loss as to where to look and what to look for. Levin advises having a trusted resource – whether a geriatric care manager or a senior care services advisor – can help caregivers make informed decisions faster which helps both the caregiver and the loved one find *home sweet home* for a lifetime.

In Joan's case, she encountered what so many caregivers do who are unaware of the variety of senior living options. I call it the *Goldilocks Syndrome.* She chose a series of different living arrangements for Gladyce before finding the right fit that satisfied both of them. However, that journey was long and fraught with some not-so-great choices that were actually negatively impacting her mom's health.

When Joan realized her mom could not live on her own, she set about finding the best next home for her. "I found a very *shmancy fancy* senior living facility – it was the chic place in town, the dining room was beautiful and she had a great apartment where she could retreat to."

Joan also was impressed the facility seemed bright and nice, and it was a large place with a lot of people where her mom could socialize and make new friends. Joan says she was finding a home for her mom that would have been perfect 30 years ago, but the reality was the person she remembered – Gladyce Blunden – was not the same woman. Joan had found the perfect home for someone who no longer existed.

Dr. Rosemary Laird, a gerontologist and medical director for Health First Aging Institute in Florida says you have to thoughtfully consider a loved one's current and future care needs to minimize the moves you may have to make. The more moves the more harm than good for both your loved one's physical and mental health. She also cautions a pitfall for many caregivers when reviewing alternative living facilities is putting our own lifestyle preferences in place of our loved one's needs.

"We see a beautiful dining room, maybe a gorgeous view, beautiful architectural or design appointments, great social or lifestyle activities such as free transportation to malls or church; when instead we should be asking more questions about staffing such as how often do nurses or health care workers check on loved ones and what is the professional to residents ratio?" says Dr. Laird. She also says caregivers should educate themselves about care transitions. This will help you and your loved one make better decisions – both health and wealth-wise – in the long run when it comes to where and how older loved one's will live out their lives. (See the chapter The Three Faces of Eve for more about care transitions).

What Joan did not realize is Gladyce needed more than a sunny dining room and a nice bedroom suite. While Joan was concerned about her mom's sundowning, she started to realize there were more problems caused by dementia. Her mom had started calling everyone she knew at all hours of the night to say "come get me and take me back home." Joan finally had to have the phone disconnected. Also, Gladyce's balance issues were starting to cause her real harm. She got up to go to the bathroom and fell and broke a toe and later a rib. Then she fell and hit her head and had to have staples for the wound. Each injury had Joan jumping on a plane to fly from her home base in Connecticut to California.

"Each step was like uh oh, this is a lot worse than I thought." It was finally Gladyce's neurosurgeon who told Joan her mom needed a small residential care facility for four or five people where someone could literally watch over her mom 24/7.

As Joan started doing her investigative journalism yet again, she continued to discover how much she never knew. "For instance, when I realized my mom was not doing well in the senior living facility, I found out there are eight levels of assisted living choices – none of the health care professionals I was dealing with at that time ever told me this."

Joan's situation is not unique. Many caregivers struggle to make good decisions for a loved one but are not armed with all the information they may need. Professional support is dependent on the situation and with many social workers and hospital dispatch personnel overwhelmed with case loads and patients, they don't spend a lot of quality time walking caregivers through their options. If a caregiver does not know the questions to ask, they are left to making decisions which can lead to the Goldilocks Syndrome. This *testing* of different facilities and moving your loved one until you find one that is just right is to be avoided as it can add to your loved one's physical and mental health issues. Lack of good research and making uninformed decisions will lead to the Goldilocks Syndrome. Secure a geriatric care manager, who is an expert in finding the right facility and will continue to work with you after your loved one is moved in; or use a matchmaking service to connect you to a facility or service that meets your loved one's needs. Finding a professional guide is the best way to go. You can read more about these GCMs and matchmaking services in the My Man Godfrey chapter.

The social worker at the hospital where Gladyce was treated for her falls was helpful and put Joan in touch with a senior care facility advisor organization called A Place for Mom. This Seattle, Washington-based nationwide service provides a local expert who can guide caregivers to the home care service or alternative living option best suited for their loved one at no cost for the service. The database of facility and services include more than 18,000 options. The advisor assigned to Joan assessed Gladyce's needs and then took Joan and Gladyce on a tour of several facilities in the Sacramento area she thought would suit their needs. They settled upon a small residential care facility with just six residents in a large home setting.

At first glance, Joan felt this home environment – the facility was located in a residential neighborhood – seemed inadequate to care properly for her mom. She worried about safety and good clinical care if needed in an emergency. What Joan came to realize was not only did her mom get more personalized, supervised care 24/7 but her mom was much happier in an environment that reminded her of her own home.

"It was really my mom who made the final decision," says Joan. "She is so much happier coming downstairs to a small living room rather than a large dining room in the other facility." This is home to her, and she is thriving whereas in the other "beautiful facility" Joan had chosen, she was rapidly declining.

When we think of a safe place for a loved one to live it might appear a large facility with a lot of staff, residents and activity would be safe, but in actuality the size of the facility does not make a difference. Hiring criteria, staff training and specialized systems are the biggest contributors to a safe community. Loren Shook, CEO of Silverado Senior Living, which offers a continuum of care from communities to hospice and in-home care services that specialize in dementia care, says many health care professionals and assisted living staff may be trained in the technicalities of caring for a person with dementia, but, "You cannot train people to have a heart." While Silverado's communities are located mostly in California, Illinois, Texas and a handful of other states, the Silverado model is one used by numerous organizations including the NFL and provides telephonic assistance for anyone in the U.S. to help with care transitions or moving a loved one to any facility.

When it comes to ensuring you have helped your loved one make the best choice in alternative living choices, Joan says, "You should ask yourself these two questions about the care of your loved ones: 1) Are they safe and well-cared for? 2) Are they happy? If you can answer 'yes' to both questions then you have accomplished your goals as a caregiver." After feeling so satisfied with the service provided by A Place for Mom, Joan became their spokesperson in 2012.

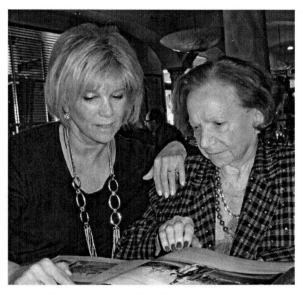

Photo: Courtesy of Joan Lunden

Joan and her mom Gladyce

Stay Connected

One of the strategies Joan uses to ensure her mom is well cared for even from a distance is to maintain contact with the staff and administrators at her mom's residential care facility.

For long-distance caregivers, the guilt of not being by your loved one's side every day can be overwhelming. Finding peace of mind your loved one is happy and well cared for is essential, and Joan advises the best way to do this is to stay in touch.

One of the things caregivers need to remind themselves of is just because you have found a facility and dropped off your loved one does not mean you drop out of the care team. At times caregivers may find themselves at odds with facility staff – blaming staff for something their parent is not doing. The reality is blame is often a cover-up for guilt – your guilt.

It is critical you keep an open mind and open lines of communication with facility administrators and staff. Get to know these people by more than just their names or their titles.

Ask a lot of questions and share a lot of information. If your mom has a ritual of always having ice cream on Sunday evening – talk to staff to see if that can be arranged. Also alert them to special occasions. If your mom has trouble on the anniversary date of a spouse's death or perhaps her wedding anniversary date and you cannot be there, ask the staff to pay a little more attention on that day. Let staff know when you will be out of town and how to reach you. Ask the staff when you visit how things are going, what is working and what may be difficult for your loved one.

Staying connected lets the facility staff know you are someone to be brought into the loop sooner rather than later, which also makes them more vigilant about your loved one's care. By being an active part of this essential care communications team you will ensure your loved one is getting a better level of care and your guilt will be greatly diminished.

In addition to staying in communication with staff, it is also critical to stay in touch with your loved one. This may seem obvious at first – of course you are going to call your loved one frequently to check in or visit as often as you can. But staying connected is more than just visits or phone calls. You need to connect with her on another level.

We know as we age we become more nostalgic. How many times have you heard dad's story about the hole-in-one on the golf course or mom's reminiscence of the high school prom where she met your dad? While we get a little exasperated hearing the story for the 40th time, it should also be a clue as to what is important to your loved ones and typically this has to do with their earlier lives.

Joan told me at first, she was putting photos of her young twins and her older daughter's college pictures in frames for her mom. While her mom would smile she was not *connecting* to the photos. Joan said these memories were after her mom lost her short-term memory. She finally realized Gladyce was living in the past.

With dementia and Alzheimer's patients, though short-term memories evaporate, they can connect back to earlier times of pleasure and happiness. Every person afflicted with dementia is different and long ago memories might be painful for your loved one but sometimes older memories are all they have. In other situations, some Alzheimer's sufferers may not recognize a wife of more than 50 years – as was the case for Nancy Reagan where her beloved Ronnie did not know who she was the last few years of his life.

What Joan found helpful to Gladyce is when she began to put photos of her and her brother when they were very young in the picture frames. She found photos of her parents before the family lost her dad, and collaged those onto an old tea tray. She made a calendar entirely of photos of her mom when she was a young girl. It made all the difference in the world to Gladyce.

One of Joan's older daughters, Lindsey, also had a great idea. When they moved Gladyce from the assisted living facility into the residential home, Lindsay took pictures of her grandmother's old bedroom – every detail. Then, when they unpacked and started putting things up in Gladyce's new room, they tried to recreate the scene as much as possible to match the old bedroom. They looked at Lindsay's photos and put everything back in exactly the same place – books stacked in the same order on the shelf, the same items on the nightstand in exactly the same place. Joan says this helped Gladyce adjust to her new environment by making it look like her old room.

Dr. Laird says particularly with dementia patients, you need to create consistency to avoid some of the paranoia and fearfulness of something new for them.

Beth Kallmyer of the Alzheimer's Association advises when considering a move for someone with Alzheimer's or another dementia, limit the moves to as few as possible. She cautions our loved ones may become angry or scared over not being able to find a bathroom or bedroom when they are in a new place. Eventually they will likely settle in but be prepared for this initial disruption. Multiple moves will only disrupt your peace as well as that of your loved one.

They say that home is where the heart is. In Joan's case, her heart is where her mom and her husband and children are happiest.

Joan's Lessons Learned

There are many lessons to be learned from Joan Lunden's story. Here is a quick recap and some additional insights from Joan:

1. Have the Family Meeting

"Caregiving sneaks up on you," says Joan. If she could go back and change anything, she says she wishes she had had the caregiving conversation with both her brother and her mom. "I'm very organized and I'm a planner; I just cannot believe I did not plan for this."

2. Be a Journalist

If there is anything Joan Lunden is great at (and there are many things believe me!) it is being a journalist. Yet, when it came to her own caregiving future – she had not prepared. You read how she had to spend endless hours researching things and asking a lot of questions – all in a time of crisis. As a reporter, Joan had to do research on the person she was interviewing, know the smart questions to ask, listen to her guest to make the interview interesting for the audience.

The same holds true for caregiving. You need to educate yourself about what your caregiving future may look like, interview your loved ones, listen to their needs and their wishes and communicate with everyone involved: your loved one for whom you are caring, their health care professionals and if needed the facility administrators and staff, your other family members, etc. Having the conversation and making the plan are essential as you will read in the C-A-R-E Conversations chapter.

3. No regrets

With any caregiving situation, but particularly for those who do not live close to their loved one there is one universal emotion: Guilt. I have not yet met a caregiver who does not suffer from some measure of it. You feel you are not doing enough, you are not spending enough time, you may not be making the right decisions, etc. Guilt and regret are very common for long-distance caregivers.

Joan and her family live most of the year in Connecticut and spend their summers in Maine where her husband operates camps for children. Joan knew her mom was a sun-lover, so being on the East Coast she would not be able to see the sun every day. Joan also knew many of her mom's oldest and dearest friends for over 50 years – people Joan's dad, who had been a doctor and had brought young doctors to Sacramento – continued to circle around the woman they call "Glitzy Gladdy." They told a worried Joan, "We visit her all the time." She also realized her business required her to travel a lot. If she removed her mom from this caring community to be close to her and when she isn't home a lot – is it better?

"I actually see my mom more now than I have in all my adult life," says Joan. "I see her every 5-6 weeks, but in my mind it's not enough, so it's hard to overcome the guilt." The residential facility administrator told Joan her mom probably doesn't realize how long it is between visits. Joan also sees her mom is happy and Gladyce has told Joan she loves her new roommates and home.

Joan told me, "I always think the really good caregivers are the ones who have their loved one living in their home with them, but caregiving is different for everyone."

Gladyce's friends could fill in for Joan with frequent visits which helped her mother stay connected to a past life she loved. Joan and her mom recently celebrated her 93rd birthday at her residential facility she now calls home. "Glitzy Gladdy" was surrounded by friends as Joan watched her mother blossom in the friendly celebration. Joan came to realize her guilt was not practical and she has no regrets when she sees how happy her mom is in her new home.

Sherri Snelling

How Joan Finds Her "Me Time"

"You're in total control of your life and then caregiving can make you cranky, unconfident and fearful," says Joan.

It is for this reason Joan advises us to tap into our inner child. When she travels and speaks to caregivers, she says she always asks, "What did you like to do when you were a kid?"

Joan loves to not just walk her dog but *play* with her dog. Seeing unbridled joy as your pet chases its favorite chew toy and lovingly looks at you with those eyes that say "more please" is a great elixir for dealing with caregiver depression and burn-out. Joan also found herself watching from the sidelines when taking her daughters to horseback riding lessons. One day she thought, "Why am I sitting here watching? I loved horseback riding as a kid; I should get out there with my girls." And from then on that is exactly what she did.

Another childhood activity is camping – something her entire family still enjoys. Joan decided to turn her love of camping into a place of renewal for women and started a camp called Camp Reveille. For four days during the summer in the Maine woods, women of all ages come to refresh and reinvigorate. While campers range in age from 22 to 72, Joan has noticed many of the women, particularly the baby boomers, are coming to get a respite from caregiving. Husbands or sisters are worried about them and send them to camp to get the break they so desperately need.

In addition to tapping into your inner child, Joan believes in living healthy. This is more than just a philosophy for Joan who has turned it into a business under the Joan Lunden Healthy Living brand with cookware, books, DVDs and more.

As host of *Good Morning America,* Joan was always an adventurous spirit where she climbed mountains and participated in a professional baseball spring training camp. She now brings that adventurous spirit to her *me time* strategy which she calls her *move and groove* strategy. Joan says she does best when she has a pal or a group of friends to motivate her to get moving. She often invites friends over and they mix it up – zumba one day, boxercise another day. It provides the camaraderie of girlfriends with the physical benefits of a fun workout. Joan has also added caregiving to part of her plan to broadcast to her female audience about how to plan ahead to care for our aging parents. She co-authored the book, *Chicken Soup for the Soul – Family Caregivers* along with Amy Newmark which is part of the popular *Chicken Soup for the Soul* series. The book includes a compilation of 101 short, inspirational stories from real-life caregivers.

"I believe you are 100 or 1,000 times more likely to do something when you do it with a friend or a group," says Joan.

It is all part of the baby boom mentality to not be in age denial but embrace age defiance. And Joan does this better than most with an added bit of humor. One of my favorite examples of Joan's fun yet defiant attitude toward getting older is a recent blog post on hair color where she advised, "Dye until you die." As a fellow *bottle blonde* I laughed out loud when I read that.

In the end, Joan says caregivers need to stop seeking permission to care for themselves.

"Caregivers almost need to be told by someone they respect and trust they need to have 'me time' – they need the permission to focus on themselves. You have to look inside and find yourself – the me is still in here and when you realize that, it will be a revelation."

Marg Helgenberger

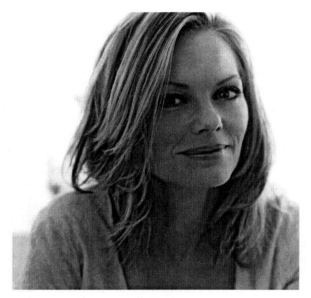

Photo: Courtesy of Marg Helgenberger

The future can be fearful or full of promise.

— Horton Foote
Main Street

Marg Helgenberger

Collecting Clues on Caregiving

Marg Helgenberger became a household name starring as one of America's most iconic TV characters, Catherine Willows, solving criminal forensic mysteries on the top-rated TV show, *CSI*. However, long before the Emmy and Golden Globe Awards, the glamour and the fame of being a respected film and TV actress, Marg was a small town girl just starting her life and acting career when she encountered caregiving.

When I met Marg she is a warm, inviting person who as a 50-something woman is stunningly youthful and beautiful. While years of life experience have made her strong and capable, as we spoke about her early years in Nebraska and the devastating illnesses that rocked her family when she was just a young woman – with both her mother and father battling a different chronic illness at the same time – the strong and steady Marg seemed all at once that vulnerable girl again.

She is full of Midwestern modesty, down-to-earth openness and has a *just do it* attitude, which underscores a tremendous work ethic she says she learned from her parents. As we talked, she took me back to the early '80s as she remembered the tough years as a caregiver both near and far to her family.

Marg, born Mary Marg Helgenberger, grew up in America's heartland in North Bend, Nebraska. A town of about 1,200, it was a place where fields, farms, family and friends abounded. Her close knit clan included an older sister, her younger brother and her parents. Her mom, Kay, was a nurse and her dad, Hugh, owned a butcher shop. Growing up in the rural Midwest, Marg originally thought she might become a nurse like her mother.

But, it was in high school she got the acting bug, and after playing Blanche Dubois in a college stage production of *A Streetcar Named Desire*, she was hooked. She told *The Hollywood Reporter*, "I've always been a shy person. Acting gave me the opportunity to express myself."

From that moment onward, Marg set her sights on the bright lights of big city Manhattan – but not before finishing college at Northwestern University outside of Chicago, keeping her close to her Nebraska home. It was while she was a junior in college Marg learned her mother had breast cancer.

A Case of College, Chronic Illness, Career and Caregiving

Back in the early 1980s, any type of cancer, including breast cancer, was still something to stop you in your tracks. People still believed a cancer diagnosis was terminal. This was before Susan G. Komen for the Cure, founded in 1982, and other organizations created a movement to improve the preventative measures, early detection, diagnosis and drug therapies. Today 90 percent of women diagnosed with breast cancer will survive at least five years or more. In fact, statistics tell us 1 out of every 8 women will be diagnosed with breast cancer, but survival rates have improved dramatically over the last 30 years with more than 2.5 million breast cancer survivors today.

In the early '80s, Marg's mother had found a lump in her breast and she knew this was not a good sign. While she did get it checked by a couple of doctors, they told her not to worry – she had cystic breast tissue – and sent her home. It was only after getting another opinion from a third doctor she was diagnosed with breast cancer. She wound up having one mastectomy only to have the doctor advise her a few days later she would have to have the other breast removed as well. In addition, she faced months of painful radiation and chemotherapy.

Marg remembers her mother's treatment was "really intense for the first three years; it was so intense the treatment almost killed her." She recalls her mom losing her hair but not her faith or her *never give up* attitude. While it took a physical and emotional toll on her mom, Marg never wavered in her belief her mom would survive. As a young college student she would come home to help care for her mom in-between classes. Marg believes her mother's Midwestern work ethic, her stoicism and her strong faith made a huge difference in her beating breast cancer.

"She was only home for a day or two, and she was actually back out on the lawn the next day with a push mower," Marg chuckles as she recalls her mom's tenacity. In an interview with author Karen Karbo, Marg's mom said, "I didn't want everyone to think I was going to die. Because I wasn't."

In Marg's mom's case, despite the missed early diagnosis, she has beaten the odds considerably, and today she is a 32-year breast cancer survivor. Because of her mother's history with breast cancer, Marg began getting mammograms at age 30 and then every few years until recently when she gets them annually and does consistent self-exams. Marg cites her mom's battle with breast cancer as an inspiration for her co-starring role alongside Julia Roberts in the 2000 film, *Erin Brokovich*. In the movie, Marg plays a cancer victim who has a positive outlook for her future, and keeps a stiff upper lip and the family together – something her mom did during her clash with cancer.

The Helgenberger clan had survived a scare, but it was just one short year after her mom's cancer went into remission her father was given a devastating diagnosis that rocked the rock-solid family yet again.

Marg had always been close to her dad, and family friends say she looks just like him. At first, her father originally attributed the tingling and numbness in his arm to his physically intensive job carrying sides of beef around and constantly chopping and cutting. However, as the symptoms progressed and persisted, he was eventually given the diagnosis of multiple sclerosis (MS) – and the prognosis could not have been worse, as it was an extremely rare and progressive type of MS.

Multiple sclerosis is one of the numerous chronic illnesses for which there is still no cure, although according to the Nancy Davis Foundation for Multiple Sclerosis recent research is encouraging. Today, more than 400,000 people in the U.S. and 2.5 million people worldwide live with this insidious disease that attacks the central nervous system. Twice as many women as men are diagnosed with MS, and it is typically uncovered when patients are between 20-50 years old.

There are four different types of MS, a disease that creates lesions and scar tissue on the protective covering of the nerve fibers of the central nervous system. The scars cause nerve signals to slow down or stop. Those afflicted have unpredictable and often debilitating symptoms that can range from blindness to partial or full paralysis. Marg's father had progressive/relapsing MS – the most rare of the four types of the disease. He was diagnosed when he was only 45 years old.

"I think it was a hard diagnosis because he owned this butcher shop and because of him having to lug around these sides of beef – the paralysis he felt – he thought maybe he just had a pinched nerve or something," says Marg. She also believes he had so much going on in his life dealing with her mom's illness that a serious problem with his own health was not a real priority at the time.

Marg says, "It was very bad…he was healthy at 45…and by the time he turned 50, he was dead."

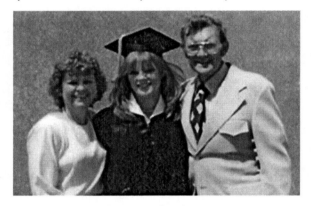

Photo: Courtesy of Marg Helgenberger

Marg and her parents at her Northwestern University graduation.

Little House on the Prairie

As both her parents faced major health scares, Marg was trying to stay focused on graduating from Northwestern University and was wondering what would happen to her plans to pursue her acting dreams in New York. Marg made frequent trips home to help both her parents.

"It was a very challenging time in our family's life," remembers Marg. "My mom was just finishing up treatment from chemotherapy and then my dad was diagnosed with MS."

While her mother became her dad's primary caregiver, Marg believes this role as caregiver to her husband helped her mom focus on his illness instead of her ongoing recovery from cancer, which actually made her mom stronger. She feels her mom "willed herself" to get better to care for her husband. Meanwhile, Marg was torn on whether or not to move to New York. This is where the Midwestern work ethic kicked in once again. Both of her parents were supportive of their daughter, and encouraged her to pursue her acting passion in the Big Apple.

Approximately 7-8 million caregivers are caring for a loved one living at least one hour away – many much further than that. In Marg's case, she was prepared to put her dreams on hold to help hold her family together, but her parents did not want their health challenges to have that impact on Marg's future.

"This is the dilemma that has plagued caregivers over the years," says Nora Jean Levin, executive director of Caring From a Distance (CFAD), a nonprofit organization dedicated to long-distance caregivers. "The guilt over whether you should move closer to your parents or have your parents move closer to you is one of the reasons CFAD was started – you have to realize you are not alone, and you have to reach out for help."

While Marg went to New York, she came home as often as she could. She was starting to make headway in her acting career and landed roles on popular shows like *Spencer for Hire* and ultimately a key role on the soap opera, *Ryan's Hope*.

After his diagnosis, her father kept his job running the butcher shop. Shortly thereafter he had to start using a cane, and the physical aspects of his job became too difficult. Eventually, her dad was confined to a wheelchair, with her mother trying to care for him and continue her job as a nurse. But ultimately even this was not enough. Marg remembers the day her mom called to say they were going to need more help for her dad.

"One day my dad's wheelchair got stuck in a hallway and he could not get it around the corner, so he was stuck there for hours while my mom was at work," says Marg. "We lived in a small house, and it just wasn't set up for wheelchairs and the space he needed to maneuver." That is when the family knew having more help more often was going to be necessary. They hired a nurse to come during the day to ensure her dad would be OK, but this put even more financial strain on the family.

Many caregivers find themselves struggling to help cover care costs for a loved one. While our expectations are that Medicare or Medicaid will cover the costs of caring for a loved one, more often than not, caregivers are digging into their own pockets. According to the National Alliance for Caregiving, 47 percent of caregivers have used all or most of their savings to cover care-related costs and 4 out of 10 are taking on more debt or borrowing money for caregiving.

With money tight, Marg, her mother and her brother formed a caregiving *tag team* (her sister had moved away) with her mom and brother performing the physical care and Marg providing them with emotional support and the family with a lot of the financial resources. Marg says her brother is "salt of the earth, funny, dependable," and since he was the one still at home, she believes of the three siblings he felt the biggest toll. Marg was dedicated to doing whatever she could to support both her mom and brother in whatever ways she could. She traveled home as many weekends as her job would allow.

One of the most difficult emotions for long-distance caregivers is the guilt over not being there every day. "I have to say there were a lot of days when I would feel guilty; it wasn't a particularly happy time for me at all," she remembers. Marg wanted to be excited and upbeat about her career, but being far away from a family that was struggling was really tough for her and gave her many moments of pause. She coped by working.

As her father's MS was quickly taking over his deteriorating body, there wasn't anything anyone could do to stop it. Marg provided her mom and brother with the emotional outlet for what they were witnessing every day with her dad. She was also called upon by her mom to help make some of the difficult medical and financial decisions about his care, which Marg found particularly tough. Marg could come home to be with her father and give her mom and brother a break, but having to face some tough decisions for him, especially for end-of-life issues, was extremely hard on her as a young woman.

"It was in rural Nebraska, so his options were limited to begin with," says Marg. "He would go to the hospital and they would give him these super-charged doses of cortisol, and he would feel better for a little while." While the shots provided some temporary relief from the persistent pain, they would also leave him bloated, unable to sleep and miserable.

Even though Marg recalls her dad had symptoms for a period of time prior to his diagnosis, she is not sure anything could have been done anyway. In the 1980s, the therapies and medications for MS we have today, didn't exist back then.

According to the Nancy Davis Foundation for Multiple Sclerosis, there are now seven MS drugs available with three more being approved by the FDA. And more information is available about how diet and exercise can tame or alleviate some symptoms. In addition to drug therapies, gluten-free diets – which eliminate the protein gluten found in grains such as wheat, barley and rye – are beneficial for those with MS according to the Mayo Clinic. One of the latest trends for MS sufferers is adopting an alkaline diet, which involves eating certain fresh citrus and other low-sugar fruits, vegetables, nuts and legumes. The diet recommends avoiding grains, dairy, meat, sugar, alcohol, caffeine, and fungi.

It Takes a Village

As her father's disease progressed, Marg came to appreciate even more her small town, rural America upbringing. Her parents had been very involved in the local community, and at one point her dad had been the head of the local Jaycees (also known as the United States Junior Chamber), a civic organization for leadership training for those ages 18-41. When her father's illness had progressed to the point he was now wheelchair-bound 24/7, the current president of the Jaycees contacted Marg in New York and said they wanted to hold a fundraiser to buy a wheelchair-equipped van with a lift for her dad and family. They were able to raise enough funds that Marg could match the amount they raised and they could purchase the vehicle.

"It was just so sweet they would help my family in this kind of situation and this is what the community wanted to do for him," says Marg. "And I remember my dad was just so thrilled to have that van; it was kind of an honorary thing for him. I realized it really does take a village to care for someone who has a disability or illness."

Caregiving Clues for our Children

According to the National Alliance for Caregiving, there are more than 1.5 million youths – those under age 18 – providing primary care to a parent or grandparent who is ill or diagnosed with a disease such as MS. While in Marg's caregiving situation, she was in college and then starting her career, she was still a very youthful caregiver supporting a mom *and* a father who faced traumatic health issues.

"All of us kids were so young when my parents become ill – I was in my early 20s," says Marg still amazed at how this all happened to her family at ages when everyone should be healthy. She also says there are days when she reflects on the fact that at her age now she has outlived her father. She believes when you are young, you don't give your caregiving role a lot of thought.

"So much happened to our family in such a short span of time we didn't have time to stop and think about it – whatever important tasks needed to be accomplished, we accomplished them."

"Caregiving youths can have a very tough time," says Connie Siskowski, founder and president of the American Association of Caregiving Youth (AACY), the nation's only organization focusing on caregivers under age 18. "When they are in school, they are expected to be kids but when they come home they have to be adults with little or no help and guidance."

Siskowski says while this has negative impacts such as contributing to high school drop-out rates, there are some benefits to being a youthful caregiver. "They learn early on about empathy, time management, organizational skills and multi-tasking – all of which can benefit them in their adult lives."

Marg believes if you were to ask her and her brother now, they would probably say they were both in denial about their caregiving roles to a certain degree. But now she thinks more about her own son and what he may face in caregiving for her.

Because Marg was so involved in helping make tough decisions about her dad's care, she has ensured all of her legal and financial paperwork are in order, so her young son, now at the same age as Marg was when she started caring for her parents, doesn't have to go through the same struggle. "I don't want to leave that responsibility on my son." And she has talked to her son about it, so there are no mysteries about her wishes for long-term care.

She has also advised her son to not have the fear and anxiety that comes when a parent becomes ill. "I told him to reach out to my family, friends and others who can help him. We never had that conversation in my family because again, everyone was so young you just don't anticipate anything will happen. But being open with your kids and having that communication is critical."

Marg is a great role-model for all caregivers. Having the conversation with our children about our wishes and plans is essential. It eliminates the guess-work so many caregivers face when caring for a parent or older loved one. I give you an overview of how to get these C-A-R-E Conversations started in that chapter of this book.

The Rewards of Caregiving

"Most of my work in the past had been with breast cancer awareness and support in honor of my mom," says Marg. In 2002, she was the host of the Susan G. Komen Race for the Cure event in Los Angeles; she also hosts an annual celebrity charity golf tournament in Council Bluffs, Iowa – about 60 miles from North Bend, Nebraska. The funds raised support cancer research and programs at two local hospitals, one in Council Bluffs and one in Omaha.

"I am so proud of the progress made in breast cancer treatments and breast cancer events get an enormous amount of attention now – thank goodness because the disease is so prevalent," says Marg. "But multiple sclerosis just doesn't get the kind of attention as other diseases so I want to shine a spotlight on this disease, which is so devastating for families."

While she has always supported MS fundraising events, Marg has more recently gotten involved in the Nancy Davis Foundation for Multiple Sclerosis. The foundation has created Center Without Walls which provides the funds to facilitate the medical community linking together multidisciplinary scientific programs and expertise across the country. The Center's network of the top six MS institutions that have established leading, innovative research programs include: University of California at San Francisco, Harvard, Yale, University of Southern California, Johns Hopkins and Oregon Health Sciences University. These six leaders are dedicated to understanding the cause of MS, advancing the development of new treatments and ultimately leading the race to find a cure for MS.

Nancy Davis told me, "It just didn't make sense to me to have these wonderful research teams duplicating effort – if we want to find a cure faster, we have to work in cooperation and share information so we get there in 10 years instead of 20."

Marg wishes the Center had existed when her dad was diagnosed. "All the medical breakthroughs and new therapies – maybe he would be here today if we had this kind of research back then." She told me, "I adore my father - not a day goes by that I don't think about my dad." Now her advocacy is bringing more awareness to finding a cure for MS.

While she helped collar serial killers on TV's *CSI*, it was as a caregiver and now an advocate that Marg is chasing down new serial killers – breast cancer and multiple sclerosis. For this star who blends vulnerability and strength – I have no doubt she will be helping to lead the teams to find the clues and the cures.

Marg's Lessons Learned

1. **Dig Deep**

    When it comes to battling a chronic illness, Marg says what she has learned from her parent's experience is "you have to go deep."

    "When you get a diagnosis and know you are going to climb an uphill battle, and there may be pain or physical issues, and you have fear and anxiety – for yourself and how it affects your family – you just have to dig deep inside yourself to fight it," continues Marg. She feels it is not different for the caregiver – finding inner strength is critical to keep going to provide the care.

    Marg says she knows her mother's strong Catholic faith helped her win her battle with breast cancer. "I would swear on the Bible her devotion and belief in God saved her." But Marg believes whether or not you are religious, you can find spirituality and strength in things like meditation and keeping yourself in a positive environment. "It's important at times we *lose ourselves* in things like nature and things that make you feel lighter and happier." She is a believer in gratitude journals and music that can help to heal.

2. **Envelop Yourself in Family and Friends**

    She also believes surrounding yourself – whether as the patient or the caregiver – with loved ones and friends is essential. "For anyone battling a disease and for the caregiver – having your family and friends around you is so important. It will keep the fear and anxiety at bay."

    She says just spending time together – being there to just watch TV with a loved one or a friend who is a caregiver is helpful. She says caregivers spend so much time going to and from doctor appointments with their loved one that burn-out can sneak up on you.

    What she found when she would come home from New York to be with her dad was just laughing at silly TV shows or movies did as much good as the doctors. She feels these times when you can "escape together" can really help both the patient and the caregiver.

    "Nobody signs up for this illness," says Nancy Davis. "A diagnosis of MS is not just about the person with the disease, it is about the family and you have to lean on each other to carry on."

3. **You Can Have It All If You Don't Try to Do It All**

She feels many women believe they can do it all – children, career, caregiving, marriage or partnership, friendships. But eventually, she says you come down off that high and it can be a painful re-entry.

"For a while you can work off of adrenaline – it's amazing what you can do that you never thought you could get done." This is not unlike caregiving – finding the balance while you're in it is essential, so you don't crash and burn when the caregiving is over (or even before it's over.)

You have to find time to relax, and she advises caregivers not to forget to find time just for them. "Take a walk with your dog, take a soak in the tub, do something just for you once in a while."

4. **Talk To Your Kids**

In Marg's story, she was a young caregiver when her family was blindsided by illness for both parents. While we need to have the conversation with our aging parents about their long-term care and end-of-life wishes, it is never too soon to talk to our kids about those same things. We believe we have time – we're still relatively young and in good health. But if Marg's story teaches us nothing more, it is that devastating illness can strike at any time, any age. Plan ahead and have the talk with family.

Sherri Snelling

How Marg finds her "Me Time"

Marg is a devoted fan of yoga and she was way "ahead of the curve" in this fitness trend having practiced it for more than 30 years. She also believes in meditating and walking with her dog, a rescue mutt mix of German Shepherd and Akita breeds. She also believes in getting outside and enjoying nature – she says it clears the mind.

When she gets the time, she loves to read. She says she has to read so many scripts for work the guilty pleasure of reading a good book is a real escape.

Lately, she has also taken up the guitar and occasionally will play the piano. She believes music is meditative, and can have a powerful impact on our lives. She has used music to inspire her in various work projects.

Jill Eikenberry and Michael Tucker

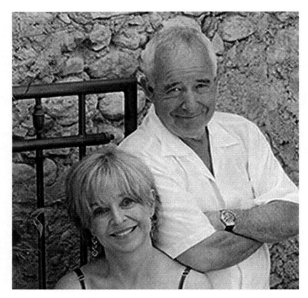

Photo: Kristine Walsh

"Cooking is like love; it should be entered into with abandon or not at all."

– Julia Child

Jill Eikenberry and Michael Tucker

Cooking Up a New Caregiving Recipe

What struck me the most when I spoke to Jill Eikenberry and Michael Tucker – co-stars in marriage, career and life – was in all things they are a team. I even did the interview with the two of them together, at their suggestion, and it gave me a glimpse into how their special bond of support, respect and caring for each other is a recipe for all couples who face a tough caregiving situation. In fact, their story is about love of family and food and the ingredients needed to keep it all cooking. Jill and Mike are like salt and pepper shakers – two distinct personalities and characters – but you never pass one without the other.

We all watched them as one of our favorite TV couples in the '80s and '90s in their roles on the Emmy-winning series *L.A. Law* (what baby boom-age woman can forget the famous *Venus Butterfly* episode?). Since then, both Mike and Jill have thrived as solo artists – Mike as an actor and acclaimed author, and Jill as a continually sought-after star on stage and screen, with her latest turn in the movie, *Young Adult*. However, it is when they are performing together – whether it is playing the couple in Broadway's *Love Letters* or caring for Jill's mother with dementia – they really are at their best.

Our House in Umbria

For many years, New York City-based Jill and Mike, have been vacationing with friends – sometimes for weeks, other times for months – in the lovely Italian countryside in the Spoleto Valley of Umbria. This is where the couple recharges – the sumptuous food infuses Mike's meals, the chilled wine, the warm people, the beauty of the olive trees and the vineyards versus the urban jungle – it is their version of *Cinema Paradiso*. They love this escape so much they eventually found a little vacation home where they planned on spending months out of the year.

It was on one of their Umbrian escapes about six years ago Jill and Mike went from the calm of their Italian reverie into the storm of caregiving. Jill's mom, Lora, was 87-years-old at the time and had been living in a Santa Barbara, California assisted living facility for several years with her husband, Ralph. Although Lora had been hard of hearing for over 50 years and had been experiencing some memory lapses, she was in pretty good health for an octogenarian.

But Jill had recently grown worried. According to Ralph, Jill's mom had started having paranoid fantasies and she had survived a fall, which according to the Centers for Disease Control puts 2 million seniors into emergency rooms every year. In addition, Ralph was not in good health. Jill was confused about her mom's behavioral issues and wasn't sure Ralph was capable of making a fair assessment. And the falls had Jill concerned for her mom's physical safety. She worried about leaving for their Italian getaway at this time. Mike assured her everything would be all right. But sure enough, just a few days into their latest Mediterranean sojourn, Jill and Mike got the call Ralph had died.

"All of a sudden I felt so far away," says Jill. Her anxiety about leaving while she was so concerned for her mom now became waves of guilt washing over Jill for not being by her mom's side. Mike became travel agent extraordinaire, making calls late at night to get them on a plane to California the next day.

After Ralph's funeral, Jill and Mike returned to New York, assured Lora would be fine surrounded by friends and the facility staff she had grown close to. As the weeks rolled by, Jill's daily phone calls to her mom could no longer bridge the 3,000-mile distance and the constant concern toying with her mind. After a few in-person visits and more falls for Lora, it became clear to Jill her mother needed more care. But moving her into the facility's dementia care center seemed wrong. Jill still was not sure Lora was "there yet." She felt Lora would be isolated from neighbors and friends and as Jill says, "It just wasn't family."

Dementia affects more than 5 million Americans and 36 million worldwide according to the Alzheimer's Association. While Alzheimer's disease is the most common form of dementia accounting for 60-80 percent of all cases, there are other forms as well including vascular dementia, Lewy bodies, frontotemporal, Creutzfeldt Jakob disease and others. While the symptoms of dementia vary widely, most signs include memory loss, confusion with language and communication, inability to focus and pay attention, trouble with reasoning, judgment and visual perception. Jill's mom was showing many of these signs in varying degrees.

Jill also says she felt "in shock because I always believed my mom would live out her days in this beautiful facility we had found for her in Santa Barbara that she loved. I had thought this would be an idyllic way for her to live this last chapter." However, what Jill found was "long-distance caregiving gives you blinders."

While Jill debated what course of action to take for her mom, Mike was feeling a pinch of resentment his Umbrian dreams were going to be put on hold indefinitely. However, his overriding concern was about the toll this would take on his wife. He says, "Jill's focus was on her mom, but my eye was on Jill. My new job was to help her do the right thing."

Mamma Mia!

One of the toughest decisions for caregivers, especially those 7-8 million long-distance caregivers of older parents, is wondering whether it is better to have them live in a special facility that can provide the care they need or move them into your home or closer to you so you can care for them.

Nora Jean Levin, executive director of the nonprofit organization dedicated to long-distance caregivers, Caring From a Distance, says, "This is the dilemma that has plagued caregivers over time." She advises if you are caring for a loved one but you do not see their daily behavior and activities, it creates a lot of anxiety in helping to make the right decisions for their care. "It is hard to spend only two or three days with a loved one and really know what is going on with them."

In Jill's case, she is an only child, which can make caregiving both harder and easier. It is harder because there are no other siblings to share the caregiving burden or commiserate with you on an emotional level. But in some instances, it can be easier because you are not dealing with sibling conflict. Jill told me so many of her and Mike's friends who were also going through caregiving situations told Jill how *lucky* she was to be an only child and not have to constantly battle a brother or sister over decisions for her mom. Mike said they witnessed situations where caring for an older parent "immediately makes the adult children three years old again – 'Mom loves you more' and comments like that – unbelievable."

But, whether benefit or burden, Jill's concerns were mounting over her mom's increasingly erratic behavior. Jill originally thought the staff at the assisted living facility was providing adequate care, but it was becoming apparent Jill's mom really needed 24/7 care.

"My mom was calling people at all times of the night, wandering off and eventually got to a point where she was physically attacking the nurses caring for her after a bad fall," says Jill. "It became clear the facility was not prepared to take care of her; the writing was on the wall.

"One night we went to dinner with our son Max, and he said what I had been in denial about, 'You have to move her to New York City. We're her family.' At that moment I looked over at Mike and he just nodded, and I knew this is what we had to do."

Many caregivers of older parents, even those who are married or who have siblings who can help, often tell me they feel "all alone." While Jill is an only child, the secret ingredient in her caregiving situation is she never had that feeling – she had Mike.

"It was a huge moment in that restaurant when I looked at Mike and I just knew no matter what, he was going on this journey with me," says Jill. "Believe me, the last thing Mike wanted to do was have my mother in our lives every minute. Even though he loved her, Mike felt my personality changed, and not for the better, when I was around my mother."

Now, not only would Mike have Lora in the same city but he would have to live with the *two Jills*. But they both realized the best thing for Lora was to be closer to family. Little did they know moving Lora closer would bring their entire family together. But first they had to get Lora to New York City.

La Dolce Vita American Style

What came next is something almost all caregivers face because so few families have that essential caregiving conversation before a crisis hits. In fact, only one-third of all caregivers have had any conversation with their older loved one about long-term care. Jill and Mike had to first become like two knights searching for artifacts during the Crusades. They had to search high and low for the paperwork to close Lora's bank and other accounts, they had to deal with Lora's expired passport and driver's license needed to get her on the plane to New York, and they had to find a memory care facility in New York City. And that was just the start.

Mike had promised Ralph before he died they would look after Lora financially and ensure her safety and comfort. Ralph was concerned there would not be enough money to ensure Lora would be all right after he was gone. But when Jill and Mike asked Lora to sign a Power of Attorney that would grant them financial decision-making on her behalf, she balked. She was certain they were trying to steal her money.

"We were so lost in the beginning," says Mike. "First of all, we had no idea how bad Lora's condition had become, but it quickly became clear something had to be done. When we got to that point, it was all done in a panic. I was just tap dancing, and you learn quickly you have to be able to move in any direction."

In retrospect, Mike advises future caregivers the conversation, especially about finances, should be had long before there is a crisis. While Ralph and Lora had both ensured their end-of-life wishes were intact and they had given copies of their Living Wills to Jill and Mike, the financial end of their long-term care planning was flawed.

"Ralph feared he had not made the right decisions about his veteran's benefits for Lora after he was gone, and he was right," says Mike.

Similar to so many caregivers who don't know where to begin, Jill tapped into her network of friends to find some pointers about how Medicaid could cover some of the costs they were facing. As Jill says, "I was getting worried watching the money spill out of her bank account and knowing there was going to be a dry well soon."

Mike had been wise about planning his and Jill's financial security but he was not expecting they would also wind up covering many of Lora's care costs. Even with Medicaid, not all costs are covered. Mike says he had promised Ralph they would help take care of Lora but this situation is not uncommon for caregivers.

According to the National Alliance for Caregiving, more than half of all caregivers spend on average 10 percent of their annual income on care-related costs for a loved one. Knowing ahead of time what your loved one's long-term care plans are will help you avoid the caregiving cost drain.

Jill was also overwhelmed with all the paperwork required to simply provide proper care for her mom. "I can't imagine with someone who is elderly, this is the level of paperwork they have to wade through." An Elder Law attorney became Jill's best counsel on how to ensure all the documentation was done correctly. One thing Jill does note is the Alzheimer's Association and her own network of friends were the best resources she turned to for help.

After they convinced Lora to allow them authority to be able to help her if she could not make decisions on her own, they then had to convince her to move to New York.

Originally they thought they had found an excellent solution. The nice-looking senior living facility was only a few short blocks from their apartment in New York City. It housed quite a few retired intellectuals – Jill knew this would be an added bonus that would make her mother happy. But ultimately it became clear although Lora needed almost constant care, the facility Jill and Mike chose for her was more like the prison in Shawshank Redemption than the wonderful Shangri-La they had thought they found.

And Jill had to face the sad fact her mother was increasingly belligerent and many of the professional care workers did not want to deal with her. "It was hell," says Jill, and I can hear the beleaguered tone in her voice. She was frustrated, angry, fearful, and felt powerless in how to deal with her mom's situation. "I was at the assisted care facility almost every day yelling at the administration that they needed to find me someone who knows how to deal with this kind of behavior. I was at my wit's end."

Beth Kallmyer of the Alzheimer's Association says, "Sometimes moving a loved one to a new facility is frightening for the person with dementia. She doesn't understand why she is in a new place, she can't remember new things such as where the toilet is – this can make her lash out or become hostile because the fear is taking over."

Kallmyer says the Alzheimer's Association also tries to counsel caregivers through what they are experiencing – depression, sadness, feeling overwhelmed and mourning the loss of the relationship they had with the person with dementia who no longer exists. "We coach them this is normal."

In many ways Jill had a role as her mother's protector and caregiver ever since she was a young girl. Lora had her hearing disability since she was in her 30s, which was around the same time Jill's father walked out on his wife and young daughter. In her words, "I was always the one who was going to save her." Yet she found herself in a situation with Lora's dementia where *saving* was not possible. Now, it was creating a new reality where Jill found herself trying to *cope* rather than *save,* and it wasn't going well.

Eat, Pray, Love

The first saving grace for Jill and Mike was a home health aide named Marcia. "Marcia actually knew my mom better than I did because Marcia knew the disease." Marcia, who was born in Jamaica and had grown up watching her mom care for her grandfather who had cancer, came to the U.S. to train to work in geriatric care. What they found was Marcia combined her trained home health aide skills with an uncanny ability to "read people." She had Lora's number from the get go and her way to care for Lora was through humor. She also renamed Lora. It was Marcia who came up with "Lolo." It was intuitively representative of the fact the *other Lora* had been transformed through the dementia. This was a new person. Lora liked the new name, and it helped Jill to understand the mom she once knew was another person now. Lolo was her name.

Marcia helped Lora accept her condition, which took an untold burden off of Jill. She also helped wean Lora off of some of the many medications she was taking. Mike writes in his book, *Family Meals*, which chronicled their journey with Lora, Marcia was responsible for helping to remove Jill's mom from taking anti-depressants, anti-psychotics and sleeping pills. In addition, after Lora passed her doctor's test, they also removed her from her heart medicine. Mike writes it was like night and day; Lora had "instant improvement in energy and well-being."

Prescription medications can be a double-edged sword for many caregivers. While a lot of drugs are helpful in managing the symptoms of chronic illness, there is a two-fold problem. Carol Levine, director of the Families and Health Care Project for the United Hospital Fund cautions first of all, medications are often managed by the caregiver unless you have 24/7 nursing care, and even then it is good to check up on your loved one's medication compliance – this can become a tedious and time-consuming task. Secondly, doctors often over-prescribe drugs, particularly if a patient asks about a new drug she had heard about, and the doctor believes it cannot hurt to write the prescription.

Levine says, "An older loved one's resistance to taking medications is a caregiver's biggest challenge." She also adds that too often, she sees many people on too many medications.

As a caregiver, trying to manage all these medications and be compliant with the instructions can become unwieldy – particularly if you have a loved one who is fighting you on taking them in the first place. Levine advises caregivers to always ask a physician when a new medication is being prescribed as to whether the drug is really necessary. And she adds, always ask the doctor to review the entire list of medications to see what can be removed from the list.

Just as Marcia has become a ray of light in their lives, another funny thing happened. They originally hired Marcia to replace the care workers in the facility where Lora lived. But shortly afterward the apartment literally across the hallway from Jill and Mike became vacant. After some soul searching on whether this was a solution or marital suicide, Jill and Mike consulted with Marcia, and all agreed this would be Lora's new home. They find the cost of having Lora live across the hall was actually half the cost of the senior living facility, allowing Jill and Mike to hire two additional home health aides to give Marcia a break.

Around the same time both their son, Max, and their daughter, Alison, from Mike's first marriage, found themselves making their way back to the Big Apple. Alison, who is a chef and personal caterer, actually took over the meal planning and cooking for her grandmother – consulting with Lora's doctor on dietary needs and doing what she does best – making it all delicious. Max, a musician, added the spiritual and therapeutic element of music into his grandmother's life. With Alison and Max only a few blocks away, Mike's dream of an Italian lifestyle was becoming a reality on the Upper West Side.

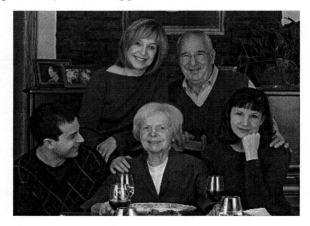

Photo: Kristine Walsh

Jill and Mike with Max, Lora and Alison from the cover of Mike's book, *Family Meals*

In *Family Meals*, Mike writes, "The difference between the American and Italian attitudes toward family and the care of aging parents is not just cultural or traditional – it's the law." He points out the Italian Constitution states the basic unit is the family not the individual. It didn't take a constitutional order for the Tuckerberry (which is the name of their web site) family to come together in the Italian tradition of *la famiglia*.

"Our kids were amazing," says Mike. "Everything came together and it became very Italian."

Originally everyone was all over the country and Mike said family gatherings were sporadic and they only saw each other when they could. Now it is more like the Mediterranean way of life where family sees each other every day. This became the great blessing of caregiving that Mike says was "completely unplanned."

"Our daughter, Alison, was truly incredible; she moved from L.A. to New York with the idea she would become the cook for our little nursing home across the hall," says Jill. "She is really my right hand in terms of all this stuff."

Jill says without Alison, Umbria may have only remained a dream of hers and Mike's. But because Alison "really stepped up," she has made it possible for Mike and Jill to finally get back on track and take some time to make their treks to the Italian countryside that feeds their souls. Max also gives his parents some respite by playing companion to his grandmother (when he is not playing drums in his jazz band).

It's not just the kids and Lora who make up this little Italian band of love. Marcia and the other two home health aides, Buela and Kethleen, have become part of the family, too.

Besides the familial ties, Mike believes his gifts from caregiving are he and Jill have become even closer, and he is now more realistic about his future and how he will want his family to care for him. Jill told me she feels caregiving has taught her to "just let things happen and to not be in denial because it doesn't serve you." She also feels it has improved the communication between her and Mike. And his support has allowed her to really discover who she is through this experience.

I've Got You, Babe

One of the things that really helped Jill and Mike through this caregiving journey is they were a team when it came to making decisions about Lora's care. Many partners whose spouse takes on a primary caregiving role for someone often become angry or resentful over their mate spending so much time and attention caring for someone else. This situation is particularly difficult for men who watch their wives get sucked into the black hole of caregiving.

Not so for Mike. His attitude was he was there to support Jill, help steady her, be her rock. He also kept an eye on her in terms of her health and wellness. He cooks for her, ensures she gets some downtime while he watches TV golf with Lora – one of their shared pastimes. And he is the shoulder always there for Jill to cry on when she feels so helpless in what to do next.

"Even to a fault I was supporting Jill in her denial," says Mike. "If Jill declared her mom was going to recover in three weeks, I would agree she would recover in three weeks, and that is not always good but I wanted to be supportive." Mike credits Jill's therapist for really helping Jill see through the denial to reality.

The most important element of their caregiving journey is they were together. One of them wasn't always flying off for a new role in another city, and Mike never looked at the situation as *Jill's problem*. It was their life together that had a new ingredient thrown into it and together they would figure out how to make it all blend perfectly.

One of Mike's passions is cooking – a passion also embraced by his daughter, Alison (she writes a great blog about cooking at awonderlandofwords.com). He sees caregiving like cooking – you are nurturing and feeding the soul of someone you love.

As the Tuckerberry family gathered recently for another family meal – this time to celebrate Lora's 93rd birthday – Jill and Mike have proven successful as both co-stars on screen, in life and in caregiving. When I think of Jill and Mike, I think of Julia Child's quote, "…nothing is too much trouble if it turns out the way it should."

Jill's Lessons Learned

1. **Explore Who You Are**

Jill had actually been a caregiver for her mother long before Ralph died. Because Lora had been hard of hearing for most of her adult life, Jill as the only child was her interpreter to the world. But along with that responsible role comes conflicted feelings. Jill also says she believes she may have felt a little bit of shame about her mom's dementia. "I didn't want people to see her that way, I didn't want people to talk about her in that way and I know she wouldn't want that either."

However, Jill tells me caregiving has made her "grateful." When she became a caregiver to her mom, Jill says, "There is so much that comes up around who I was as a child and who my mother was – every day as this drama unfolds I learn more." She found the exploration of both herself and her mom interesting and fascinating. She embraced the good with the bad. This is how most people find tremendous wisdom in their lives and I would definitely label Jill *wise*.

2. **Don't Dwell in Denial**

Jill found caregiving helped her to learn a valuable life lesson. "Allow things to happen as they happen rather than making them happen the way you think they should happen." It really comes down to learning to trust yourself, your loved one and the natural order of things.

She also feels by letting go it actually also helped in her communication with others, especially with Mike. At times, fear will keep us silent and leave us feeling isolated. Through communication and opening up, you can improve all the relationships around you.

Another recommendation Jill makes to all caregivers is to "be present, see the truth of the situation and don't pretend it's not happening." She strongly believes you have to find ways to leave denial as fast as you can. Mike adds sometimes it's difficult to even see you are living in denial. He says the hardest thing for adult children caring for a parent is to admit your parent is changing, and changing in ways you may not want to be happening. This is where Jill believes professional help can hold the mirror up for you and help you see clearly.

3. **Ride the Rapids with Professional Help**

Jill says it is helpful to find a professional therapist who can help you understand the deeper meaning in these parental relationships.

She makes a comparison between caregiving and being in a canoe among the rapids. "I cannot stress enough that if you can do it, you should try to get a professional who can be objective. These waters are the most basic but they are the trickiest waters you have to navigate. You feel like you are in the rapids and it never ends."

What Jill also found surprising to admit to, which so many caregivers feel, is anger. Jill had spent so many years adjusting to her mom's need to "put on appearances" because of her hearing disability. When Lora came to a point in her later life when it wasn't just her hearing problems but it was also the dementia taking over, Jill's pent up anger came to the forefront. Some of the anger was based on guilt. Jill felt as her mom's lifelong savior, maybe she should have done more.

Again, with the help of therapy, many caregivers can better understand caregiving emotions are not just about the current situation – often they are about a lifetime of emotions that have not been dealt with. A professional therapist can help you sift through these caregiving emotions.

As much as Jill is grateful for the love and support of her family, she is a huge believer having a professional who is outside the family dynamic to see things with the wide angle lens and not just a telephoto lens can do more for your wellness than you can imagine. "Having this professional help has gotten me to calmer waters. I don't know if I could have done it without the professional help."

4. Don't Let Caregiving Consume You

Jill does credit her husband for ensuring caregiving did not become their entire life. Jill was often focused only on the responsibilities of caring for her mom but Mike was also saying, "Yes, but we have to have a great life," says Jill. While it is hard to find balance in life, Mike says, "The answer is you have to do both."

This makes me think of the Broadway play and movie, *Barefoot in the Park*. One partner is always focused on playing by the rules and being strait-laced (Robert Redford's character in the movie, which in the Tuckerberry version would be played by Jill) and the other partner is full of *la dolce vita* kicking up her heels and experiencing the joys of life (played by Jane Fonda in the movie and in our version would be Mike's role). In the end, they switch roles and come to a better understanding of how to blend *responsibility with a little regale*.

Mike's Lessons Learned

1. Caregiving Can Bring You Closer to Your Spouse

If Mike could impart any wisdom to other husbands and partners who have a mate going through a caregiving situation, he advises, "It is the greatest opportunity you have in your marriage to get to know your wife and to let her know you are going to support her." He also says more than any other event in their lives, the caregiving of Lora "really made us learn to trust each other. We had never been tested before." Even though they are still on their caregiving journey, this whole experience has "deepened our marriage."

2. It's Your Choice but You Have to Have "The Talk"

Mike believes our generation needs to learn from our own caregiving experience to be responsible for making sound long-term care plans and initiating the conversation with our children.

"We've seen what the fall-out can be, so it's our responsibility to put this in place and talk to our kids. We're not going to ask the kids what they think – it's our choice – but with that choice comes the responsibility of conversation among family."

He also believes going on this caregiving journey with Jill and her mom, "Made me more realistic about my own future."

3. Beware Caregiving Can Make You Childish

Mike says when it comes to caregiving, especially caring for a parent, it is not unusual to revert back to being a child. Eight years before the caregiving crisis occurred with Lora, Mike had lost his mom to Alzheimer's so he knew the signs and some of the bumps in the road. He often found himself becoming his mother's *little boy* again, trying to please her.

I agree with Mike's assessment on reverting to being a child again when we become caregivers. So often, I have seen the primary caregiver, let's say it's the wife, become a frightened little girl. She needs to be held, consoled over her grief, her fears, her guilt. The person receiving the care – typically the parent – can also become childish. He is vulnerable, afraid and angry over losing his independence and often becomes obstinate and throws temper tantrums just like a two-year-old. And the spouse or partner of the caregiver can become a *big baby* – no longer getting the amount of attention he was used to. Sharing the love of a mate with another person who may be getting more attention because of the level of care needed is a difficult transition. This can make the spouse, whiny, jealous and resentful – in other words, *childish*.

Most of us are adults when we are faced with caregiving but some may revert back to the childhood sandbox in emotional dealings.

4. Live, Love, Laugh

Mike also believes, "In humor, there is truth. And in any life situation, including caregiving, it is invaluable – you cannot live without it." Jill adds her mom has been a great source of material for Mike's humorous writing.

How Jill Finds Her "Me Time"

Jill is devoted to activities that help clear and calm the mind. She has twice battled and won her fight with breast cancer – first in 1986 and then again in 2009. She eats a healthy diet, practices daily yoga, meditation and Pilates. In fact, Jill was gifted a Pilates reformer which she says she dragged from Los Angeles to New York only to realize she had nowhere to put it. Since the live-in health aides like to sleep in the same room as Lora, a bedroom opened up in the "little nursing room across the hallway," and Jill was able to set up her equipment in that room. Every morning, she rises, greets her mom and spends time in the Zen zone. She says, "It's really wonderful because I realized I would not have that room for me across the hall if it were not for my mother."

How Mike Finds His "Me Time"

Mike is a truly passionate writer – perhaps even more a passion than his acting these days. His book, *Family Meals*, is a poignant, humorous look at the dilemma of caregiving. If this chapter has whet your appetite for more of Jill's and Mike's caregiving story I highly recommend you read his book. Just be forewarned – you will laugh out loud and you will want to go have an Italian dinner afterward.

His writing did not end with pouring his observations about caring for Lora onto the page. His first novel, *After Annie,* was published in 2012. It is the story of a man who loses his wife after a few years and has to explore whether he can live without her. Mike takes ordinary situations – whether real or fictional – and finds the funny bone in life.

Mike says, "I have to write every day or I'm just not happy."

How They Find Their "We Time"

Date night in New York City. As much as Jill and Mike loved their time in Los Angeles during their heady *L.A. Law* years and they love their Italian getaways, they say Manhattan is their kind of town. They love strolling the streets or walking in Central Park, visiting museums, finding a great little restaurant, visiting friends, performing in and attending Broadway performances. Whatever they do, they do it together.

Sylvia Mackey
"Mrs. 88"

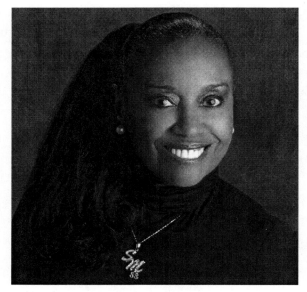

Photo: Courtesy of Sylvia Mackey

The two most powerful warriors are patience and time.

— Leo Tolstoy

Sylvia Mackey – "Mrs. 88"

A Football Wife Tackles Dementia and the NFL

When it comes to the gladiators of the gridiron, he was the Charlton Heston or Russell Crowe of his day. But in the end, it would be his wife – on the sidelines of his entire career – who would become the warrior at the center of the action.

I first met Sylvia when she invited me to her Baltimore home to talk about her caregiving journey. Reminders of John Mackey – one of the NFL's greatest players and Sylvia's husband of almost 50 years were everywhere – photos of his football days, family photos, a bust of John and even his trademark cowboy hat. Sylvia, who is still model-slim, was a gracious hostess and full of energy and passion as she talked about being a caregiver for her husband. It is this energetic spirit which gave her the strength to face her husband's dementia and win.

When John Mackey, No. 88, was inducted into the Pro Football Hall of Fame in 1992, he was only the second tight end to receive the honor. He was and still is considered one of the best tight ends to ever take the field. In fact, Mike Ditka, himself a Hall of Fame player and the first *pure* tight-end to be inducted into that rare club of exceptional players, stated Mackey should have been first.

As a Baltimore Colt, where he played all but the last year of his career, John scored one of the most famous plays in NFL championship history. In Super Bowl V played in 1971, John scored a touchdown by catching the nail-biting pass from quarterback Johnny Unitas that first careened off the hands of the opposite team's player, grazed the fingertips of his teammate and finally wound up safely in the arms of John who ran it for a then-record 75-yard reception. It was this decisive play that helped the Colts beat the Dallas Cowboys and won John his coveted Super Bowl ring. He also started wearing what would become his trademark – a cowboy hat – to commemorate his victory over the Cowboys.

Twenty-one years later, as John took his place in football's pantheon of great players for his Hall of Fame induction ceremony, right by his side was the woman who had been in the same spot since his college playing days, his wife, Sylvia. Theirs would prove to be a true love story, challenged only by a devastating medical diagnosis.

Little did either John or Sylvia know that day in 1992 that 14 years later, John's toughest battles would be fought off the football field with his lovely wife serving as both tackler and blocker.

For Love of the Game…And the Man

As we sat talking over coffee, Sylvia told me the story of how she first met John Mackey as a beautiful model and co-ed at Syracuse University.

"It was right before school officially started and I was walking across campus and this car pulled up with four of the school's football players – John Brown, Ernie Davis, Art Baker and John Mackey – who offered me a ride to my dorm."

It was 1959.

While Brown had his eye on Sylvia, she had her eye on the quiet John Mackey. It wasn't until football season ended they were walking to a class in January and Sylvia finally asked John why he and the other football players never seemed to date any of the college girls.

"John said to me, 'Why? Do you want me to take you out?' And I said, yeah. He always says I asked him out but I guess it is however you want to look at it."

She recalls Mackey was going to cancel the date because he didn't have any money or a car. It was roommate Ernie Davis who saved the day giving John his car and $5.

"And that was it," she says.

It had only taken one date for the quiet yet mesmerizing college football athlete to win her heart. From the start, they were a team. Knowing John would be playing in the big leagues of professional football, after graduation they planned their lives around his career when he was drafted as a Baltimore Colt.

For more than 40 years they had a wonderful life. Football victories, three beautiful children – Laura, Lisa and John – a career with their beloved Baltimore Colts (1963-1971) and San Diego Chargers (1972). After John's retirement from the NFL in 1972, he went on to become the first president of the NFL Players Association. As he had done on the playing field, Mackey fought hard winning pensions and benefits for players.

It took four years of Sylvia recognizing small things weren't right with John before he was diagnosed in 2001.

"One of the first things I remember is when we were at a golf tournament and John had not taken a shower," says Sylvia. "I asked him why and he told me he had but the shower and towels were dry and I thought that was strange to fib about taking a shower particularly since John was so adamant about taking his showers."

She says gradually his behavior became strange, suddenly out of nowhere he was warning people about cheese – about how it was bad for them. He was a lifelong avid reader and he stopped reading all together. He would sit on cross-country plane trips with a blank stare the entire hours-long trip, never looking at a magazine or engaging in conversation. He was a snazzy dresser who now wore the same outfit day after day. He would sit all day long in front of the TV just watching the weather channel. Sylvia started keeping a list of these things that were out of character for John.

Friends now tell her they were noticing things with John as far back as 1997. But none of them said anything at the time fearful of what it might be and not wanting to upset Sylvia. One friend, a doctor, mentioned to Sylvia he thought John should be checked for Alzheimer's and Sylvia recalls becoming really angry. Deep down inside Sylvia knew something was wrong and her husband was slowly slipping away.

"The first thing I remember feeling when I took John to get tested and they told me John had frontotemporal degeneration, was relief," remembers Sylvia. "I finally knew something was medically wrong with him and it wasn't just him getting crotchety or strange."

John was only 60-years-old.

Frontotemporal degeneration (FTD) is also known as frontotemporal dementia or frontotemporal lobar degeneration (FTLD). Not unlike Alzheimer's disease, it is a neurodegenerative disease that affects the frontal and anterior temporal regions of the brain. These areas of the brain control personality and social behavior, speech and language comprehension, reasoning, decision-making and planning. According to the Association of Frontotemporal Degeneration (AFTD), this is the most common dementia among a younger population, and represents about 10-20 percent of all dementia cases. It is sometimes misdiagnosed or mistaken as a psychiatric problem, Alzheimer's disease, or Parkinson's disease.

In his book, *The Alzheimer's Prevention Program*, Dr. Gary Small, director of the UCLA Longevity Center, says getting knocked out for an hour or more can double your risk for developing Alzheimer's disease. He states professional football players have higher rates of dementia at earlier ages in life because of the repeated minor concussions they can suffer during games.

When John was tested at the UCLA Medical Center by neurologists he had no idea why he was there – he thought they were there for Sylvia to get some tests.

"By the time he was diagnosed, he had no idea what was happening to him, we did not have a chance to discuss it."

One incident that highlights the special challenges FTD caregivers face was during a simple football game on TV. A few years ago, Sylvia and her husband were watching his beloved Baltimore Colts take on the New England Patriots. While watching games on TV was actually enjoyable for John, this game was suddenly different. At first John was excited. He saw the familiar 88 jersey of his Baltimore Colts on the screen and thought they were re-running one of his famous plays. But as they showed a close-up of the player's jersey, it was not the number 88 with Mackey's name on the jersey but that of the current player using the same number, Marvin Harrison.

Mackey grew confused then agitated. He could not understand the person on the screen was not him. Even with his wife's explanations he could not grasp someone else was wearing his jersey and it had been more than 30 years since he took the field. He continued to be bewildered about why the TV showed the jersey with the wrong name.

"He simply could not differentiate between the reality of today and more than 30 years ago when he was playing," says Sylvia.

Sylvia faced what so many caregiving spouses of someone with a dementia or Alzheimer's diagnosis do. It starts with denial, followed by an almost obsessive need to learn everything you can. Finally, you encounter fear for the day you know will come when your loved one's memory – including possibly not recognizing you – will be gone.

What makes Sylvia's story one of inspiration is this diagnosis could have sacked her (in football jargon) but instead she did not let this devastating news knock her down. She was determined to create a new way for their lives to remain as normal for as long as possible.

Tackling Dementia

"John and I were on our way to an autograph signing – we never missed one – and I was determined this was something we were going to continue to do," says Sylvia. "It always made John happier as we got ready for these trips – he never once turned down anyone who wanted his autograph."

But this year was different. There was an incident with TSA airport security that almost took them both down – literally.

Her husband, proudly wearing his Super Bowl ring and trademark cowboy hat, refused to remove these items and place them on the conveyor belt to be scanned. He did not understand there had been a 9/11, he did not understand why they did not recognize him, and ultimately he thought they were trying to rob him of his precious possessions.

As he grew more frustrated with the TSA agents who, unaware of his diagnosis, thought he was just being a belligerent traveler, the agents grew increasingly irritated. As John looked ahead at the metal detector people were passing through, his dementia caused him to be confused and think the detector's overhead archway was a goal post. Summoning the ironman speed and agility he displayed on the football field, John charged through the scanner archway with several TSA agents now in full pursuit. As he had done in so many games and Super Bowl match-ups, John knew he could outrun the defense and get to the goal line. Unfortunately, this was not a field of play but a crowded airport, and the sight of the six-foot two-inch, 220-pound former football great who was dragging the agents several feet through the airport until they finally tackled him, handcuffed him and called an ambulance to take him to the hospital for evaluation was almost more than Sylvia could bear.

During this dramatic episode, a tearful and frightened Sylvia was trying her best to explain to the agents and the curious onlookers her husband was the NFL great and one of Baltimore's favorite sons, John Mackey, that his illness meant he had no ability to understand what was happening. She was frightened the exertion and trauma of the incident might stress John's heart too much or confused TSA agents might shoot her husband who was violating federal travel regulations. They could have had John taken to jail. However, because this was Baltimore and they finally recognized the famous tight end, they offered to have John released to the local hospital. She collapsed while they escorted her confused husband away, and thought to herself, "I don't know if I can do this anymore."

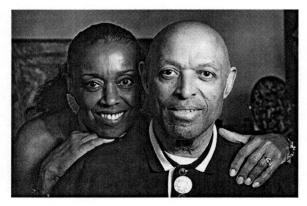

Photo: Jerry Jackson

Sylvia and John Mackey

Hemingway wrote, "Courage is grace under fire."

Once at the hospital, Sylvia was trying to recover from the anguish of their ordeal, but John was back to his typical, jovial, social self – signing autographs for many of the doctors and nurses who instantly recognized the NFL great. It was at this moment as her husband basked in the bright light of his fame, she realized she could not give up on her husband or herself. This is when her courage took flight.

Instead of deciding that attending future autograph signings, their annual Super Bowl trip or other travel would be out of the question, Sylvia got to work contacting the head of TSA at the Baltimore/Washington International Airport. She explained her situation and asked the TSA executive for his help to allow her husband to travel, especially to the sporting events and autograph signings he truly lived for and were important to maintaining some type of normalcy in their lives.

The TSA executive designed a plan with Sylvia to have John brought through a private area where they could scan him without incident and without his having to remove items precious to him. In addition, the TSA executive also contacted his TSA counterpart at the arrival airport to explain how similar treatment of John upon his return flight out of their airport would be helpful to avoid any similar, dramatic incidents neither party wanted.

These special plans are not just for those with famous last names. One lesson all caregivers can take from Sylvia's travel strategy is to plan ahead and ask a lot of questions. All airports will work with caregivers on the special travel needs of their loved ones but do not wait until you get to the airport. Call ahead and make plans – take names so you can reference the details of the plan when you arrive at the terminal. Sylvia advises making these arrangements at least one month in advance of your travel and then calling the week of travel to confirm the details.

For years, John and Sylvia were able to travel with no drama and no more hassle than the rest of us face as we navigate airport security in this new era of heightened safety rules.

Running Interference with Incontinence

One of the least talked about issues of caregiving – especially for someone with dementia or Alzheimer's – is the uncomfortable reality of incontinence problems. In the later stages of dementia, almost all patients suffer from varying degrees of incontinence which is the inability to control one's bladder or bowels.

Beth Kallmyer, vice president of constituent services at the Alzheimer's Association, says incontinence happens when a patient is not very mobile, they forget they have to relieve themselves, and it happens spontaneously; or they cannot remember where the bathroom is located. Urge incontinence – the strong, sudden need to urinate due to spasms or contractions, typical of dementia patients with neurological issues – can result in confusion and sometimes humiliation for the sufferer. It can also create a constant burden on the caregiver who has to change adult diapers, a loved one's clothing and bed sheets.

Lynn Wilson, founder of the Caregiver Partnership, which is an online site dedicated to incontinence products and caregiver support for the issue, says, "Incontinence is one of the toughest issues caregivers face." She advises many diseases and disorders can cause incontinence – diabetes, Crohn's disease, dementia, multiple sclerosis or even a bad hip or knee. It is the inactivity of the patient that makes incontinence worse over time.

The Caregivers Partnership offers more than 400 incontinence products in its online store, and its customer service team is 100 percent staffed by former caregivers, so they understand your issues.

"When it comes to talking about adult diapers, it's about denial, discussion, dignity and decisions," says Wilson. The patient is often in denial about the problem, but the discussion has to happen. Wilson advises caregivers to appreciate the dignity of your loved one, and she says many of the newer products on the market help.

"Some of the latest products are cloth-like, which eliminates the embarrassing noise of the plastic on former adult diaper models," says Wilson. "There are also full body fabric suits now." Caregiver Partnership will actually ship you a free sample, so your loved one can try on several styles before you have to purchase the product in bulk – saving a caregiver not only cost but also the time to try out different models.

Incontinence, while a common symptom of those with neurological disorders or diseases, can also be a normal part of aging. What is encouraging is this once taboo, sensitive and uncomfortable topic is making its way into mainstream media and marketing campaigns. Husband and wife acting duo, Lisa Rinna and Harry Hamlin, who both look at least 10-15 years younger than their real age, star in a new TV commercial for Depends, and actress/comedian, Whoopi Goldberg, and actress Kirstie Alley have both recently been spokespersons for Poise brand incontinence products.

In Sylvia's case, she was having problems getting her proud husband to try the adult disposable diapers that became an unwelcome side effect of John's dementia.

"He just did not want to admit this was his life now," says Sylvia. Even though he did not entirely understand he had dementia and his illness was causing this, he was either in denial it was happening or denial he had to do anything about it. "Well, the reality is, he wasn't the one doing the worrying and cleaning up – I was and I needed to solve this."

Her plan played off of her husband's loyalty to the game and the league he had served so faithfully for years. She simply put the diapers, as well as the incontinence medication John (who shunned all drugs) refused to take, and a letter she wrote with NFL logos into a box with NFL labels on it, and set it outside their front door one night. The next morning she got the box and told John a special package had arrived from the NFL. John asked her to open the box and read the letter. She told John the NFL was requesting all retired players, especially those in the Hall of Fame, were to wear the special men's underwear they were researching. In addition, she told John the enclosed pills were vitamins they recommended for aging players to stay fit.

Mission accomplished. John never questioned the instructions and Sylvia smoothed the way to solving his incontinence problems in the same creative way she had solved their travel challenges.

According to Beth Kallmyer of the Alzheimer's Association, for many caregivers, incontinence becomes the tipping point at which they feel they can no longer manage their loved one's care at home. However, with the constant improvements in product offerings, medications and in new experimental treatment of controlling incontinence through Botox injections, many caregivers have hope of turning this *mission impossible* of incontinence into mission accomplished just like Sylvia.

Taking Her Game Plan to the NFL

In the last couple of years of her husband's life, even the resilient and resourceful Sylvia could not manage her husband's care at home any longer. While she was managing the incontinence, Sylvia says the dementia would sometimes keep John up all night and on more than one occasion, Sylvia would wake up to find John dressed with his cowboy hat on walking out the door at four in the morning. She also struggled getting him into and out of cars. While she would drive, John, who still weighed in at about 200 pounds, would refuse to get out of the car.

Sylvia says, "After a while, as a caregiver, you just can't survive like that."

At one point, John, who also suffered from diabetes, had a diabetic attack and had to be hospitalized overnight. Amazingly, Sylvia had finally gotten a full night's sleep. She also realized John was being taken care of by professionals and that is when Sylvia says she realized maybe having John in a facility would be best for everyone. Making the decision to have a loved one moved to a facility is one of the toughest decisions of a caregiver's life. For Sylvia, there was relief in finding the best dementia care facility about five minutes from their home where Sylvia knew he would be safe and cared for and she would literally be down the street.

What became very important to Sylvia is the staff at John's assisted living home had no turnover while he was there the last two years of his life. She was also impressed with the bright, uplifting atmosphere; the food which always looked attractive and the friendly staff who really became an extension of family.

While Sylvia knew this was the best decision for John and for herself, she worried about the cost of John's care. During his decade-long run in the NFL as one of the league's most valuable players, John made less than $500,000 – a salary most back-up players make in one season today. Despite his NFL Players' Union pension of $2,500 per month, costs were escalating. John needed special care and 24-hour supervision, requiring he and Sylvia live in separate places – costs his pension could not cover. To supplement his pension, Sylvia went back to work taking a job as a flight attendant at United Airlines – a career she still has today.

Sylvia became frustrated a superstar like her husband should spend his final years with his family struggling just to survive. But as with every other hurdle Sylvia encountered in this caregiving journey, she decided she would clear this one as well. She wrote a poignant, heartfelt letter to then NFL commissioner Paul Tagliabue who was ending his career with the NFL. Sylvia had met both Tagliabue and his wife, Chan, years earlier and decided to throw the proverbial *Hail Mary* pass. She pleaded with Tagliabue that helping the retired players and their families with home care and care facility costs would be a legacy that would make a difference long after his tenure as commissioner was over.

Both Tagliabue and his wife embraced the idea, and incoming commissioner Roger Goddell became its ongoing champion. There were several months of negotiations and planning with the NFL Players' Union, but eventually Sylvia received a call with some heartwarming and fulfilling news.

The NFL called Sylvia with the news they decided to cover some benefits and costs for former players who qualified with a diagnosis of dementia or Alzheimer's (later expanded to include Parkinson's disease and ALS), and even better news, the plan would honor her husband and her advocacy by naming it the *88 Plan* for the jersey number Mackey had worn throughout his entire career in both college and the NFL. The landmark insurance benefit would allow qualifying retired players and families to receive $88,000 for nursing home or day care or $50,000 to secure care at home annually.

The Final Play

In his final days at the assisted living facility in Baltimore, Sylvia visited her husband every day. Her loneliness was assuaged by the fact John was getting the best care possible – care she could not possibly handle at home as capable and courageous as she is. Even though her daughter, Laura, had quit her job to move back to Baltimore to help her mom and give her a break in caring for her dad while he was still at home, both women knew this situation could not go on forever.

John Mackey lost his battle with FTD on July 6, 2011. Sylvia has taken his place among NFL players and wives both current and retired. She attends every Super Bowl, and has represented her husband at numerous NFL-related events. She proudly wears a beautiful necklace with her initials and the number, 88.

But perhaps her starring role is as a passionate advocate for FTD and for understanding the plight of caregivers like herself. In 2009, Sylvia was named to the board of the Association of Frontotemporal Degeneration (AFTD). As their best cheerleader for awareness and education, Sylvia tours the country speaking to caregivers and support groups about the impact on families living with FTD. She also participated in the NFL sponsored *NFL Community Huddle*, a free town hall-style forum to help communities develop strategies for preventing and reducing the risk of dementia and stigma related to mental disorders. These events bring together community members, health providers, experts, NFL players, alumni and concerned advocates to discuss the mental health challenges faced by athletes, their families and people in the community.

Her husband was considered one of the NFL's best tight ends who ever played the game – maybe *the best* – earning credit for his Baltimore Colts' Super Bowl win and a place in the Football Hall of Fame. When knocked down by dementia, his resilient wife came up with a decade-long game plan to keep life as normal as possible for her college sweetheart and life's partner. From her caregiving experience she lobbied one of the most powerful organizations in sports to care for its own, resulting in security and support for former players and their families when it comes to brain-related illness.

Her husband was a superstar on the field and her superman. But it is Sylvia Mackey who deserves our praise in the Caregiver Hall of Fame as a superwoman.

Sylvia's Lessons Learned

1. Don't be an Accidental Tourist

As you just read in Sylvia's story, traveling with a loved one with dementia or other health-related issue is not impossible; it just requires a lot of preparation. In fact, Sylvia's mantra for caregivers is: "Prepare, Prepare, Prepare." Understanding the challenges of your loved one is essential in planning ahead.

Talk to TSA agents or other travel customer service if you are traveling by train or taking a cruise or checking into hotels. Learn what accommodations there are if your loved one is in a wheelchair or needs special assistance or help. And again, Sylvia's tip is make these accommodations at least a month in advance – do not wait until the last minute in case there is more for you to do before the trip can happen.

Another great resource is the Society for Accessible Travel and Hospitality or the Automobile Club. Both offer support to caregivers who travel with those with special needs or disabilities. You will find their contact information in the Resources section.

2. Get Creative

Understanding your loved one and what motivates him is the key to making your lives more manageable. In Sylvia's case, knowing anything required or requested by the NFL her husband would agree to became her golden ticket to solving the incontinence issues he faced.

Because dementia and Alzheimer's patients have more difficulty with short-term memory, meaning recent learnings are lost, it may help to try to find things that tie them to the past.

Again, in Sylvia's case, John had not played football for the NFL in more than 30 years, but it was this tie to his dedicated past career that enabled her to solve her caregiver's dilemma. They also moved back to Baltimore after living in California so they could return to the city they both loved and where John was happiest.

3. Come Fly with Me

Although Sylvia went back to work as a flight attendant during John's illness – partially as financial support for the family – she truly enjoys her career in the air. She credits her work with keeping her grounded during caregiving and giving her something to look forward to. In fact, if you are a frequent United Airlines traveler, you might be lucky enough to have Mrs. 88 taking care of you as a passenger.

How Sylvia Finds Her "Me Time"

While caregivers need a break and can sometimes find help from family or friends to get this respite, it is critical to have some balance in your life as a caregiver. Sylvia found this by keeping up with friendships and her family. She and John have several grandchildren from their two daughters and son, so having time to be a grandma and not just a caregiver was essential to Sylvia's survival during caregiving.

In addition, her daughter Laura and other close friends kept Sylvia in good spirits and got her mind off of her worries about John – even if it was just for a few minutes or an hour to grab lunch or dinner. This kind of break from caregiving duties – called respite – is essential for caregivers to continue to keep going.

One of Sylvia's passions in life is dance. She loves salsa, disco, anything where she can get out on the dance floor and feel the music transport her to a different place. The therapeutic effect of music and the physical benefit of dance for core strength, improved balance and a heart-healthy cardio workout, make dance one of the best things a caregiver can do to care for themselves. Even if you cannot find a good night club or get to a dance studio, turn up the radio or put your iPod in its docking station and let your inner *Dancing with the Stars* performer take the floor (even if it's just in your living room).

Alan and David Osmond

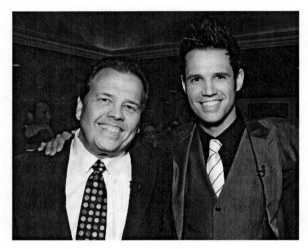

Photo: Courtesy of David Osmond

Life is one grand, sweet song, so start the music.

— Ronald Reagan

Alan and David Osmond

Like Father, Like Son – In Perfect Harmony

They say lightning never strikes twice in the same place yet this is exactly what happened to Alan Osmond and his son David Osmond of the famous entertainment family. Their lightning came in two forms: great musical and performing talent as well as a gift for songwriting; but also something less glamorous: a diagnosis of the autoimmune disease multiple sclerosis (MS).

I first met David Osmond and his wife, Valerie, at the Nancy Davis Foundation for Multiple Sclerosis Race to Erase MS Event. His positive energy and youthful, healthy appearance belied the fact his legs are in almost constant pain from MS. What struck me the most when I asked him what helps him fight his battle with MS was his exuberant response, "Family – the family is everything."

A couple of weeks later I followed up on his comment when I spoke to both David and his father, Alan, about living with a chronic disease. Their story looks at caregiving from a different perspective – that of the person with the condition and they provided insights as to how essential the love of family caregivers can be to someone with a devastating disease.

As I talked with both father and son, it became clear family, faith and the power of positive thinking is what is helping both these men to thrive in their lives while at the same time battle an unpredictable chronic illness.

The Entertainer

Growing up Osmond means you know how to be at the pinnacle of the entertainment world – you sing, you dance and no matter what the show must go on. Back in 1958, Alan was the oldest of the performing Osmond brothers, which also included Wayne, Merrill and Jay. The young brothers, ages 9, 7, 5 and 3 respectively, began as a barbershop quartet, singing at local events and contests in their hometown of Ogden, Utah. The performances originally began as both fun and fund-raising efforts to help the family afford hearing aids for the two oldest Osmond sons, Virl and Tom, both of whom were born deaf.

On a trip to California to audition for the *Lawrence Welk Show* (which they did not get), their father, George, decided to treat the disappointed boys to a trip to Disneyland. As they strolled through the theme park, the Osmond boys joined an adult barbershop quartet who were performing on Main Street, and curious visitors stopped to listen to their youthful glee and harmonies. Disney executives hired them on the spot, and they were soon performing in Disney televised specials.

During one of these TV appearances, Andy Williams's father was so impressed he called his son, one of the most famous crooners of that era, and told him to hire the boys for his *Andy Williams Show* on TV. The boys performed on the show during the '60s with younger brother, Donny, soon joining the group. Beyond the TV show the boys also began live tours performing both domestically and internationally in Europe. In the early '70s the Osmond boys decided they wanted to evolve from variety performers into a pop rock band. It was this crucial decision that brought them a lot of fame and attention and Alan managed most of the group's decisions and songwriting. In fact, Alan wrote most of the lyrics to the 39 hit songs resulting in the 102 million albums the Osmond Brothers have sold.

Although younger brother Donny broke away from the group to start a solo career and soon joined sister Marie in their still ongoing brother-sister performing act, the family stayed close, and the brothers continued to perform and entertain for 40 years with Alan at the helm. However, it was during a stage performance in 1987 Alan noticed the first signs of what would be an unbelievable diagnosis for someone with such energy and gusto for life.

"I began to trip on stage, clumsy stuff, but when I looked down to see what I tripped on nothing was there," he says. As he continued to stumble and fall both on and off stage, he also noticed when he played the trumpet or guitar, the fingers of his right hand were not as fast. It took a few years for doctors to diagnose him with multiple sclerosis. He was only 37 years old.

Multiple sclerosis (MS), which affects 2.5 million people worldwide, is an autoimmune disease that attacks the central nervous system and is incurable. Essentially, the myelin, which is the protective covering for the nerve fibers in the central nervous system, become inflamed or damaged, and through this inflammation the myelin becomes scarred, thus forming *sclerotic patches*. These multiple scars or lesions interfere with the transmission of signals to the brain and spinal cord causing the unpredictable and often debilitating symptoms MS patients experience such as numbness, tingling and searing pain in the extremities, with periods of partial or full blindness, loss of sensory function such as taste or smell and in some cases even full paralysis.

There are four types of MS based on the progression of the disease. Alan's was the rare primary progressive type – a diagnosis only 15 percent of all MS patients receive. With primary progressive there are no flare-ups or periods of remission, and this type means there is a slow degeneration of the body's functions.

While Alan stopped performing regularly with his brothers in 1996, he stayed behind the scenes managing the business side. In addition, he and his lovely wife, Suzanne, were raising eight sons and managing Alan's disease with grace and resilience.

As Alan told me, "I had been in the army and we [the Osmond Brothers] had always danced in our performances, so I felt I was very strong physically. I was raised to have a *can do it* attitude, so I was strong mentally. When I learned more about what MS would mean to my physical abilities, I thought, I may have MS but MS does not have me."

It is clear positive thinking and humor are part of Alan's daily medicine. He joked when he was first diagnosed with MS he thought MS must stand for *many sons*.

Family Ties

Growing up second generation of the famous Osmond clan has always been a blessing for David Osmond, one of eight sons born to Alan. As a torchbearer for the Osmond dynasty, David, age 32, has a successful solo career, still performs as the lead singer for the Osmonds - Second Generation, is hosting a new TV music competition reality series and participated in the eighth season of *American Idol*. The apple did not fall far from the tree.

As a young boy he watched his father cope with the impact of MS, and what he saw was this amazing strength of spirit that unbeknownst to David would become a beacon in his own journey with this disease.

"Pretty much my entire life I knew my dad had this thing called MS," recalls David. "You hear about it; you see it, but it never really made sense to me until I was diagnosed with the same disease."

Imagine if, as a young person in your 20s, you woke up and found you could not walk, you could not hold a guitar, you could not sing, because the pain in your chest and paralysis in your body reached from your toes to your diaphragm making it hard to breathe. This was what David Osmond faced in 2005 when he was diagnosed with multiple sclerosis and went from a promising entertainment career into a wheelchair.

"It started when I was playing a round of golf. I've had perfect 20/20 vision my entire life, but all of a sudden I could not see the ball in front of me – it felt like I was staring right into the sun, and I would turn my head and objects would pop or flash in front of my eyes."

Even though he had grown up watching his dad encounter similar physical difficulties, David says he looks back and cannot believe he did not go to a neurologist right away. A few weeks later, his feet were in excruciating pain – he chalked that up to being tired after a long performance that night. Just a few short weeks later, the persistent pain had not gone away and in fact was traveling up his leg, to his waist and finally his chest, making his breathing labored while his vision remained impaired. Three short months after his first symptoms, he found himself confined to a wheelchair.

While researchers feel there may be genetic predictors for MS, the National Multiple Sclerosis Society states siblings or children of those with MS have a 1 in 40 risk of also having MS. David also advised recent research has uncovered even more evidence that siblings of those with MS may have a higher risk factor for being diagnosed at some point in their lives. While there is no clear connection one generation passes it to another, what Alan did pass to his son David is a *can do* rather than a *can't do* attitude towards living with MS.

"When I originally received the diagnosis, I had tested positive for West Nile virus but some of the symptoms did not match up," says David. They [the doctors] thought I had a pinched nerve or a problem with my spine."

David wasn't thinking MS and neither were his doctors. "Finally, they tested for MS and found I had the relapsing/remitting form of this disease, which my doctors believe may have been dormant in my system but was triggered by the West Nile virus," says David. "I was in complete denial – I had grown up watching my dad battle MS and my symptoms were not exactly the same so I just could not believe it."

Most MS patients fall into one of four categories of the disease: 1) Relapsing/Remitting (the most common with 85 percent experiencing flare-ups with periods of remission); 2) Primary/Progressive (continuous worsening of the disease with no flare-ups or remissions); 3) Secondary/Progressive (begins as relapsing/remitting but left untreated becomes primary/progressive); and; 4) Progressive/Relapsing (the most rare with continuous decline and increasingly intense flare-ups). While Alan has Primary/Progressive, David was diagnosed with Relapsing/Remitting.

Originally, David was devastated and he had the typical reaction people have when faced with a difficult diagnosis: "Why me?"

He relates how one day while in a wheelchair he watched his brother playing on the floor with his son and wondered to himself, "Will I ever have that?"

You can hear the emotion in his voice as he continues, "I'm almost embarrassed to admit that is how I felt, because when I looked from my brother and my nephew to my dad, I realized, here is this man who has lived with this disease for 20 years, and he has never complained and he has never asked that question. I realized life can go on and you can find ways around this disease just like my dad did."

Alan said he has always tried to raise his boys with an attitude of "What's next?" instead of "Why me?'" He is proud of David's accomplishments through his struggle with the disease and indicates he is inspired by his son's positive attitude about life. If there is an Osmond prescription for helping to tame the symptoms of MS, it is simply *family and faith*.

Both Alan and David credit their wives, Suzanne and Valerie respectively, with the kind of unconditional love so essential in a spouse when someone is facing a chronic illness. According to the National Health Institute Survey conducted by the Centers for Disease Control, 75 percent of marriages among those couples dealing with a chronic illness end in divorce – 50 percent higher than the overall national divorce rate.

In contrast, a 2012 survey conducted by the National Alliance for Caregiving (NAC) about caregivers of those with MS showed that half of those caregivers stated their relationship to their loved one improved and 75 percent said becoming a caregiver to their loved one made them closer to that person. This is certainly the case in the marriages of Alan and David.

"There is a good side to every challenge in life," says David. "With the right perspective, good communication and the unconditional love you get from your spouse, it can bring you closer together."

David says as he was struggling in his wheelchair and trying to figure out his disease, his wife lost her mom who had battled breast cancer for many years. The double blow for her was "tough and really terrible." The fact that she remained steadfast in her love for David when she could have easily left to avoid any more pain in her life is what he says "buoys me up – it makes me stronger to think she's by my side and we're in this together."

Alan agrees it was Suzanne who has been right by his side fighting this disease and helping him seek the alternative remedies that have helped him defy the odds of his prognosis. All doctor predictions pointed to Alan being in a wheelchair by now, but instead Alan travels with Suzanne, and is walking with only the occasional use of a leg brace or cart when he has to walk long distances. Alan says, "It is not just one person who gets MS, it is the whole family."

That is one of the reasons why Alan created his web site, TheFamily.com, which addresses family issues around chronic illness and other life lessons.

Healing Powers

Both Osmonds have made transformational changes in their lifestyles to find ways to deal with MS and overcome the many obstacles and the dire prognosis of their disease.

David was able to get up and out of his wheelchair with powerful steroid shots that helped him walk down the aisle with his beautiful bride, Valerie, a few years ago.

"I proposed to her from my wheelchair and she said, 'Yes!' Being able to walk down the aisle with her was something I just knew I had to do." He has not been back in his wheelchair since.

David tells me when he was first diagnosed and dating Valerie, his neurologist said she felt so sorry for him as a young man with this disease, but she felt even worse for his young fiancée. David says his doctor thought to herself this young woman had no idea what she was getting into. However, it is the strong faith of this Mormon couple and the belief that together they will battle this thing called MS that has ruled the day.

Today, David and Valerie have two beautiful daughters, ages one and three, and recently danced together onstage at the Race to Erase MS Event to benefit the Nancy Davis Foundation for Multiple Sclerosis, for which David serves as a board member.

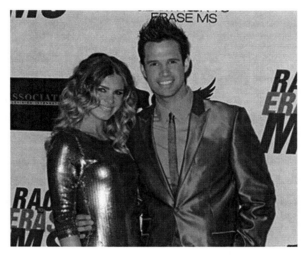

Photo: Courtesy of David Osmond

David and Valerie Osmond

For Alan, he originally followed doctor's traditional orders but quickly found there had to be another way.

"I was given a cortisone shot when I was first diagnosed in 1987," says Alan, "and it just about killed me. It was right then I decided there has to be a better way, and I started investigating alternative medicine that would not have the side effects of traditional drugs."

While there are currently seven drugs available today that help MS patients (with three more drugs about to be approved by the FDA), both father and son have turned their efforts to all-natural and alternative therapies to combat their MS. They embrace all-natural homeopathic remedies: David takes up to 50 all-natural supplements a day, including fish oil and calcium, and both men add a daily dose of 2,000-5,000 IUs of Vitamin D. The power of Vitamin D has been proven in several studies to improve bone density and strength, since it helps the body absorb calcium needed for strong bones. Known as the *sunshine vitamin,* Vit D has been shown to reduce the risk of falling by 17 percent, fall risk being a huge issue for those with MS, since balance is compromised by the disease. Researchers are now feeling it also helps combat other symptoms of MS as well. David says he follows information from a web site called getnumune.net, a biolab that provides the latest information on using peptides to improve immune system function.

The Osmonds also expound on following a healthy diet based on gluten-free (wheat-based products) and casein-free (milk protein) foods with limited meat and other proteins. Alan and David talked about their belief in *raw food* preparation which stipulates foods – mostly vegetables, fruits, nuts, seeds and beans – be cooked no hotter than 116 degrees so essential enzymes are not destroyed. Those who eat at least 75 percent of their meals raw are considered *rawists* and they report having extraordinary energy. The strict adherence to an all-natural diet which Alan blends into most of his meals has helped manage his MS symptoms and helped him lose 30 pounds. In fact, blending is another way to get the most nutrients out of food and has shown to make those who adopt blending to feel stronger mentally and physically.

"I recently had another set of MRIs, and I believe the changes I made to my diet have really helped contribute to the fact I have had no new lesions in the last four years," says David.

In addition, both Alan and David avoid stimulants such as cigarettes, coffee, tea or caffeinated sodas, which are part of their Church of Latter Day Saints faith but also has huge impact on their ability to fight their MS. Alan says many problems with MS and other diseases come from dehydration. He advises everyone should drink at least eight glasses of water daily. He feels it has eliminated a lot of his problems with MS.

The power of aromatherapy is something Alan is very enthusiastic about. He believes in using essential oils, such as frankincense, to cope with his MS. The MD Anderson Cancer Center at the University of Texas in Houston has done research into the benefits of aromatherapy. They have found simple things such as bubble bath scent improves memory, other scents such as lavender calms patients who are fearful or fitful; the scent of typical kitchen cleaners actually helps cancer patients avoid nausea during and after chemotherapy.

The use of aromatherapy in health care has been in existence since the ancient Egyptians. Researchers know rosemary relieves muscle pain, spearmint aids digestion and bay laurel and ylang-ylang can help treat rheumatism, skin rashes and stomach ailments. In Alan's situation, the frankincense oils he uses are shown to promote regeneration of healthy cells and keep existing cells and tissues healthy, and he knows it's working.

"Recently I had a check-up with my doctor who takes the traditional path of pharmaceutical medicine, and he said to me, 'What are you doing?' and I asked him, What do you mean? and my doctor said, 'Well, you're supposed to be getting worse but you are getting better.'"

When it comes to exercise, many MS patients struggle with finding a physical activity that does not require strong balance. In addition most exercise increases body heat, which can exacerbate MS symptoms and increase fatigue. However, current health care professionals feel it is essential for MS patients to find physical outlets to help improve balance and maintain core strength in order to combat the progression of the disease.

Alan, who is affected mostly on his right side, chooses hydro-exercise as his physical outlet – the buoyancy of the water not only takes the pressure off of sometimes painful joints but also helps with balance while practicing movements. In addition, water helps keep the body's temperature cooler so heat does not become a barrier to exercising. And David says yoga and acupuncture have helped a lot of people he has talked to who have MS.

Both men also appreciate the power of music as therapy, which has been at the core of their lives and careers. Alan says music can feed your soul, and David says studies have been done on musical tones that can help with meditative healing.

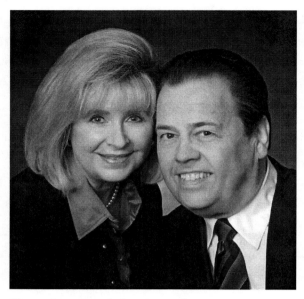

Photo: Courtesy of Alan Osmond

Alan and Suzanne Osmond

Mostly, both Osmonds attribute their amazing progress in the face of a degenerative disease with the power of positive thinking, prayer and the amazing love of their wives and family.

"One of the most important things whether you have a disease or a disability is your mental attitude – you become what you think about," advises Alan. "If you say to yourself, 'I'm sick' then you are."

Alan shares after he was diagnosed with MS, a friend of his called and said she had received the same diagnosis. She told Alan her husband wanted a divorce, because he told her he couldn't be married to a cripple. Alan was sad for his friend but so grateful for his wife Suzanne, who upon hearing he had MS told him, "OK, this is something we can deal with – we can live with this."

"Your spouse and your support system is the most important weapon in battling any disease," says Alan.

David, who travels the country talking to groups about MS and the power of positive thinking as a healer, says he is also grateful for his wife who is his biggest champion and best friend. He says, "Whether it's a spouse or a sibling or a friend, you have to have love and have someone on your side who is fighting with you – it keeps you going."

Having someone you can lean on is critical. In the NAC study of MS caregivers, those caring for someone with MS provide care for twice the duration of general caregivers – on average nine years as opposed to 4.6 years.

While both men are modest about talking about their religion, they quote scripture as a natural part of the conversation and they are very engaged in their church and the *giving back* ethic that is part of many religions. It is clear their devotion to God and their faith have been among the key prescriptions in their successful battle against an otherwise devastating diagnosis.

The Show Goes On for the Osmonds

Alan admits at first he was embarrassed by his MS. There was so little known about the disease in the '80s and '90s but Alan was encouraged to share his story so it would help remove the stigma surrounding MS. In fact, Annette Funicello, who at the time was probably the most famous person with MS, encouraged Alan to share his story to help others. Since then, increased awareness, ongoing research and therapeutic options have given those with MS hope. And people look at Alan, David, Nancy Davis, country music star Clay Walker and Ann Romney, wife of Mitt, who have not let MS hold them back or keep them down.

"I know it's crazy to say, but it is actually a great time to have MS," says David.

When his father was diagnosed more than 25 years ago, there were not a lot of options, but today David says, "The numerous choices we now have to attack this disease that is attacking our bodies – especially with the education about alternative, all-natural choices I have made for my lifestyle – are encouraging. I truly think we are going to lick this disease, and the great research minds agree – they believe MS is one of the chronic illnesses I may see a cure for in my lifetime."

What makes this story so inspiring is for the Osmond family, whose longevity in show business is legendary, both Alan and David are not only *living* with MS today, they are actually *thriving*.

"You can live a great life and still have these struggles," says Alan. "I look at it like a test. If you're a weightlifter it may be hard to lift those weights and it may hurt, but you get stronger the more you do it."

While their strength is inspiring, both men admit to still having to find ways to adapt to and cope with their disease. Alan says he admires his son for continuing to have the strength to perform even though he knows David's legs are in constant pain, especially while he is on stage entertaining thousands.

David jokingly told me his urologist told him he has "the bladder of a very old man," so David says the first thing he does when he goes to an event is scope out how far the restrooms are, so he can be prepared at all times. And David credits his father for giving him that will and that drive to persevere – that *you can do it* attitude, which has been part of the Osmond genes for generations.

Alan says he occasionally has to wear a leg brace on his right side to maintain balance to walk, and he often sleeps with a C-PAP machine to help him breathe at night. Suzanne and Alan travel in style using a cart when he may be faced with walking long distances such as in airports. He says many people would avoid the trip all together, but for Alan that is not an option. He simply uses the tools available to do what he wants to do.

And the humor is always there. He tells me he is always brainstorming on new ideas. It's gotten to a point his family says a lot of the ideas are "nuts" so he's thinking of changing his name to "Alan Almond."

Both men say what makes it all work is family, faith and a belief in yourself.

As we finish the interview, David is eager to get back to playing Legos and watching Disney movies with his two young daughters – a scene he was not sure he would enjoy just a few years ago. He says he wears a ring on his right hand engraved with ETTE – Endure To The End. He says he has had the ring since before his MS diagnosis, so today he adds, "Endure to the end…of the day."

With his girls calling for daddy from the other room, we say our "so longs." A couple of days later, I have to laugh as I see a tweet from David that sums up the Osmond positive approach to adversity and MS.

It says simply, "Going to make t-shirts for my girls that say 'Having MS gets on my dad's nerves.'"

Alan's Lessons Learned

1. Get T-U-F-F

"I have a motto I live by – you have to be TUFF," says Alan.

"It stands for:

T = Target what you need to do.

U = Understand everything you can about the challenge you face.

F = Focus on how to live with or beat that challenge.

F = Fight, Fight, Fight – you have to have the drive and desire to keep living and keep fighting for yourself and those around you."

Alan remembers when he was a young boy just starting out in show business with his brothers. He said they had to learn to play instruments and learn to dance; he says they even had to learn how to ice skate for one of Andy Williams's TV shows. And right behind them was Alan's father, who had been an army sergeant saying "you can do it." When Alan received his MS diagnosis, he says, "I heard in the back of my mind, my dad whispering in my ear, 'you can do it.'"

Alan advises this is a philosophy he has tried to instill in his boys, and he believes it is how caregivers can find their strength. He says, "No matter what stage you are on – this is your show – do what you can, seek help and higher powers to guide you and you will succeed."

2. Patience and People

Alan believes his MS has taught him about patience but also about people. By talking to others about his challenges, he has learned so much he felt he never would have if he had not been given this life challenge. He has also met so many people who have touched his life in a positive way. This is one of the reasons he started his web site, so he could share all he has learned on this journey.

For caregivers, having faith will help your patience and having others you can talk to will help you cope and keep going.

3. Look for Choices and Listen to Your Instincts

Alan's advice to those struggling with a disease or disability and to their caregivers is to seek out as many options for treatment as you can. Don't get stuck in traditional ways of doing things – alternatives are out there, and they just might work for you.

You are your own best advocate, and if you are caring for someone, you have to push the envelope. Ask questions, do research and don't be afraid to try new ideas.

4. Faith and Family

Alan credits his faith as a member of the Church of Latter Day Saints and his upbringing with that intense work ethic as the drive behind fighting this disease with the tenacity he does. Having his family to support him, having his faith to give him hope – he says these are probably the two most powerful prescriptions you can have in facing any challenge.

He says his faith is about "forever." It is not just about this life and ultimately transitioning to something else – it is a graduation and your spouse is your partner through this entire journey. Alan says in working with the National MS Society, he has learned of studies showing those who pray daily do better in managing their disease or caring for their loved one than those who don't have this spiritual, meditative outlet.

"When you have this long-term view, not a shorter version of just this life here today, it gives you encouragement and hope." Alan says everyone needs to find for himself who he really is inside; and find that inner peace to help you keep going whether you are the person with the disease or you are the caregiver.

David's Lessons Learned

1. No Pity Parties

David feels it is hard to think about your father and yourself having a debilitating illness. He told me, "Just the other day I was looking at old videos of my dad performing when he was my age. It's hard to see how great he was on stage and even though he is doing great today, he doesn't have the chance to perform anymore." However, David says the big lesson he has learned from his dad is to never feel sorry for himself. He isn't sure he would have learned that lesson as poignantly if he hadn't been diagnosed with the same disease. He says he doesn't look at MS as a burden but rather a blessing in disguise.

He also believes no matter how hard you think you have it – don't complain because others can have it worse. David tells me about a recent visit he made with his church group to an assisted living facility. While most of the residents were in their 70s, 80s and 90s, David saw a young man of 24 in a wheelchair and went over to talk to him. The man told him he had been in a car accident – his cousin had fallen asleep at the wheel and rolled the car, and this young man was now paralyzed from the neck down.

David, who remembers what it felt like to be in a wheelchair, says, "I thought to myself, how can I ever complain about anything when I meet someone like that? I got to drive my car here today – this young man will probably never do that again."

Learning to find gratitude in your caregiving role is critical to your ability to keep going.

2. Focus On Your Ability Not Your Disability

David says there is so much he is still able to do in life, and that is what keeps him positive and able to push away the *woe is me* attitude. He says because of MS he is leading a richer, fuller life and there aren't a lot of barriers he can't overcome.

He says, "We all have struggles, we all have challenges and you learn suffering is optional." He says his younger brother has diabetes and his wife lost her mom to breast cancer. David says he realizes everyone has something they are facing so it is best to get on with your own battles and learn to live the best life you can.

3. A Diagnosis Is Not for One – It's For All

David says when anyone is diagnosed with a disorder, disease or has a disability; it is not just that person who is affected.

"I have MS but in reality my wife and kids have it too, because they have to live with me and this disease every day," says David. He believes taking that team approach can actually bring everyone together.

This is a great lesson for all caregivers. Don't be an outsider – learn everything you can, get breaks for yourself so you can keep going, do what you need to do to be there for your loved ones. He encourages caregivers and those with the diagnosis to reach out to organizations like the MS Society and the Nancy Davis Foundation for MS. "You will find love, and you will find acceptance, support and hope."

4. Power of Prayer

Having a belief in a higher power is essential. David says he spent a lot of time praying about his disease, how it was affecting his family and what his future may hold. Having faith is critical if you are facing adversity. Studies have shown faith is part of the program when it comes to surviving and coping with life's challenges. I told David I had seen a quote, "Science will take you so far and then comes God." David laughs and says, "God is the greatest scientist of all."

One thing caregivers have told me over and over again is they feel all alone. David believes if you have faith in your life and in your heart, you are never alone.

How Alan and David Find Their "Me Time"

When I asked both Alan and David what are their private passions – both responded almost simultaneously with "spending time with family." Alan says, "I love my wife and my family – having them around me makes me whole." David says being with his "girls," including his wife, playing and laughing with his daughters is pure "magic." It is truly where the Osmonds rejuvenate – with each other.

When it comes to solo endeavors, David enjoys sports like skiing or golf, even though his balance and agility are not what they used to be because of the MS. Alan loves to continually learn new things and brainstorm on ideas – like teaching himself html code, so he can build web sites.

Whatever they do they always have a song in their hearts.

Alana Stewart and Farrah Fawcett

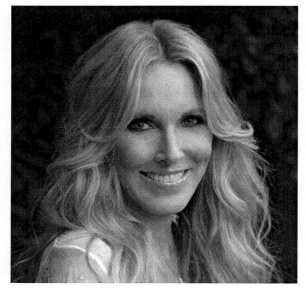

Photo: Courtesy of Alana Stewart

Friendship is a single soul dwelling in two bodies.

— Aristotle

Alana Stewart

Caring for an Angel

Some friendships last a lifetime. And then there is Alana and Farrah. For Alana Stewart and the late Farrah Fawcett the friendship continues even though Alana lost her dear friend of more than 30 years in 2009. Theirs is a true love story – it's about sharing your innermost secrets, having each other's back, laughing when you want to cry, taking the good with the bad, never giving up on each other. This kind of friendship is rare.

When it comes to caring for an ill friend, many people will bake a casserole, visit you in the hospital or help by picking up your kids at soccer practice. Not many will put their own lives on pause for almost three years to chase promising new cancer treatments half way across the world, be your advocate with health care professionals, hold your head and hand while you spend hours with nausea from chemotherapy. And even though Farrah is gone, Alana continues to honor Farrah's memory by carrying out her wishes for the foundation Farrah created before she died to help others struggling to beat cancer. That is love.

When I told Alana how rare her friendship with Farrah is, she responded, "I didn't think it was so rare, it was just the thing to do." She says she considered Farrah to be her soul-sister. When Farrah asked Alana to accompany her to Germany and U.S. medical centers while she sought treatment, there was no question in Alana's mind she would be there for her best friend.

"It is a really rare friend who steps in like a family member to be a primary caregiver," says Dr. Rosemary Laird, medical director at the Health First Aging Institute in Florida. In fact, the National Alliance for Caregiving reports that only 11 percent of those caring for someone with a chronic illness or disability are friends.

Ryan O'Neal, Farrah's longtime love and companion writes in Alana's memoir, *My Journey with Farrah*, "The bond between women friends is all-powerful and not to be taken lightly. But the bond between Alana and Farrah is like nothing I've ever seen between two women. They grew together like vines."

To understand the special bond between Alana and Farrah you have to take a look back over a friendship that lasted 30 years.

Gentlemen Prefer Blondes

In Hollywood in the 1970s, every young model or waitress hoping to be a starlet was blonde, tan, lean and beautiful. It was hard to stand out in this Amazonian village of blinding white teeth and lioness manes but two women seemed to hold Hollywood and its men in the palm of their hands.

Born in San Diego, California, Alana Collins was raised in Nacogdoches, Texas, making her a Texas gal at heart. Her best friend-to-be, was born Ferrah (she changed the "e" to "a" later) Fawcett in Corpus Christie, Texas. Both of these Lone Star state women can claim American Indian ancestry – Alana is ¼ Cherokee and Choctaw mix and Farrah was part Choctaw. It may be these genetic ties that later gave both Alana and Farrah the spirituality to face Farrah's ordeal battling cancer.

Both Alana and Farrah took the typical road to Hollywood at that time – beginning as models and then landing roles in commercials and as extras in TV shows. Alana was one of the famed Ford models of the '70s alongside other big names such as Jerry Hall (Mick Jagger's long-time girlfriend and wife), Lauren Hutton, Kim Basinger and Christie Brinkley. Farrah's modeling was actually in TV commercials including turns as the Breck Shampoo Girl and the woman who gave football hunk Joe Namath a shave in a Noxzema TV ad.

They both did guest spots on TV shows at the time: *I Dream of Jeannie* and *The Partridge Family* for Farrah and *The Bionic Woman, Hart to Hart* and *Fantasy Island* for Alana.

In 1972 Alana married George Hamilton, the habitually tan actor and legendary playboy. The following year, Farrah married Lee Majors, star of the top-rated TV series *The Six Million Dollar Man*. But it wasn't until 1976 when Farrah posed for the now iconic red bathing suit shot – which became one of the best-selling posters of all-time reaching 12 million copies – that Farrah stepped into the never-ending glare of the Hollywood limelight. In fact, the poster is so much a part of our American pop culture it now hangs in the Smithsonian National Museum of American History in Washington, D.C. It was later that same year Farrah would star in the first season of *Charlie's Angels*, the TV show for which she is still most closely associated. Although she was only on the show for the first season, her indelible image remained associated with the series long after she left.

It was during this period Alana and Farrah found themselves at a crossroads in their personal lives and when their friendship seeds were planted. Both women endured some tough times weathering the pain of divorce. Alana and George Hamilton called it quits in 1975 after having one son, Ashley. For Farrah and Lee Majors, cracks were showing in their marriage as well. Farrah's career took flight and Lee's took a nosedive. While most gossip columnists blame the demise of the Fawcett-Majors marriage on Ryan O'Neal who was friendly with the couple, Fawcett did an interview with *People* magazine in 1979 that told a different story and showed her fearlessness and feminism.

Because Farrah had taken a lot of industry flak for leaving *Charlie's Angels* after one only season, many in Hollywood were not willing to give her serious acting career a chance. She called herself "poison" in the industry. She faced her critics and the sting of being a Catholic who was seeking a divorce with the same determination and fight she would later show in her battle with cancer.

"You can't survive that kind of crushing attack and still be an innocent," Fawcett told *People* reporter Sue Reilly in 1979. "I had to grow up and I did. I began to think about what I wanted, and needed, for myself… In some ways I'm much happier than I used to be when all I ever thought about was pleasing everyone else… I came dead last… [now] I'm determined to survive."

It was this survival instinct Alana would see again and again over the three years Farrah fought cancer.

"She had such amazing courage, she remained hopeful and she had incredible faith," remembers Alana of her friend. "We never even talked about the possibility of it [the treatments] not working."

At a dinner party in the late '70s the two women found themselves seated together with their significant others and instantly hit it off. Alana was remarried to British rock star Rod Stewart, and Farrah was with Ryan O'Neal, whom she had an *on* and *off* relationship with spanning 30 years. Over the years the girlfriends would share cooking recipes, especially the pair's favorite pies and downhome Texas dishes, support each other through their mutual children's substance abuse problems, weather the realities of going from ingénues to sophisticated Hollywood insiders.

Both women loved the beach and often found themselves gathering at Farrah's home in Malibu sharing life's intimate secrets and just being there for each other. Their California lifestyle was sunny, happy and full of promise. Until that October day in 2006 when Alana first heard her best friend had cancer. Suddenly their friendship entered its most poignant period – with one friend helping another to survive.

Beaches – Forever Friends

"Men come and go – God knows they certainly have in my life – but girlfriends are forever," writes Alana in *My Journey with Farrah*. In her book, Alana writes it is as much "a celebration of friendship as it is a chronicle of cancer treatment." It is this concept that some friendships are forever that propelled Alana through a three-year odyssey helping Farrah fight cancer.

When Alana first learned Farrah had cancer, she was stunned and in denial. Her first thought was, "not athletic, healthy Farrah." It is the typical response of many caregivers and friends when they hear the *C-word*. Cancer has a stealth effect on those diagnosed. Very often symptoms are subtle or non-existent until they pop up like Freddy Krueger in the *Nightmare on Elm Street*.

"One day you're fine and the next day you're fighting for your life," remembers Alana.

In Farrah's case, her type of cancer – anal cancer – is particularly rare. According to the American Cancer Society 2008 data (the latest year statistics are available), the prevalence of all Americans diagnosed and living with cancer – lung, pancreatic, lymphoma, breast, etc. – was almost 12 million people. Comparatively, in 2012, there were 6,230 new cases of anal cancer and approximately 780 deaths. Anal cancer strikes more women than men typically in their 60s. However, in African Americans, more men than women are diagnosed with this type of cancer. Farrah was only 59 years old.

Your anus is found at the end of your rectum, and it is this anal canal, about 1 to 1.5 inches, where stool leaves your body. While many people with anal cancer have no predictable risk factors, the American Cancer Society says most squamous cell anal cancers seem to be linked to infection by the human papilloma virus (HPV), the same virus that causes cervical cancer. In fact, women with a history of cervical cancer (or pre-cancer) have an increased risk of anal cancer. HPV is a group of more than 100 related viruses that can be passed from one person to another during skin-to-skin contact with an infected area of the body. HPV can be spread during sex, but sex doesn't have to occur for the infection to spread. The Mayo Clinic states risk factors for anal cancer include HPV, smoking and lowered immunity, sometimes from medications or long-term use of corticosteroids.

If found and treated early, the survival rate can be good. In Farrah's case, her cancer was extremely rare and very aggressive.

"Farrah was very positive she was going to beat this and I was positive along with her," says Alana. She recalls her friend always remained upbeat, even when she was in pain and tired. "She would have moments of feeling down," Alana says, "but it never lasted for long; Farrah was a fighter and we never addressed the possibility of a different outcome."

"Her whole life changed overnight," Alana says somewhat wistfully remembering those tough days. "It's the last thing anyone expects and when you go through something like this you learn to really value life, you learn to value your friends and the people you love."

Something else Alana learned through this journey is sometimes it isn't even about the cancer. Farrah had problems with blood clots in her IV line and she was so weak she could not walk and would have to use a wheelchair after painful treatments. To the athletic and fit Farrah, this was a cruel turn of events. To be vulnerable and frail was not her nature according to Alana. In addition, radiation and chemotherapy create a situation where as the medicine is trying to kill the cancer, it is almost killing the person receiving the treatment in the process. Alana remembers Farrah's radiation treatments were so intense she had bright red burns and blisters all across her buttocks and the insides of her thighs. She could barely sit or lay down for the excruciating pain. In addition, the chemotherapy left her frail and weak. She would curl up in a ball huddled over a trash can vomiting all night for hours.

While the cancer was invading her body and stalking her night and day, Alana remembers Farrah was also stalked by the omnipresent, intrusive paparazzi.

Farrah was in pain and feeling at her worst, and there they would be – in the parking garage of the medical center, chasing her car down the street, trying to climb the walls surrounding her home – waiting like vultures. The exploitation of someone's pain and suffering is the lowest depth of human depravity. And while many people suffering with cancer and other illnesses go through what Farrah was and have caregivers like Alana doing their best to help and protect them, most of us don't have to do this while being hounded by obnoxious photographers – this is one of the downsides of fame.

Alana says the turning point for Farrah was when one tabloid blasted the headline, "Farrah Says: I Want to Die!" She'd had it.

When Farrah was originally diagnosed, she wanted to document everything the doctors told her. She felt the best way to do that was to videotape the discussions. This is an excellent idea for caregivers. Taping – whether it is video or audio – all the discussions with doctors will help you keep details in order. Sometimes when we are in the middle of an emotional ordeal, we might hear what is being said but we don't process what we're hearing at the time – we might still be in shock from the devastating news. In these instances, you can forget or mix up the details of a discussion. If you have recorded information to return to it will be extremely helpful to your peace of mind and help you get an action plan together when your emotions have calmed a bit.

In Farrah's case, she chose videotape and she asked Alana to be the cameraman. After the tabloid attacks, Farrah's videotaping took on another mission. Since her diagnosis was made public, Farrah had received thousands of letters from people wishing her well but also from people battling cancer as she was. She wanted to show those people her will was still strong and she was determined to beat the C-monster. She believed the way to do that was to show the world the real truth of her ordeal. What started as a video diary of medical information eventually became the Emmy-nominated NBC-TV documentary, *Farrah's Story* which eventually aired one month before Farrah's passing in 2009.

Alana recalls how hard it was to watch her friend go through painful treatments that were helping her fight the cancer but were also beating down her immune system and making the athletic Farrah so weak. On several occasions Alana wanted to turn the camera off but Farrah insisted on capturing everything.

"It was very hard – sometimes unbearable – to watch my friend suffer, but I was in awe of her ferocious determination," writes Alana in her book. She also called Farrah's cancer "the terrorist." Indeed, both women became warriors in a war on this terrible intruder.

As is typical in caregiving situations, Alana became Farrah's protector and advocate. They created intricate plans to ensure no paparazzi caught a photo of Farrah in a wheelchair. Alana explains this wasn't vanity on Farrah's part; it was her not wanting other cancer patients to feel she was losing the fight or that she was weak – she wanted to be strong for the people who had written to her.

Another thing Alana did for Farrah was to really encourage her to seek as many opinions and alternative treatment options as possible. Alana recalls how Farrah would frequently ask Alana what she thought she should do. In addition to holding the video camera, Alana listened intently to what the doctors would tell Farrah, and would write down notes later in her room. She also helped Farrah by asking a lot of questions of the many health care professionals that Farrah saw. Alana says the decisions were always Farrah's, but Alana was the counselor on making sure they had covered all their bases and left no therapy or option undiscovered.

"When she would say, 'What do you think I should do?' I would tell her she should talk to other doctors and talk to Ryan because I don't want to encourage you to do this in case it doesn't work," says Alana. Alana says Farrah would often make the decisions about her care with Ryan but she valued Alana's encouragement to always seek as many opinions as practical.

This type of inquisitive advocacy is so critical for caregivers. Often our loved ones are tired or feeling so frail from treatments and tests it is hard for them to be focused and clear about what to ask and how to continuously pursue all the options. In the end the decision on their care is theirs, but your role can be the one to ensure there are as few *what ifs* after the fact.

Wind Beneath My Wings

When I spoke to Alana, she told me, "Love is a very healing energy." I could tell she was still wishing there was something more she could have done for Farrah as she continued, "They've done studies that people who have love in their lives, including that of a close friend, have a better chance of recovery. Knowing someone is really there in your corner when you are battling something as devastating as cancer, or any illness, is really important because it makes you feel like you are not alone."

During the course of the three years Alana was by Farrah's side, Farrah's cancer would have short periods of remission – a few months at a time. What was devastating for both Alana and Farrah was how every celebration over her remission periods would be replaced with discouragement when the cancer would return. Both Farrah and Alana had to stay strong in the face of these setbacks.

Always by her side, Alana and Farrah traveled from Los Angeles, seeing doctors at UCLA and City of Hope, to the Leonardis clinic in the Bavarian Alps known for cutting edge cancer treatments. During this time, Alana faced her own cancer scare.

It was while Alana was in Germany with Farrah she received the results of tests that had been done at UCLA in the U.S.

Alana had to have a biopsy and later found out it was Stage 1 cervical cancer. Subsequent check-ups have confirmed it may have been pre-cervical cancer, but the irony that both she and her good friend would face cancer at the same time was unbelievable to Alana.

According to the American Cancer Society, although cervical cancers start from cells with pre-cancerous changes (pre-cancers), only some of the women with pre-cancers of the cervix will develop cancer. The change from cervical pre-cancer to cervical cancer usually takes several years, but it can happen in less than a year. In Alana's case, the doctors in Germany performed surgery, and assured her they removed all the cancer cells.

When it comes to the power of friendships, the book, *Connected: The Surprising Power of our Social Networks and How They Shape Our Lives* by Nicholas Christakis and James Fowler, illuminates how friendships can impact and even revolutionize our lives. These researchers from Harvard University and the University of California at San Diego say friends can hold sway over us (and us over them) in both good and bad ways – and this influence can extend to three degrees of friendship. One intriguing statistic is having a first-degree friend who is happy increases the likelihood of your happiness factor by 15 percent. Their study showed happiness is like a virus that spreads through social networks – your friends' happiness and even their friends' happiness can affect (or infect) you.

While the reason for Farrah and Alana's journey was not a happy occasion, they made it a journey they took together and found "a lot of laughs" along the way. After Farrah died, Alana struggled as so many caregivers do with feelings of guilt and loss. Alana's voice grew wistful as she tells me, "I felt like I failed her, it took me a long time to get over it."

A Cast of Caregivers

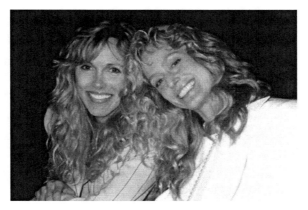

Photo: Courtesy of Alana Stewart

Alana and Farrah in happy times from the cover of Alana's book, *My Journey with Farrah*.

Hope and Healing

Alana says the caregiving experience with Farrah completely changed her life. Since she had never been a caregiver – both Alana's parents died suddenly, and she had never gone through a long illness with anyone – she says she learned so many things caring for Farrah.

Looking back Alana says, "I always felt like maybe I could have done more or maybe there was something we overlooked." This is a refrain I have heard from so many caregivers, and Alana admits in retrospect it is an unnatural emotion; we don't have the power to play God.

"I didn't have the power to save her, but I was so committed, we were both so committed, to her beating this disease that when she didn't beat it I kind of felt like I had failed her in some way."

Alana's guilt takes the form of regret. She told me she and Farrah spent so much time together the last three years of Farrah's life, especially the last year, it makes Alana look back over the whole 30 years of their friendship and wish she had spent even more time with her friend when she was well. We talked about how difficult it is to reconcile how you sometimes rush to do things with someone only after you learn you may lose her.

It was only the last month of Farrah's life Alana worried maybe her friend would not make it. Alana says this may be the toughest point of the journey for caregivers. You have been by your loved one's side, fighting with her and never giving up hope, but now you are fearful.

"You have to be strong," advises Alana. "I had to be strong for her [Farrah], because she was still strong so I couldn't afford to just go in my room, shut the door and cry," although Alana says there were several times she did just that – out of sight from Farrah. "In the end, you have to just suit up and stay strong."

It was after Farrah was gone that the loss really hit her hard and Alana says it took a year for her to start to recover.

"I didn't realize it had taken so much out of me physically and emotionally," remembers Alana. She suffered from chronic bronchitis and other lung problems. Alana, who has been a health enthusiast her whole life and is very informed and intelligent about how stress affects the body, says she was so engrossed in focusing on helping Farrah she wasn't paying attention to the signs of stress that were hurting her health. After Farrah was gone the stress was replaced by grief.

"For many caregivers, the risk of stress is invisible," says Dr. Rosemary Laird. "As a caregiver you have to pay attention to your vulnerabilities and know your risks." Dr. Laird says the cumulative effect of chronic stress can eventually suppress your immune system.

"There is a chance it [chronic bronchitis and lung problems] was grief since all my physical ailments were in the chest and lung area – right near my heart," says Alana. She finds it interesting and not unrelated that was the part of her body to be so affected.

Two of the most common emotions associated with caregiving are guilt and grief. Typically you want to control your loved one's illness or disorder, and you want to solve it. What we find is we are powerless and guilt sets in. Eventually we become fearful, because we realize we may be facing impending loss.

When facing both guilt and grief, Vic Mazmanian, director of faith outreach for the Mind, Heart & Soul Ministry of Saddleback Church and Silverado Senior Living advises, "God is not intent on inflicting pain. Caregivers need to realize the pain of a loved one will be removed and while we may lose them today, we will be reunited with them." He feels this belief brings peace to many caregivers and allows them to accept the situation and be more present with a loved one at the end of life. Or as Alana wrote in her book, "Let go and let God."

In Alana's situation, she embraces a strong faith and spirituality, and Farrah was a lifelong Catholic. This strong sense of faith brought peace to both of them at the end.

Farrah lost her valiant battle with cancer the morning of June 25, 2009. Ryan and Alana were by her side. While her friend may be gone, the memory and mission of Farrah Fawcett lives on with Alana.

"I used to have this belief that people who were famous or bigger than life were immune from these kinds of things, but I've watched too many people who I thought were invincible, who seemingly had it all, experience life's hardships and tragedies just like everyone else," writes Alana.

Imprints in the Sand

Alana continues to carry out Farrah's wishes as president of The Farrah Fawcett Foundation, a nonprofit organization dedicated to providing funds for alternative methods of cancer research, clinical trials – such as gene therapy and targeted therapy – and providing early detection, preventive programs and awareness with an emphasis on anal and pediatric cancers. If Farrah could not find the cure in her lifetime, she wanted to ensure the foundation created in her name would do it for others after she was gone – and Alana is the keeper of that flame.

Alana told me Farrah established the foundation after her cancer diagnosis and had every intention of running the foundation herself. One of the things Alana hopes for and supports as head of the foundation is to encourage new directions in treatment beyond the traditional radiation and chemotherapy employed in the U.S. today.

"Hopefully we're going in a new direction with cancer treatment, because the old treatments – the standard chemo and radiation – are so debilitating," says Alana. "They have such terrible side effects, and I watched Farrah go through it and it was just horrible." Alana laments the suffering people go through is awful, and so many times these harsh treatments don't work. She believes the new direction researchers are taking for cancer treatment and cures is going to be so much better.

While many cancer sufferers find positive outcomes and remission through radiation, chemotherapy and other traditional treatments, Alana remembers Farrah's doctor in Germany, telling them one day chemo would be obsolete as an effective cancer treatment. She also recalls Farrah had entered a chemo trial study in the U.S., and it was after that trial study Farrah began to "go downhill."

Alana is dedicated to continuing dialogue among the world's leading researchers for new ways to fight cancer. She hopes the message that not all cancer patients are the same resonates with both the medical community and those future patients and caregivers. For instance, research on chemotherapy sensitivity testing was the main topic of leading cancer researchers and experts around the globe, who gathered at a recent conference held by The Farrah Fawcett Foundation. Chemo sensitivity testing and findings are a particular passion of Alana because of Farrah's experience.

"The first time she [Farrah] was given chemotherapy it was a type that didn't work on her type of cancer," laments Alana. While she realizes the process for drug approval through FDA regulations is lengthy but necessary, Alana is hopeful many of the non-standard treatments, including those Farrah sought in Germany, result in more clinical trials in the U.S., and she wants the foundation to continue to help promote awareness of these issues.

In addition, Alana is following the wish of Farrah to help families directly with the challenges that come with a cancer diagnosis. The Farrah Fawcett Patient Assistance Fund provides support for families struggling with financial and other challenges. Alana says while insurance may pay for patients' cancer treatment, it doesn't cover the travel and related costs for the caregiver or family to be with them while they seek treatment – often at leading institutions far from where they live.

"Whether it's meals or hotel bills or even parking costs for every day when you are at a medical center while your loved one gets treatment, our program provides direct financial help to those families in need who qualify for assistance," says Alana.

In addition to the conferences to explore new therapies and promotion of methods to prevent and detect cancer, the foundation worked with Urban Outfitters to sell a vintage T-shirt depicting the iconic Farrah red bathing suit shot from the 1970s with a portion of sales proceeds benefitting the foundation.

Being at the helm of the Farrah Fawcett Foundation has helped Alana rechannel her feelings of guilt she could have done more for Farrah by continuing to make Farrah's wishes to help others and to find a cure for cancer come true.

"For me it's really important to not only carry out Farrah's wishes for the foundation to help people, but I want to keep her legacy and her memory alive, I want to keep the flame burning about what she stood for," says Alana. "Every time I have to make a decision with the board for the foundation, I think to myself, what would Farrah do? I just want to make her proud."

Alana's Lessons Learned

Alana talks about how many things she learned walking this path with Farrah but here are the big lessons:

1. **Give Back**

Alana says one of the biggest lessons she learned in her experience with Farrah was how important it is to do something for another person.

"Getting out of yourself and your own problems and showing up for someone," advises Alana helps both others and caregivers. She believes giving back, whether it is to an individual or the world, is important. "I think a lot of us forget that, I know with myself, I focus so much on my own life, sometimes I would forget to look at the bigger picture and say what can I do?"

Because of Farrah, Alana says showing up and giving back is now a much bigger part of her life than it was before her experience of giving to Farrah.

2. **Appreciate Every Day of Your Life**

"Life can just take a turn and it can change in a heartbeat, as it did for Farrah." Alana feels she values people and loved ones more since her journey with Farrah.

3. **Value Your Friends**

In many ways, action speaks louder than words. If you have a friend going through an illness, give her primary caregiver a break or create a team with her spouse or partner to take on the burden of supporting her through an illness. Alana says we often take love and friends for granted. Once they are gone we may wish we spent more time with them. Don't let regret happen – make the time today, be there for people you love. Alana says, "I don't always do it but I try to keep it in mind – it's a valuable lesson."

4. **Find Humor Everywhere You Go**

"Laughter is the best medicine" is an old expression popularized by Norman Cousins's book *Anatomy of an Illness*, in which he describes his battle with a degenerative disease of the connective tissue and how he "laughed" his way to recovery.

Alana says one of the things that kept her and Farrah going through the ordeal of cancer was their ability to laugh along the way. Laughter is a great tension-releaser, pain reducer, breathing improver, and elevator of moods. Humor is a great elixir to get us through difficult or stressful times.

Make sure you find your own laughter to keep smiling in your own life. Your energy for others will only happen when you energize and empower your own life force today. You can read more about the healing power of laughter in the Cue Cards chapters.

How Alana Finds Her "Me Time"

While Farrah is gone, Alana's caregiving journey continues as the head of the Farrah Fawcett Foundation. She may not be caregiving for a loved one every day, but she works every day to help those who are caring for loved ones and the work keeps her constantly busy and traveling on behalf of the foundation.

After a life spent at glamorous affairs with glittering people, Alana says what she likes to do the most is curl up at home and catch up on some missed TV. When we talked she was engrossed in DVDs of the hit PBS series *Downton Abbey* and AMC's *Breaking Bad*. She is also a devoted cable news viewer and admits to the guilty pleasure of watching *The Bachelor*. You can tell in talking with Alana she wants to be informed and uplifted – it's her positive energy that encircles everything she does.

She also reads as much as she can and these days it is mostly articles, research and books on cancer treatments and clinical trials that may provide the elusive cures for cancer or at least provide better relief for sufferers today. And while she is reading she is also writing. Her second book, *Rearview Mirror*, touches upon her friendship with Farrah, but is more an autobiography of Alana's life in full.

When it comes to her own health, Alana is devoted to meditation and yoga, which she practices every morning and evening even if for just 20 minutes a day. She believes this centers her for the day's challenges and then relaxes her so she can get a good night's sleep.

Mostly her life is centered around family including her adult children, Ashley, and her kids with Rod Stewart, Kimberly and Sean. And she gets to play *grandma* (although no one would ever look at the perpetually gorgeous and youthful-looking Alana and think *grandma*) with Kimberly's new baby.

It was summertime when Alana and I talked and this evokes memories of Farrah for her. Her idyllic days spent at the beach with her friend have left imprints on her heart forever. This summer she was spending a few days respite from foundation work to be with friends enjoying the beach and sun that was so much a part of her life with Farrah. While friendship is still essential in Alana's life, the special bond she shared with Farrah will never be replaced. But the footprints in the sand are still there – in Alana's memories and in her work for the foundation created in her friend's memory.

Act II

The Role of a Lifetime: Caregiver

All the world's a stage, and all the men and women merely players: they have their exits and their entrances; and one man in his time plays many parts.

—William Shakespeare
As You Like It

Casting Calls – Which Caregiver Role Will You Play?

I longed to break out of the system and do different roles.

– Leslie Caron

Of the many roles we all play in life – someone's son or daughter, someone's partner, wife or husband, someone's mother or father, someone's boss or employee – the one we can all expect to play is the role we are least prepared for: caregiver.

Over the last decade I have spoken to hundreds of family caregivers and they all had a similar response when I anointed them with the caregiver title. "Oh no, I'm just a daughter caring for my mother," or "I'm just a wife caring for a husband with cancer," or "I'm just caring for my son – yes he has Down syndrome but I'm just a mom trying to manage it all." While we all have many roles in life, becoming a caregiver needs to be on the list.

> **The role we are least prepared for: caregiver.**

Today, there are more than 65 million Americans caring for a loved one who has a chronic illness, a disability or is simply getting older and needs more help. This represents almost 1 in 3 U.S. households (31%) who have at least one person who is a caregiver and the numbers are only growing. Most of the caregiving discussions focus on caring for parents as they age. And in fact, 80 percent of the long-term care provided in this country, especially to keep an older loved one living at home, is provided by a family caregiver. According to the U.S. Census Bureau, today we have 40 million Americans who are over age 65 – in 20 years that number will almost double to 70 million. Basically by 2020 1 in 5 adults will be over the age of 65 and in 2025 our society for the first time in recent history will have more parents than school-age children needing care.

The other reality is with today's technology and drug and other therapies, many illnesses or diseases that were fatal 20-50 years ago are now simply a chronic disease that can in many ways be managed with help. When you combine our longevity factor with our growing older population, what we are creating is a new class in society called caregivers who face a potentially later life-long commitment to care for a loved one.

There is no *one size fits all* for caregivers. As you will read in these Casting Calls chapters, the role of caregiver crosses all economic, geographic, gender, age, racial, ethnic, cultural, sexual preference boundaries – caregiving is the true *rainbow coalition*. You can suddenly be caring for a spouse with a chronic illness like Meredith Vieira who cares for a husband with multiple sclerosis. Or, you may be a mother who has a child with special needs – this catapults you into a new category. You are a special kind of mother and yes, you are a caregiver like Holly Robinson Peete who cares for a son living with autism. And as Holly gets older, she worries about what will happen to her son – who will look after him when she is gone? And in each caregiving situation, the solutions, the conversations, the journey can be very different.

Preparing for caregiving is a tough task. After all, we are a nation with mixed reviews when responding to a crisis – look at 9/11 (good job) or Hurricane Katrina (poor job). We can rise to the occasion and we can triumph over our challenges. But when it comes to long-term plans, whether retirement or caregiving, we often fail to make the necessary preparations. Maybe this is denial about getting older. We do not like to face death – whether it is our parents, our spouse or ourselves. But like taxes, death is not a choice.

What is your choice is how your last wishes and days will play out. The ability to exit life as you wish with as little emotional and financial drain as possible on the loved ones you leave behind is a true legacy. As a caregiver, knowing the long-term care wishes of your loved one or making plans for a child with special needs after you may be gone is essential. There are legal and financial implications with end-of-life and perhaps most importantly, there are emotional implications.

If you are an actor, you need to read through your script for a new role. If you are a caregiver, you need to understand your script such as the legal and financial documents for your loved one's care wishes. You need to know where these documents are located and what they say and ensure the whole family understands these wishes to avoid as many family conflicts as possible. You also need to understand the *context* for your character role of caregiver. Actors want to understand what motivates their character, what is their life about in order to nail the role. Caregivers need to understand all the aspects of caregiving you may be facing – money, housing, food, transportation, etc. And you need to talk over these issues with your loved one. This is the conversation aspect of caregiving and I will coach you on these conversations in the chapter called C-A-R-E Conversations[SM].

While end-of-life seems to only apply to aging parents, think about yourself and your family members as well. If you are one of the baby boomer generation you are most likely a current caregiver, have been one recently or will be stepping into the caregiving role soon. As former First Lady Rosalynn Carter, known as a pioneer in the world of caregiving, famously said,

"There are only four kinds of people in this world:
Those who have been caregivers,
Those who are caregivers,
Those who will be caregivers; and
Those who will need caregivers."

"We are a society increasingly dependent on caregivers," says Dr. Leisa Easom, executive director of the Rosalynn Carter Institute on Caregiving (RCI). As a member of the national task force that created the report, *Averting the Caregiving Crisis*, Dr. Easom advises that public and private sector organizations must come together to educate the public, advocate for better support and access through policy changes, turn good evidenced-based research into real programs and make investments in sustaining funding for programs. Most importantly Dr. Easom says caregivers must self-identify to get the help they need.

"Caregivers are often invisible and selfless which make them an overlooked group," she cautions.

AARP in collaboration with the Ad Council launched a public service awareness campaign aimed at helping those Americans who are in a caregiving situation to see there are resources and solutions but it starts first with understanding the critical role you play in our society: caregiver.

We know caregiving is something we all face – so having these plans and conversations in place for ourselves is essential as well. In becoming a caregiver for an older loved one, we are getting a dress rehearsal for becoming someone who will be cared for in our own future. Our lessons learned in caregiving today are providing Cliff's Notes for the next generation on how to care for us.

When I spoke to Marg Helgenberger, she talked about how caring for her parents at such an early age made her more aware of the issues her young son, who is now at the same age she was when she cared for her parents, may face as both she and her son grow older. We have seen the future and hopefully it makes us more aware of how to prepare. And if you are caring for a sibling or child with special needs – the same planning needs to happen so you have the things in place to care for this loved one in the event something happens to you or your spouse or partner.

Some caregiving is impossible to plan: car accidents that create physical disabilities; sudden strokes or heart attacks that create loved ones who now may need help dressing, bathing, eating; wives or husbands of veterans who return home with post-traumatic stress disorder (PTSD) or traumatic brain injury (TBI). How can you plan ahead for these situations? In many ways, you cannot. What we can plan for is getting older and what will happen to our parents, ourselves and our children as we age and approach those end-of-life choices.

Actors and professional athletes know how to prepare for a role or the big game. It typically takes months or at least weeks to get in shape, know their part, understand the strategy, research the role or the opposing team and get to a mental and physical place where fame and victory can be theirs. And as Spencer Tracy famously once said of what actors can do to prepare, "Know your lines and don't bump into the furniture."

Caregiving is really no different. If we know something is coming – taking care of an older parent, a partner or sibling with special needs – then we need to know the basics we can plan for now so when the situation arises, we are not caught like a deer in the headlights.

Studies by the National Alliance for Caregiving show 75 percent of all caregivers felt they did not have a choice to provide the care their loved one needed and most of us do not think about caregiving until a crisis forces us into service.

Imagine Eli Manning not practicing before the Super Bowl or Meryl Streep just showing up on the film set without having read the script or understanding her character (OK she could probably still pull off a great performance because she is Meryl Streep but you get the drift). That is the equivalent of not taking the time to understand the general basics of caregiving. Every actor, athlete, musician, news anchor or person in the spotlight needs to prepare. As a current or future caregiver, you need to prepare to care.

Your caregiving situation will be unique to you and your loved one. However, there are some basics to help create a foundation for the long-term care you will be facing so you will not feel like *Titanic* passengers, Leo and Kate, going down with the ship with no life boat in sight. This book will inspire you to think about what caregiving entails and you will become empowered as you read about these celebrities and their lessons learned on how to become a caregiving superstar.

What type of a caregiver will you be? For actors, there are those who specialize in comedy (Lucille Ball) and those who are known more for drama (Al Pacino) and then there are those who are great cross-over artists (Alec Baldwin who crosses over from comedy to drama and TV to film effortlessly – and who was a caregiver to his mother who successfully battled breast cancer).

The pitfall for many caregivers is they become enablers or co-dependents. Many of the caregivers and experts I have interviewed over the years have a tendency to *over-care* – whether it is an older parent, an ill spouse or a child with special needs. It is easy to typecast your loved one as someone completely vulnerable who cannot live without you. But it becomes critical to understand boundaries – both theirs and yours – and allow for a level of independence while still stepping in when more care may be needed.

In some instances, your loved one may become more dependent than necessary – the more care provided, the more care requested. In other situations, your loved one may resent you hovering over them all the time. They feel they will let you know what they need and when they need it and until that time, they want you to back off. But as caregivers, we believe we know what is best for our loved ones. This is a delicate tightrope to walk for many caregivers but learning how to find your balance will help you avoid feeling like a martyr or victim in your caregiving role. This is why having the C-A-R-E Conversation is so important.

One thing is certain: the No. 1 challenge caregivers face is dealing with the stress of caring for a loved one. Stress comes in many forms and it is not always the same type of stress. As you read through the various Casting Calls of Caregivers, you will see I put a Spotlight on Stress – how it differs for the various caregiving roles you may play. In the Stressbusters chapter, I will give you tips and recommendations on how to conquer stress so it does not conquer you.

Following are some of the profiles in caregiving. You may find yourself in one or more of these roles someday. This overview will help you understand the difference in these caregiving situations and how to best prepare for each role.

And lastly, as I stated in my Preface, my concern is about you – the caregiver. Almost without exception, every caregiver I have spoken to says, "Everyone always asks about [my mom, my husband, my child, etc.], how is he/she doing? No one ever asks how I am doing."

This book is for you – I want to know how you are doing. Because in the end, it is about you. Caregiving is about caring for a loved one but it is also about self-care. Think of it like a sports team – you cannot have a quarterback without a receiver, you cannot have a pitcher without a catcher. You can also think about it as a great comedy team – where would Laverne be without Shirley? Abbott without Costello? Rowan without Martin? You are not only valuable but you are essential so finding the balance to care for yourself is what this book is all about.

Trading Places

Caring for a Parent

In the 1983 comedy film, *Trading Places*, movie stars, Eddie Murphy and Dan Aykroyd, literally trade lives with each other to hilarious effect. When we think of caregiving, the typical scenario we think of is an adult child trading places with their aging parent. And while many may describe this type of caregiving as a role reversal, in actuality, our aging parents do not become children. They still have choices, they still strive for as much independence as possible and they need to be considered and consulted – things we typically do not have to do with children.

Statistics from the National Alliance for Caregiving show almost 44 million Americans are caring for a loved one over age 50 and 36 percent of all caregivers are caring for a parent. If there were any caregiving role you will play – caring for an older parent is it. According to the U.S. Census Bureau, over the next 20 years the population over age 65 will double what it is today. And while we currently have 80,000 centenarians in this country (those who live to reach the 100 milestone), by 2040 – around the time our grandchildren are our age – there will be 580,000 centenarians who need care. The aging trend pundits are saying the future will bring us not only

> **36 percent of all caregivers are caring for a parent**

more parents to care for than children, but we will be caring for those parents longer than we cared for our kids. In fact, because we are all living longer and the 78 million baby boomers – the largest segment of our population born between 1946 and 1964 – started turning 65 last year, preparing to care for a parent is not something you can put off like Scarlett O'Hara who famously says throughout *Gone With the Wind,* "I'll think about that tomorrow."

And this situation is not unique to Americans. There is actually a worldwide aging phenomenon: Great Britain mirrors the U.S. growth spurt of the baby boom generation and the Soviet Union calls its baby surge, which happened after 1957, the Sputnik Generation. Japan faces one the largest aging population increases. Today, its citizens have an average lifespan expectancy of 81 years – one of the oldest worldwide. And while its overall population numbers will fall in the coming years (due to falling birth rates and low levels of immigration), 40 percent of its total population will be over age 65 by 2060. No wonder they lead the world in robotic technology for assisted living.

"Global aging and replacement birth rates are what demographers use to determine a whole host of issues facing societies – Russia, Ireland, Japan are just some of the countries with a decreasing population," says Jeff Cole, executive director for the USC Center for the Digital Future. "Where the impact of all this will really be felt is when you have certain programs such as Social Security in America where you had approximately five people paying into a system where two people were using those funds and when that equation reverses, which is happening now with aging baby boomers where you have two people paying into a system and five people using the benefits, all of a sudden economically the math doesn't work."

The takeaway from all this is family caregivers are not only being called upon to provide the hands on physical care for an older loved but they are also stepping up more and more to financially support the longevity of a loved one when other benefits are depleted. To not understand this economic situation can spell disaster for families.

Parenthood

Caring for a parent often accentuates the relationship you had with your parent growing up. If it was a loving, nurturing upbringing then you want to give that same love and nurturing back to your parent. If it was dysfunctional or problematic in your house growing up, then those feelings come surging back and make caregiving more a burden than a blessing.

Whether it is positive or negative, parental caregiving creates a role reversal that is hard for both the adult child and the parent. As your mother once bathed you as a small child, you may now find yourself needing to bathe her. As you begged dad to give you the car keys upon getting your driver's license at age 16, you may now have to beg dad to give up his car keys at age 86.

When you think about it – caregiving is about the circle of life. We enter this world vulnerable, bald, needing to be fed and have our diaper changed. Well, we exit life in about the same state.

Many caregivers I have spoken to have told me caring for an older or ill parent is a "labor of love." But even if your caregiving role is a chosen one, you still are fraught with anxiety over whether you are making the best decisions for your mom or dad. They may have made you promise to never put them in a nursing home but you are finding that caring for them at home is taking a toll on you physically, emotionally and often, financially.

If your relationship with your parent was full of strife, you may now resent the caregiving role you feel has been thrust upon you or you may choose to not be involved in caregiving at all, leaving your parent's care to others which can cause feelings of guilt and remorse.

These situations create untold stress, anxiety and often depression for adult children and I will address how to manage these emotions in the Refreshments chapters.

Stand By Me

The other difference in caring for a parent rather than a spouse or a child with special needs is sibling relationships are put under the microscope. In some instances, caregivers find comfort in having a sibling or many siblings they can turn to for emotional, financial and even physical support. You will read in Marg Helgenberger's story she formed a caregiving team with her brother to care for their parents. This is the ideal caregiving situation.

Your sibling relationship is the one you will have the longest (barring no tragedies) – it will last longer than that with your parents, your spouse, your children and most if not all of your friends. Through caregiving these familial bonds can become a stronger kinship built as you become a team to care for mom, or just commiserate on how irascible or stubborn dad has gotten over the years. Having someone who has not only known your parents as long as you have and has gone through those growing pains with you, but who has also known you from childhood to adulthood can result in a deeper relationship with your sibling(s).

While our sibling roles may be evolving as we grow up, get married and have our own families, the status you have among your siblings will not change and will come flooding back when a caregiving situation hits a family like a hurricane. There is a great book that will give you some insights into these sibling relationships and why caregiving may fall to one adult child (typically oldest daughter) over others. It is called the *The New Birth Order Book* by Dr. Kevin Leman and you will smile while you read it as you recognize yourself and your birth order personality traits from first born, middle born, last born, only child, twin, etc. It will also help you understand your role vis a vis your siblings when caring for a parent – why are you always butting heads with one sibling? Why kids #2 and #4 in birth order are typically united against #3? Why 64 percent of all U.S. Presidents are first borns?

In the movie, *Hangin' Up,* three sisters, played by Diane Keaton (who also directed the film), Meg Ryan and Lisa Kudrow, struggle with each other and with their terminally ill father played by Walter Matthau (in his final on-screen performance). Written by the sister team of Delia and Nora Ephron, this quirky movie explores the issues of siblings with vastly different lives and lifestyles and their common bond – a conflicted relationship with their father. It is a great example of how families can struggle when a sense of obligation outweighs outrage over familial relationships and in the end how siblings become closer over the pending loss of a parent.

Another book, *They're Your Parents, Too!* by Francine Russo takes you through the journey of sibling issues when it comes to caregiving. She writes, "We need to recognize that caring for an aging parent is not just a job to be done but a new era of family life that involves us all."

One path is for caregivers to approach siblings with the idea of splitting up the work. If one sibling is business-like and professional and either cannot or does not want to do some of the more emotional and physical aspects of caring for mom or dad, then assign that sibling the role of dealing with the legal documentation and health insurance issues. Another sibling may live long-distance and cannot be there physically to help but can contribute financially. Let everyone perform the tasks they are good at or in areas they have expertise.

East of Eden

However, there is the other side to this and some may say the above scenario is as much a fairy tale as *Hansel and Gretel.* As you go through the looking glass of caregiving, family conflicts often arise between siblings. First of all, the mortality of a parent brings the adult children's own issues on death into sharp focus.

The natural order has changed and there is no generation ahead of you to cushion the fall into the afterlife. This often creates more chaos as adult children grapple with feelings of fear and anxiety and enter into childhood wars with their sibling(s) or retreat into denial. Siblings can also start bickering with each other to avert the grief they are feeling in watching a parent decline. According to noted authors David Kessler and Elisabeth Kübler-Ross, the second stage of the five stages of grieving is *Anger*. In their book, *On Grief and Grieving*, they write, "Anger is a necessary stage of the healing process of grief which can feel like being adrift at sea. Underneath your anger is your pain but anger actually anchors you. You may turn your anger on someone, [like a sibling], but it creates a connection to that person and gives you something to hold onto. Anger is just another indication of the intensity of your love."

In addition, adult children of an ailing parent fall into their childhood roles and this can make old rivalries or jealousies resurface. In fact, 40 percent of siblings involved in caring for an older parent experience serious conflicts according to a report from Association of Conflict Resolution. The oldest sibling typically takes on the most responsibility and decision-making while younger siblings revert or feel relegated to their childhood roles.

When sibling arguments erupt, the blow-up may be over the right medical care for dad but in reality you are revisiting some old hurt or conflict from the past. Jill Eikenberry told me as an only child now caring for a mother with dementia, friends who had suffered through sibling dramas over ill parents told Jill how lucky she was to not have to deal with this added burden of sibling squabbles.

> **Siblings can also start bickering with each other to avert the grief they are feeling in watching a parent decline.**

Cinderella

Beyond the parental role reversal and potential sibling conflicts, you may also find yourself in conflict or having to navigate the relationship of an ailing parent with a step-parent or their new partner. According to a study conducted by American Association of Geriatric Psychiatry (AAGP), older widowed men were seven times more likely than similar-aged widowed women to remarry and the U.S. Census Bureau found for those over age 50, almost 6 out of 10 men and 41 percent of women remarry each year. If a parent has remarried and then becomes ill, these types of conflicts can often be difficult for adult children, especially if the step-parent relationship is relatively new or resembles Cinderella's situation with her stepmom.

The glass slipper may also be on the other foot and you may find yourself as a step-parent carrying out the wishes of an ill spouse only to face conflict with his/her adult children. A somewhat similar scenario played itself out in the movie, *Stepmom* starring Julia Roberts and Susan Sarandon. Julia played the stepmom dealing with the emotions and conflict of her new husband's ex-wife, played by Susan, who is diagnosed with terminal cancer. Ultimately it is the stepmom Julia who helps carry out the last wishes of the dying Susan for the family's sake.

Having the conversation with family is important for so many reasons, not the least of which is maintaining family harmony. I will review how to think about these *talks* in the chapter on C-A-R-E Conversations. It is also important to have the proper legal documentation in place which I review in Raiders of the Lost Ark chapter in the Rehearsals section.

One of the ways to address all these potential family conflicts is to enlist the help of a professional geriatric care manager (GCM). Trained in elder care issues, a GCM can also help facilitate or mediate family discussions around caregiving in the same way a referee ensures it is a clean fight and there are no fouls. You will learn about GCMs in the My Man Godfrey chapter of Rehearsals.

Young At Heart

Aside from all the relationship issues involved in caring for an older parent, at the center of all this attention is your older parent. For many caregivers of a parent, it is simply helping them as they grow older. They may not have a diagnosis such as Alzheimer's or cancer which requires more acute, 24/7 care – they may just be facing the challenges that come with aging.

While caregivers may encounter many responsibilities, including senior driving issues, finding alternative housing, dealing with transitions from hospital to home, one of the biggest issues caregivers face is not health or wealth connected when it comes to their loved one. It is about being alone. Isolation and its solution – companionship – are common ways for caregivers to begin their journey with an older parent. About half of all adults age 65 or older are divorced. In addition, women outlive their male counterparts on average by 3-4 years – which means having a widowed or divorced older mom is more common than we think. And while women are better at establishing social outlets to cope with loneliness, often these social outlets include their adult children and grandchildren.

While family time is precious, it can also put strain on a caregiver. Juggling *together time* with mom or dad while juggling all your other responsibilities can make caregivers anxious, resentful and short-tempered. This stress can negatively impact your relationships at work, with your kids, with a spouse or partner and with friends. Finding ways to eliminate your guilt over wanting or feeling you need to always be there for mom or dad will help. There are many alternative social activities, such as senior centers or Adult Day Care, to keep older loved ones active and engaged. It is also important to explain to your parents the stress you may be feeling over becoming your loved one's only or primary social outlet.

The American Psychological Association *Stress In America*™ 2012 survey showed the negative health impacts from stress are more pronounced for those over age 50 who are also a family caregiver. In addition, the American Academy of Family Physicians conducted a poll showing 88% of caregivers experience stress.

Other studies found caregivers who experience stress turn to bad habits to cope. The National Alliance for Caregiving says 10% of caregivers use alcohol or medications to cope with stress. Another survey, *Stressed and Strapped: Caregivers in California* conducted by the UCLA Center for Health Policy Research, found among the state's 6 million caregivers, more than 16% were smoking and 27.5% are obese — at least four percentage points higher in each case than non-caregivers. For caregivers with serious emotional distress, smoking increased by 208%.

Spotlight on Stress
Caring for Parents

The Parent Trap

Sandwich Generation Juggling Act

In the family movie, *The Parent Trap,* starring a 12-year-old Lindsay Lohan (before the drama) we are watching a reboot of the 1961 Disney movie with Haley Mills. In the film, two identical twins are raised separately by each of their parents after a divorce but meet at summer camp and hatch a plan to get their parents back together. When I think of *Sandwich Generation* caregivers, I think of them as the parents in this movie, with one twin being their children and the other twin being their older parents. They are caught in a *parent trap* caring for both generations on either side of them at the same time. This can make both family drama and comedy.

It was actually gerontologist and author Elaine Brody who coined the term *Sandwich Generation* in the 1980s included in her book, *Women in the Middle: Their Parent Care Years.* If we were casting the role of the typical Sandwich Generation caregiver it would look like this:

- 48-year-old woman
- Cares for her 74-year-old mother
- Has children under 18 at home
- Married and works either full or part-time

- Spends up to 10 percent of the household annual income on care-related costs for her parent
- Suffers from stress and burn-out and often some guilt
- Lack of time for self results in health impacts like insomnia, poor nutrition, little or no exercise, missed doctor or dental appointments and ultimately ongoing stress and even depression

The notation on this Casting Call would say "this is a potentially short term role – the star may not be able to perform long before burn-out and exhaustion force this show to close."

There has been a lot of attention focused on the Sandwich Generation – the 24 million Americans who are literally sandwiched between caring for two generations. Representing approximately 38 percent of all caregivers, Sandwich Generation members are still parenting children living at home while they also care for older parents who now need more help.

Because Sandwich Generation caregivers tend to be in their 40s, 50s and even 60s, 7 out of 10 are also juggling a career along with child rearing and caregiving. With so many balls in the air, the Sandwich Generation caregivers often feel overwhelmed, burned out and stressed to their limits. These caregivers are caught in a three-ring circus of children, career and caregiving, and they are the star juggling act. At some point, the ball that gets dropped is the one that says *self-care*.

While on average these Sandwich Generation caregivers are baby boomers, Gen Xers are not immune. Many in their 30s are encountering caregiving much sooner than anticipated. A web site started by Adina Saperstein, The Veneration Project, speaks exclusively to Gen Xers to help open this generation's eyes about the coming caregiving role they will play. She and her Gen X sister are caring for their 65-year-old mom who has a complex set of physical and mental illnesses. While Adina lives in New York she cares long-distance for her mom who is in an assisted living facility in Maryland. She calls her caregiving experience so far a game of *chutes and ladders* as she oversees a care crew to ensure her mom has affordable and dignified care. Not quite what this 35-year-old working woman thought she would be doing at this age.

> **Sandwich Generation caregivers tend to be in their 40s, 50s and even 60s, 7 out of 10 are also juggling a career along with child rearing and caregiving.**

If this were a movie, I would title it *No Way Out* (and no, you do not wind up with Kevin Costner in the end). The familial responsibilities can be overwhelming – soccer schedules and after school homework for the kids, doctor appointments or emergency calls from your mom at all hours, your husband feeling neglected, your boss feeling like you are slacking, your friends feeling like you dropped off the face of the earth (and some days you wish you could). The balls you are juggling feel more like 50-pound weights.

Two celebrities whose stories you will read in this book are classic Sandwich Generation caregivers: Holly Robinson Peete and Joan Lunden. And they are not alone – other stars and luminaries such as Brooke Shields, Caroline Kennedy Schlossberg and her cousin Maria Shriver, Demi Moore and Denise Richards are or were all part of the club we call the Sandwich Generation. Oscar-winner Diane Keaton was also a Sandwich Generation caregiver, watching the slow good-bye of a mother with Alzheimer's, which she wrote about in her poignant memoir, *Then Again.* In her book, Diane describes her caregiving role:

> "As Mother struggled to complete sentences, I watched Dexter, my daughter, and a few years later little Duke, my son, begin to form words as a means to capture the wonder of their developing minds. The state of being a woman in between two loves – one as a daughter, the other as a mother – has changed me. It's been a challenge to witness the betrayal of such a cruel disease while learning to give love with the promise of stability."

Sandwich Generation caregivers juggle children, careers and caregiving and since women are twice as likely to be caregiving as men, they are at greater risk for health impacts from stress. *So Stressed* found the evolution of women's biology over the last 100 years has not caught up with the expanded roles that women play in today's world including motherhood, career woman and caregiving. The advances of communication technology while helping us have also negatively impacted our bodies' defenses to protect and heal. The constant disturbance of our peace with texts, emails or cell phone calls puts us on high alert at all times and actually isolates us rather than connects us.

Sandwich Generation caregivers also suffer from subjective cognitive impairment or what researchers call *busy life syndrome*. An American Psychological Association study showed 36% of Americans suffer from chronic work stress. For working caregivers, it jumps to 50% according to the National Alliance for Caregiving.

Spotlight on Stress
Sandwich Generation

When Harry Met Sally

Spousal and Partner Caregiving

In one of my favorite movies of all time, *When Harry Met Sally* (written by one of my heroes, Nora Ephron), interspersed with the love story of Meg Ryan and Billy Crystal, we see a series of vignettes of older couples sitting on a couch explaining how they met and married. I often wonder if real couples (as opposed to those *reel* couples) think about what the vow *in sickness and in health* means during their wedding ceremony.

That is why I am so inspired when I hear of the commitment Meredith Vieira and her husband Richard Cohen – who has twice beaten cancer and lives with multiple sclerosis - have for each other. They have truly lived their marriage vow since they took it 26 years ago. And when you read the stories in this book about Jill Eikenberry and Michael Tucker, Rodney and Holly Robinson Peete, David and Valerie Osmond, and Alan and Suzanne Osmond, you will see how strong marriage partners can make all the difference when facing caregiving and chronic illness.

We often think the *sickness* part will come towards the end-of-life. And for many it will. While we are living longer – 20 percent of us who reach age 65 will live on to age 90 and one in every 50 baby boomer women will live to be a centenarian (100 years young) – our bodies still become battle sieged by chronic illness beginning in our 70s and 80s. In fact, 1 of every 2 Americans who reach his 85th birthday will develop Alzheimer's disease or dementia.

However, you will see when you read the story about both Alan Osmond and his son David, chronic illness can strike in your 20s and 30s – as it did with this father/son duo both living with multiple sclerosis. They both credit the love and support of their wives, Suzanne and Valerie respectively, with helping them continue to live and thrive (in fact, David proposed to Valerie while in his wheelchair but was able to walk down the aisle with her at their wedding).

The discussion about end-of-life wishes with your spouse, and ultimately with any family member who might become your caregiver, becomes imperative. The National Alliance for Caregiving estimates more than 3 million Americans are caring for a spouse with a chronic illness – heart disease, cancer, Alzheimer's, ALS, multiple sclerosis, etc.

If there is any legacy Terri Schiavo left all of us it is no matter what age you are – you need to have an Advance Directive. If you become incapacitated, which Schiavo was for 14 years, it is critical all your key family members understand your wishes. And waiting until you are older to create this legal document is folly. Schiavo was only 27 when she was put on a ventilator and feeding tube after cardiac arrest left her brain dead. She lay in a vegetative state for all those years while her husband battled her parents over whether or not to keep her alive on machines. If she had a Living Will, there never would have been a battle.

> **More than 3 million Americans are caring for a spouse with a chronic illness.**

Having the proper legal documentation, which we talk about in the Rehearsals chapter, Raiders of the Lost Ark, is essential but so is the conversation with family so there are no mysteries when the time comes and we will address those conversation tips in the C-A-R-E Conversations chapter.

Another issue faced by caregiving spouses may be the resistance the affected spouse has to being *cared* for. In the case of Meredith Vieira, she has spoken about how her husband does not want to be a burden despite some limitations of his MS. Meredith has had to find ways to be there for him when needed and remind him that sometimes he does need help and that it is OK to ask.

The same holds true for Tracy Pollan. Michael J. Fox is living with Parkinson's disease and the challenges of his disease have not put his acting career on pause one iota. He guest starred on TV's *The Good Wife* and in many articles Tracy would not describe herself as a caregiver but just a partner and wife. Do you think she had any idea her then 30-year-old husband would be diagnosed with Parkinson's disease? Yet Michael credits Tracy for not only keeping their family together but helping motivate him to live as normal a life as possible and face an unknown future with amazing grace and optimism.

Whether they want to label themselves caregivers or not, the reality is both Meredith and Tracy have had to create a new normal – a life that accommodates the complications and challenges of a spouse living with a chronic illness or disability.

One of the sad realities of chronic illness is the stress put on a marriage. A 2009 study published in the journal *Cancer* found a married woman diagnosed with a serious disease is six times more likely to be divorced or separated than a man with a similar diagnosis. Among study participants, the divorce rate was 21 percent for seriously ill women and 3 percent for seriously ill men. A control group divorced at a rate of 12 percent, suggesting that if disease makes husbands more likely to split, it makes wives more likely to stay.

In her book, *The Caregiving Wife's Handbook*, Dr. Diane Denholm, a medical psychotherapist, who is better equipped than most to deal with caregiving issues, talks about how she could not convince her husband, who suffered from Parkinson's disease, to stop driving when she knew he should. She writes, "Often, husbands do not want the illness or disease that is attacking their body to also attack their manhood. They feel helpless and it is harder for men to ask for help, which makes it imperative for a wife to create new ways to communicate and operate." Dr. Denholm recommends two things, "Have written agreements with your spouse that addresses issues on both sides; and avoid becoming an enabler."

She says instead of doing everything for your spouse, help with what they *cannot* do – not only does this allow them to still feel a sense of some normalcy but it also eliminates you from being a martyr which can lead to anger, stress, guilt, fights and even depression. If it is too hard to create better communication then it is time to call in a mediator. Solicit the help of a professional – whether that is your spouse's doctor, a geriatric care manager or another health care professional who can be an impartial party to both your issues and help you find solutions.

As mentioned earlier, the reality of caring for a spouse or partner is illness or accidents can happen at any time. Take the numerous examples of military wives and husbands caring for returning veterans who are paralyzed, suffering from post-traumatic stress disorder (PTSD) or unable to perform the typical activities of daily living because of traumatic brain injury (TBI). These caregivers of veterans – 10 million strong – are the real *Bravehearts* in this book and you will read more about them in that upcoming section.

Lastly, I return to the wedding vow *in sickness and in health*. Both Katie Couric and Lisa Niemi Swayze lost husbands to cancer. They have managed their grief with grace and carry the legacy of their loved ones forward by fighting to find a cure for this *terrorist* as Alana Stewart calls cancer.

But there are some who believe *sickness* may release you from your wedding vows. In 2011, television evangelist Pat Robertson stepped on a moral minefield when he announced a spouse of someone suffering from Alzheimer's who was "too far gone" should be free to divorce their spouse to seek other companionship. The controversy that erupted was nothing short of the Mount St. Helen's volcano blowing in 1980.

Although Robertson clearly struggled in his answer to the caller who asked this question during his *700 Club* TV show, he stated, "I hate Alzheimer's… because here's the loved one — this is the woman or man that you have loved for 20, 30, 40 years – and suddenly that person is gone." He went on to say it would be OK to divorce your spouse ensuring they have custodial care before you move on to be with someone else. When a co-anchor pointed out the marriage vow, "til death do us part," Robertson responded with "this is a kind of death."

In the end, you made a commitment to your spouse when you walked down the aisle. The only answer to this difficult situation which many of us may face is to have the conversation now, when you are both healthy, about each other's wishes in such a situation. At least you can try to make a decision together that leaves less room for anger, jealousy and the emotional agony of being disconsolate when your loved one is here in body but not in mind or spirit.

A study published in the *Journal of the American Medical Association (JAMA)* by researchers at the University of Pittsburgh showed the caregivers' stress levels rose and fell along with the stress their loved one was feeling. In another study conducted by researchers at the University of South Florida in Tampa published in the journal *Stroke,* caregivers tending to their ailing spouse where they felt *a lot of strain* were 23% more likely to have a stroke compared with their caregiving counterparts who said they felt no strain. The study also showed stroke risk was higher among men, especially African-American men. In addition, stressful events, such as the health decline and ultimate loss of a spouse has been linked to an increase in breast cancer among women within two years of the event.

Spotlight on Stress
Caring for a Spouse

Bringing Up Baby

Caring for Children with Special Needs

Bringing Up Baby was a 1930s screwball comedy starring the incomparable Katherine Hepburn and the debonair comedian Cary Grant. The *baby* in the movie was a leopard – a rare and wonderful creature – that needed special care only Cary could provide (or so Katherine thought). When you have a child with special needs – whether it is Down syndrome (DS), cerebral palsy, muscular dystrophy or autism – you have a rare and wonderful child who needs special care.

According to the National Alliance for Caregiving, almost 17 million Americans care for a child under age 18 with special needs. While caregivers of an older parent or spouse may exhibit sadness or depression over their loved one's decline – the initial sadness of the caregivers of a special needs child is typically replaced by a fierce fighting spirit that would scare any *tiger mom*. Parents of newborns are filled with future promises, but parents of special needs children are faced with health care professionals mostly telling them about the limitations for their child. However, many of these parents encounter these roadblocks and find a detour to a fulfilling life for their child and success along the caregiving road.

> **Almost 17 million Americans care for a child under age 18 with special needs.**

Renowned authors David Kessler and Elisabeth Kübler-Ross, outlined the five stages of grief in their book on the subject and wrote that the fifth and last stage is *Acceptance*. When it comes to the parents of special needs children, *acceptance* does not mean defeat but rather *rebirth*. These parents create new dreams to replace the old expectations.

In fact, many of these parents become passionate advocates for their child's disorder or disease and they become experts at finding innovative solutions – whether it is a special diet, homeopathic medicine or alternative health and wellness techniques such as music therapy. They take on schools, government agencies and care providers with the fearlessness and ferocity of Clint Eastwood in the *Dirty Harry* movies. I can just see them saying to anyone standing in their way with that steely determination, "Go ahead, make my day." It has been my experience that parents of special needs children could fix the economy, create all the jobs to eliminate unemployment and solve global warming if the same passion they have for their child were turned to some of our nation's biggest issues of the day.

However, this passionate advocacy can come at a price. Some reports show special needs parents have a higher divorce rate than average married couples – 85 percent versus the overall national average of 50 percent. While this high incidence of divorce was recently challenged by another study showing virtually no higher incidence of divorce for parents of an autistic child, there is no doubt the unique challenges and extraordinary focus of caring for a child with special needs puts added strain on a marriage. The frustrations over not being able to fix their child's challenges, the need to assign blame – which typically means the spouses target each other for this blame – the high level of attention and focus that needs to be placed on the child's needs above all else can take its toll on a marriage.

The strong survive and you will be encouraged when you read the story in this book about Holly Robinson Peete and her husband Rodney, who overcame these issues to create an even stronger family unit and strengthen their love and support for each other through their experiences with their autistic son, R.J.

The other issue special needs caregivers face is in becoming an educator and ambassador for your child's challenges. Parents of special needs children need to communicate to teachers, friends and their child's peers the nature of the disorder. They can find comfort and compassion in others when they take the time to explain why their child does certain things or has certain limitations and not just the fact their child has a special challenge. It is through this communication and education others learn how to interact with special needs children.

These parents also have to sometimes balance caring for a child with special needs while caring for their other child or children who may feel neglected. This constant balancing act can be a huge challenge for the caregiver but the positive aspect is the other siblings learn patience, compassion, sensitivity and other valuable characteristics that will serve them well in the adult world and make them more thoughtful, informed people.

Perhaps the biggest concern of parents of children with special needs is the future of their child as they age into adulthood. Twenty years ago, children with Down syndrome (DS) were not expected to survive into their early 30s – today their average lifespan is age 55. In addition, children with DS are developing Alzheimer's disease after age 40 in almost 100 percent of cases according to recent studies.

Dr. Rosemary Laird, medical director for the Health First Aging Institute, says adults with DS have premature aging. "We know Down syndrome is an accurate predictor for an Alzheimer's diagnosis in later life but earlier than in general Alzheimer's patients. DS makes the body age more rapidly."

In 10 years, one-half million autistic children will be adults with typical expectations for living into their 70s and 80s. The significant difference they face is a society that does not understand how to assimilate them and support them once their parents are gone.

And autism and DS are not the only two childhood conditions that create special needs caregivers of their parents – cerebral palsy, muscular dystrophy, ataxia, cystic fibrosis and mental health issues all require a special kind of parenting.

There is a lot of research that points to the improved therapies and the ability for parents to nurture their special needs children at home rather than being forced into institutionalizing them which some believe contributed to shorter lifespans for the child in previous decades. However, caring for a child over her or his lifespan is the dilemma that most concerns the parents of special needs children. If you are unable to continue to care for your special needs child because of your own health issues, who will take care of them? The question becomes whether this burden falls to other siblings or relatives or to the state and federal government which will already be buckling under the weight of its hefty population of seniors as the 78 million baby boomers – our society's largest segment of the population – continues to grow older and live longer.

Holly Robinson Peete, champion and advocate for special needs children – especially those with autism like her son – says the big white elephant in the room that our policymakers, health care officials and society at large are not addressing is how we will care for special needs children after their parents are gone. What these caregivers are teaching us is special needs children, most of whom will be special needs adults, can be valuable to our society if we take the time to understand them.

The stress of caring for a special needs child can have a devastating impact on your health as the primary caregiver. According to the book, *So Stressed*, a study done by the University of California at San Francisco found moms of special needs children who experienced high stress actually sped up their aging process by harming their DNA – they appeared 9 to 17 years older than their biological age.

Dr. Rosemary Laird, medical director for Health First Aging, says the risk of stress is sometimes invisible – it is not like a physical wound we can see. Therefore, we tend to ignore it until it is too late. She says not managing stress levels can severely impact your immune system.

Spotlight on Stress
Caring for a Special Needs Child

The Sons Also Rise

Men as Caregivers

The classic 1920s Ernest Hemingway novel, *The Sun Also Rises* (and 1950s movie of the same name) is about love, death, renewal and above all, masculinity. When we think of the typical caregiver, we think of a baby boomer-age woman. While women are in the majority when it comes to the caregiving role, men make up one-third of primary caregivers, typically caring for a spouse or partner, according to national surveys.

Men are also stepping up more than ever to help with the caregiving role for an older parent or play a strong supporting role to a wife who is working and is a primary caregiver for her aging or ill parent. You will read a great example of this caregiving support role in the story of Jill Eikenberry and Michael Tucker. Jill credits Mike with giving her the ability to care for her mom without falling apart.

When it comes to a few good men, the entertainment world has several male stars who are or were caregivers for a parent: Peter Gallagher, TV star of *Covert Affairs* and *The O.C.*, Victor Garber, star of TV's *Alias* and blockbuster film *Titanic*, Bryan Cranston, TV star of *Malcolm in the Middle* and *Breaking Bad*,

> **Men make up one-third of primary caregivers.**

all cared for mothers with Alzheimer's disease; and comedic actor Seth Rogen of *Knocked Up* fame supports his wife as they care for her mother with Alzheimer's. That icon of male strength, The Rock (aka Dwayne Johnson) was a pillar of strength as he helped his mom battle lung cancer.

Just as men have been recruited into the world of baby diapering, nursery school and soccer carpools, these adult sons are also finding themselves faced with taking care of mom and dad and that may include adult diapers and car service to doctor appointments or Adult Day Care.

According to the *MetLife Study of Sons At Work – Balancing Employment and Elder Care*, men are often taking on caregiving duties. This includes such activities as:

- Handling the finances for mom or dad
- Helping to navigate Medicare or Medicaid and other insurance and health care provider paperwork
- Helping with home improvements to make an older parent's home more safe
- Managing medications for a parent
- Providing transportation for a parent to and from doctor appointments
- Taking care of some household chores like mowing the lawn or shoveling the snowy driveway
- Helping to transfer a non-ambulatory loved one from wheelchair to bed

And it is not just parental caregiving. Men are also caring for spouses and siblings who have a chronic disease or sudden illness.

One of our most famous caregivers was an adored children's book author who cared for his wife while she battled several chronic illnesses including cancer. Theodor Geisel, better known as Dr. Seuss, has an enduring legacy as the author of some of the best loved and most widely published children's books: *The Cat in the Hat; Horton Hears a Who!; Green Eggs and Ham; One Fish, Two Fish, Red Fish, Blue Fish;* and my favorite, *How the Grinch Stole Christmas*. While Geisel was celebrated as the magical Dr. Seuss, he was also a veteran of World War II, which gave him the opportunity to create a documentary film about his war experiences for which he was honored with the Academy Award for Best Documentary Feature in 1947. He went on to win another Oscar in 1950 for Best Animated Short Film based on an original story he conceived during his Army days.

What is perhaps the least known fact about Dr. Seuss is he was a caregiver for his first wife. For several years during perhaps his most productive writing phase, Geisel's first wife, Helen, had major health issues and ultimately lost her battle with cancer. While he poured his passion into the writings that made reading for children entertaining as well as educational, he poured his love into caring for his ill wife. Since the Geisels did not have children, Geisel was primary caregiver for his wife during those years.

And Dr. Seuss is not alone. The sophisticated, cool star of TV's *Remington Steele* and several James Bond movies, Pierce Brosnan, cared for a first wife he lost to ovarian cancer. Veteran stage and screen actor, Hal Holbrook, cared for his wife, actress Dixie Carter, as she lost her battle with endometrine cancer. Music legend and former Beatle Paul McCartney was by his wife Linda's side for three years as she battled bravely with breast cancer before she passed in 1998. And actor, entertainer Jamie Foxx cares for a sister with Down syndrome.

There is also obviously a higher incidence of male caregivers in same-sex couples, particularly when illness such as AIDS or other chronic illness creates a caregiving situation. What is terribly difficult for these couples is the ongoing social obstacles and often family conflicts that can arise which I explore more later in this chapter, Angels in America.

While women seek social networks of friends to nurture away their stress, men act more like they are in a classic Godzilla movie with the *fight or flight* response often seeking ways to escape stress. Thus, male caregivers may never get a chance to deal with their stress – it stays bottled up inside and ultimately can lead to serious health risks.

However, a 2012 study conducted by researchers at Bowling Green State University found men tend to take the *block and tackle* approach to caregiving that actually helps them cope with stress. "Our study found women are more socialized to be nurturing and able to handle caregiving but they internalize their caregiving performance and worry, 'Am I doing well enough?' which adds to their stress levels," says I-Fen Lin, associate professor and lead researcher on the study. "Men block their emotions and take a task-oriented approach to caregiving – they are problem solving when it comes to caring for a loved one, especially an older parent."

Spotlight on Stress
Men as Caregivers

Brothers & Sisters

Caring for a Young Adult

The 2006-2011 TV series, *Brothers & Sisters*, starred Calista Flockhart, Sally Field and Rob Lowe and showcased a family of five siblings – all with distinctly different personalities – who would fight and make-up with each other and with the matriarch played by Field. Tensions and conflict erupted weekly but in the end the siblings all looked out for each other and you knew this is how it would be for the rest of their lives.

Most of us believe caregiving means caring for an older parent or maybe a spouse as we age. However, when it comes to caring for a young adult (defined as age 18-49) with a disability or chronic illness, caregiver roles tend to be managed by siblings and are longer-term and more intensive according to the National Alliance for Caregiving study *Caregivers of Young Adults*. Other studies have found as we age, 18 percent of those caring for someone over age 75 were siblings caring for siblings.

Our casting call for the average caregivers of a young adult would look like this:

- Approximately 46-47 years old
- Six out of 10 are female
- More than half care for a woman whose average age is 32

- Most of the young adults need care because they are single (60%), widowed, divorced or separated (16%)
- Four out of 10 care for their older child with special needs, while 14 percent care for a sibling
- Seven out of 10 are employed
- Has been caregiving for 7.6 years (national average is 4.6 years)
- Four out of 10 feel they have no other choice
- Approximately 40 percent live in the same household with loved one

As stated above, 40 percent of these young adults needing care are still being cared for by a parent. This is especially true in baby boomer or older age caregivers of returning veterans who are paralyzed, or have other injuries such as traumatic brain injury (TBI) or mental health issues such as post-traumatic stress disorder (PTSD).

> **Caring for a young adult tend to be managed by siblings and are longer-term and more intensive.**

But often in these young adult caregiving situations, and particularly as both caregiver and care recipient age, the caregiving is being done by a sibling, especially if an older parent has recently passed away. Slightly more than half of the young adults needing care are struggling with long-term physical conditions while almost half are challenged with emotional or mental health issues.

These young adult caregivers report they came into their caregiving role because their loved one has a mental or emotional illness (23%), developmental delay including mental retardation and Down syndrome (9%), surgery or wounds (5%) and attention deficit, substance abuse and diabetes each account for 4 percent.

Often the reasons for caring for a sibling have a stigma attached making sibling caregivers less likely to share with friends or their work supervisors their caregiving responsibilities. Two actresses have been raising awareness for disorders that in the past have been in the shadows.

Eva Longoria, best known for her role on the long-running TV series *Desperate Housewives*, has an older sister living with Down syndrome (DS). Eva comes from a very close-knit family in Texas with three older sisters who along with their strong, independent mother all look out for each other. Eva has expressed in interviews that having a sibling with developmental disabilities is a gift. She believes it helped her and her other sisters become selfless growing up and her mom made sure the girls all knew the opportunities they had in life that others did not and to learn from their sister as much as she leaned on them. Eva started a nonprofit organization to help developmentally challenged children in Texas called Eva's Heroes.

Another area of caregiving shrouded in myths and social stigma is mental illness. Oscar-nominated and Emmy and Tony Award-winning actress Glenn Close has been a champion for shedding light on the dark world of bi-polar disorder which affects her sister. Appearing on the TV morning show, *Good Morning America*, Glenn said she believes we need to be having discussions around mental illness and talk as openly as we do about other diseases such as cancer or diabetes.

According to the National Institute of Mental Health, 1 in 4 adults in the U.S. has a diagnosable mental disorder and the average age is 14 for the on-set of mental health issues. Glenn and her sister star in a public service announcement (PSA) campaign on mental health issues and Glenn formed the nonprofit organization, BringChange2Mind, to help eliminate the stigma and myths about mental illness in an effort to get more people to seek help.

You will also read in the story about Holly Robinson Peete, how she joined her daughter Ryan to write a children's book about autism to help other kids understand the disorder that affects her brother, R.J.

While 4 out of 10 of these caregivers reported an emotional toll in their role, the biggest price sibling caregivers pay is financial. Ten percent of those caring for an older loved one report a financial burden associated with their caregiving role, but twice as many sibling caregivers (25%) report the same. They also spend more time in their caregiving role than general caregivers. According to the National Alliance for Caregiving, 26 percent of caregivers of young adults provided care for 10 years or more – which makes their average caregiving duration 7.6 years compared to the 4.6 years general caregivers spend caring for a loved one. The stress of money worries over a long period of time can start to impact the sibling caregiver's stress levels and lead to their own health risks.

While most sibling caregivers reported little physical strain, they did report emotional strain with 4 out of 10 stating they found caregiving stressful. Twenty-three percent of these caregivers also reported their health had become worse since caregiving according to the National Alliance for Caregiving.

In addition, 4 out of 10 sibling caregivers felt they had no choice to become a caregiver and they become less engaged in their social networks with 57% reporting they have less time for other family or friends once they became a caregiver. We know disengaging in social outlets that can be a lifeline can add to a caregiver's stress level.

Spotlight on Stress
Caring for a Sibling

Far and Away

Long-Distance Caregiving

The 1992 movie, *Far and Away,* starring Tom Cruise and Nicole Kidman, tells the story of two immigrant Irish adventurers leaving their families to come to a new world in 1890s America. National studies show approximately 7-8 million Americans are caring for a loved one who lives at least one hour away – and for them caregiving is a brave, new world that in some cases can be cross-country or even *across the pond* such as actress Jane Seymour who cared for her mom living in England while she lived here in the U.S.

In fact, according to Nora Jean Levin, executive director of Caring From a Distance, a nonprofit organization dedicated to long-distance caregivers, there are approximately 1 million U.S. caregivers living overseas – either working for the U.S. State Department or for private corporations – who are caring for a loved one, typically a parent, still living in America.

It is hard if you only visit your parent occasionally to know if things are amiss or changed. In Joan Lunden's story you will read how she did not realize the extent of her mother's dementia until her brother passed away and Joan had to step in. Since Joan lived on the East Coast

> **7-8 million Americans are caring for a loved one who lives at least one hour away**

and her mom lived on the West, everyone put on a happy face for occasional visits. But when Joan spent more time without her brother as the protective shell around her mom, the reality hit home. The question for caregivers like Joan is whether or not to contemplate a move.

The move may be your parent's – do you remove them from the home and community they are familiar with possibly having lived there for 30, 40 or even 50 years? Or, do you decide to move closer to them possibly uprooting your family or having to change jobs in order to be the caregiver you want and need to be? In Joan's story you will read how she solved the problem with the help of a professional and was able to keep her mom safe and happy in California and her husband and children based on the East Coast.

Long-distance caregivers have to learn how to be keen observers since their time with their loved one is typically limited. It is difficult to know what may be amiss with your parent if you are only spending a couple of days with them. One tip Levin gives long-distance caregivers is to ensure you plan on attending a doctor visit with your parent when you make those short trips. Being able to talk to your loved one's doctor helps you see the bigger picture you may be missing.

Becoming a keen observer means you need to tap into your inner Dick Tracy. In other words, you need to become the ultimate detective. Often, this includes two things:

1. Observe your loved one and his/her home environment for significant changes:

Is your loved one unusually quiet and withdrawn, drinking more than usual, wearing dirty clothes or exhibiting bad hygiene? Is he/she much thinner, bruised or had recently broken bones or other accidents? Is there a lot of unusual clutter, dirty dishes piled up in the kitchen, stove left on, car has a lot of dents or dings or other signs of accidents, bills unopened or unpaid, Home Shopping Network purchases piling up in the guest bedroom?

2. Enlist the help of local neighbors or even engaging a professional care manager to help:

Since you cannot be observing your loved one every day you may need the help of your detective team. If there is a local neighbor both you and your loved one are close to, you may want to have a conversation about your concerns and ask her to observe and give you a call if she sees anything unusual with your parent. These *eyes and ears* to help caregivers can also be found through the volunteers that are part of the Village Movement which you will read more about in Cocoon chapter of the Rehearsals section.

If there is no one locally you can count on, there are professional geriatric care managers (GCMs) who can be engaged to visit your loved one and conduct a care assessment. Or if you have a home health aide, home care service person or even a housekeeper helping out your parent, you need to deputize this person to be part of your detective discovery team. This is a little trickier since loved ones can be resistant to the fact they may need care or may not want a stranger coming into their home. I review these C-A-R-E Conversations in a following chapter to help you have this discussion with your parent.

In addition to living long-distance from a loved one, some caregivers also face the impediments of having a loved one who is living in a rural area where resources are limited. Rural communities are defined by the U.S. Census to be areas of less dense population, typically under 2,500. More than 21 percent of all Americans live in rural areas. In the study, *Caregiving in Rural America*, the National Alliance for Caregiving (NAC) found caregivers caring for loved ones in rural areas had little or no options for transportation services and were less likely to use home health aides. Also daily neighbor observations are a lot tougher in rural areas where loved ones live on farms that are not close together like you would find in a suburban or urban neighborhood. For caregivers of those living in rural areas, the detective work becomes even more difficult but important.

When it comes to long-distance caregiving there is good news and bad news. The bad news is your costs will be higher than caregivers who live closer to their loved one. A study conducted by the NAC showed long-distance caregivers spent on average $8,728 – almost double the annual amount spent by caregivers who lived within one hour of their loved one.

The good news is long-distance caregivers are better at building caregiving teams out of necessity. If you only visit mom or dad occasionally because work and distance keep your visits limited, having local help becomes essential. As stated above, it might be a trusted neighbor or local home health aide who can be your eyes and ears and helping hands in caring for your loved one. This circle of care also allows the caregiver to have the breaks and respite from the day-to-day physical and emotional tolls of caregiving.

"Caregiving is a patchwork quilt of services with a lot of holes in it and not all the patches touching each other," says Levin. "This fragmented system has plagued caregivers over the years and the only way to solve it is to learn as much as you can, reach out for help and create a team to help you care for your loved one." Levin said the Internet has been a blessing to caregivers, particularly those caring from a distance. Not only can they more easily find local resources for a long-distance loved one but they can access that information 24/7 and not just during daytime hours when they may be living and working in a different time zone. Being able to do research and not have to take numerous days off work to find resources has been one cure for long-distance caregivers.

While long-distance caregivers do a better job at building care teams to manage the load – alleviating physical impacts and exhaustion – they still encounter the typical caregiver emotions of worry and stress. The road they travel is the same road all caregivers journey on and it is called the guilt trip.

Almost all of the long-distance caregivers I have spoken to bring up the *G-word* as a natural part of their caregiving role. The distance creates this gulf of guilt that is hard to overcome. Joan Lunden said it about caring for a mom across the country. Marg Helgenberger remembers it caring for parents in Nebraska while she was in Chicago and then New York. The reality is if you know where to turn for help you can help offload some of the guilt and banish the stress.

Spotlight on Stress
Long-Distance Caregivers

Bravehearts

Caregivers of Veterans

In the climatic final scene of the Oscar-winning movie, *Braveheart* about 13th century Scottish warrior William Wallace, Mel Gibson who plays Wallace, yells out before his death, "Freedom!" As Americans, we have this gift of freedom every day because of our brave men and women around the globe who serve our country and because of their family caregivers who care for our nation's veterans. We owe them a debt of gratitude and thanks as they are very special forces.

The U.S. Department of Veterans Affairs projects there are more than 23 million U.S. veterans and the National Alliance for Caregiving (NAC) reported more than 10 million Americans are caring for a veteran, and nearly 7 million of them are veterans themselves.

> **10 million Americans are caring for a veteran, and nearly 7 million of them are veterans themselves.**

What makes this group of caregivers special is how and why they become caregivers. While some are caring for a veteran who has typical aging issues such as diabetes, cancer or heart disease, many more of these caregivers are caring for a loved one who has a mental health issue such as post-traumatic stress disorder (PTSD) or physical disabilities such as paraplegia or traumatic brain injury (TBI) – all as a direct result of service to our country.

A 2010 NAC study, *Caregivers of Veterans - Serving on the Homefront* surveying the caregivers of veterans from World War II, the Korean War, the Vietnam War, Desert Storm, Operation Enduring Freedom and Operation Iraqi Freedom found 9 out of 10 caregivers of veterans are women and 70 percent provide care for a spouse or a partner. The study also found 30 percent of these caregivers are part of the classic Sandwich Generation and compared to caregivers nationally, caregivers of veterans are twice as likely to be in their caregiving role for 10 years or longer (30 percent vs. 15 percent).

As in all caregiving situations, the illness or disorder does not just affect the person with the diagnosis – it is typically a family diagnosis. For families of veterans who need care, 57 percent reported their children or grandchildren have experienced emotional or school problems as a result of their caregiving or the veteran's condition.

While many of these caregivers are the wives of former Army, Navy, Marine and Air Force servicemen, many younger veterans from recent conflicts who return with wounds both emotional and physical are cared for by a baby boomer mother. This older mom was contemplating the golden years of retirement only to have her wounded child return home facing an uncertain future and needing mom's help as much as when he/she was a young son or daughter.

And while there are many reasons these women become caregivers – paraplegia or quadriplegia, cancer from possible exposure to elements such as Agent Orange used during the Vietnam War, TBI – perhaps one of the more challenging issues a caregiver of a veteran faces is caring for someone with PTSD.

In the 2010 HBO documentary film, *Wartorn 1861-2010,* produced and narrated by James Gandolfini (of Tony Soprano fame) we learn that what we call PTSD today has been part of our military collateral damage since the Civil War. Throughout the years it has been called melancholia, shell-shock and combat fatigue and it is a mental health issue brought on by the anxiety of having been in life-threatening situations. The documentary was produced in cooperation with the U.S. military to bring awareness to the increasing rate of suicide among our service men and women and to show the devastating effects on the psyches of our veterans and the impact to their families.

And PTSD is not limited to military service men and women. Many law enforcement officers, firefighters and the first responders of 9/11, as well as other tragic situations such as those innocent people caught in the 2012 Aurora, Colorado theater spray of gunfire from a crazed gunman, have described symptoms of PTSD from their traumatic experiences.

In the same way we have stigmatized many brain-related health issues such as schizophrenia, bi-polar disorder or Alzheimer's disease, PTSD is a serious but hidden disorder. When someone who needs care does not use a cane, a wheelchair or other assistive device, most of us believe they are *fine*. But in reality those with mental health issues and their caregivers suffer in the shadows.

One young wife of a returning veteran with PTSD from Operation Iraqi Freedom (OIF) told me her neighbors did not understand why she needed help. They would see her husband and he looked just fine – he wasn't missing a limb and did not had a concave head that is typical of those with TBI. She cried as she described to me how they could not go to restaurants or even shopping with their children because any sudden movement or sound would make her husband jumpy and extremely nervous. His pulse rate would increase and he would sweat profusely. She told me how one night she awoke out of a deep sleep to find him standing over her looking odd. Terrified she did not move. All of a sudden her husband punched his hand through the wall above her head and started crying. She struggles to understand his illness, get him the help he needs and keep herself and her children safe – even from her husband. These are the wounds of war most of us do not see.

In 2010, the Veterans Omnibus Health Services Act called for the creation of more caregiver service and support through the Department of Veteran's Affairs (VA). To date, the VA has established a toll-free 24/7 Support Line for Caregivers, they have a Caregiving Coordinator in every VA Medical Center location to handle family caregiver queries and help coordinate the care necessary for caregivers to care for their veteran at home – whether it is financial support through veterans' benefits, health care services, etc. The VA benefits also provide training, counseling and a living stipend to veteran's caregivers.

In addition, there is a more flexible respite care benefit that provides up to 30 days respite care a year so caregivers can get a much-needed break to recharge their batteries.

The VA also continues its leadership in implementing technology solutions for veterans and their caregivers. There is an online tool for keeping personal health records (PHRs) to help caregivers of veterans called My HealthE Vet. And in collaboration between the Departments of Defense, Labor and Veterans Affairs, there is an online site, and smartphone app called the

National Resource Directory that puts thousands of resources at the caregiver's fingertips. The services and resources are at the national, state and local levels to support recovery, rehabilitation and community reintegration. Caregivers can find information on a variety of topics including benefits & compensation, education & training, employment, family & caregiver support, health, homeless assistance, housing, transportation & travel and other services & resources.

I call these caregivers of veterans *bravehearts* because despite their sacrifices, 94 percent of them are proud to serve. Seven out of 10 reported feeling a sense of reward from having gained knowledge and skills through caregiving; and 67 percent find caregiving to be fulfilling.

The sacrifices caregivers of veterans make are significant. They have much higher stress levels (88%) than other types of caregivers, 63% reported depression over their situation, 77% reported sleep deprivation and 43% provided more than 40 hours of care a week.

The three most effective ways caregivers of veterans can relieve stress are through support groups, through counseling and through respite retreats either alone, with other caregivers or with their spouse and family. Many veterans service organizations (VSOs) such as the Wounded Warrior Project, Project Sanctuary and Operation Purple Healing Adventures by the National Military Family Association offer a variety of caregiver respite or family social activities.

But while they report more stress, they also report being proud to serve as a caregiver to their loved one. God Bless America and God bless our nation's veterans, first responders and their caregivers.

Spotlight on Stress
Caregivers of Veterans

The Joy Luck Club

Caring for Multiple Loved Ones

In the 1989 movie, *The Joy Luck Club,* about Chinese immigrant mothers and their daughters based on the best-selling novel by Amy Tan, we follow several story lines about the sacrifices the mothers have made to give their daughters a better life in San Francisco, California. The interlocking stories of love, regret, caring and sacrifice are not unlike a rare breed of caregivers who essentially provide care back-to-back or simultaneous care for multiple loved ones over most of their lives. They get on the caregiving carousel and find the ride never ends. I call them *career caregivers.*

While there is no statistic on how many caregivers get into a cycle of caregiving for multiple family members back-to-back, the National Alliance for Caregiving reports one-third of the nation's 65 million caregivers are caring for two or more people at the same time. The study also found there are more than twice the percentage of caregivers of young adults – often siblings – caring for three or more loved ones (18%) compared to caregivers of older adults over age 50 (8%). In the stories about Holly Robinson Peete and Marg Helgenberger, you will read how they had overlapping or back-to-back caregiving situations in their lives.

> **One-third of the nation's 65 million caregivers are caring for 2 or more people at the same time.**

In my travels talking to caregivers I spoke to one woman who began her caregiving journey looking after her older parents who were experiencing the typical issues of aging that require more help from a family member. Her mother was 78 and was losing her hearing and suffering from painful arthritis; her father was 82 and had COPD (chronic obstructive pulmonary disease). She was an only daughter and had an uncle, age 85, also living alone nearby.

Her caregiving carousel ride began simply with her parents by paying their bills, ensuring their house was clean (doing the maid work herself), buying their groceries and often serving as taxi service to help them get to church. However, the day her uncle fell and broke his hip, her father asked his only daughter if she could help care for her uncle since the uncle was all alone and they [her parents] were too old to provide him much help. She took on the care of her uncle who insisted on remaining in his home alone. Her uncle passed away a couple of years later from Stage 4 pancreatic cancer.

At the same time, her father's disease progressed over the next few years until he succumbed to COPD and emphysema. Six months later her mother had a stroke. After being discharged from the hospital, she moved her mother into her home to care for her. Because this caregiver had a limited income and was divorced, she took on the physical caregiving duties of lifting and transferring her mom from bed to wheelchair to bath all alone. She pulled a muscle in her back but could not afford to take a break. Instead she took Advil and several glasses of wine nightly to cope. She also had not taken care of a chronic toothache and after ignoring her own dental needs, lost the tooth.

Five years into this phase of caregiving, her only son, who had been living too far away to help his mom in her caregiving duties, had a horrible accident and became partially disabled with some paralysis in his legs. Now having two people to care for, she moved her adult son into her home as well. It did not take long for this over-stressed, overwhelmed caregiver to be drowning in caregiving responsibilities. We will just call her daily existence, *The Days of Wine and Roses* (without the roses). This caregiver never said "no" and never was able to afford any help or back-up in her ongoing caregiving duties.

Amazingly, these types of stories are not uncommon. Former First Lady Rosalynn Carter is widely recognized as a pioneer in caregiving – leading a groundswell around caregiver awareness and advocacy. She founded the Rosalynn Carter Institute for Caregiving at Georgia Southwestern State University in 1987 and to this day it is still the only college that has a dedicated caregiving program for advocacy, research, education and programs that reach even beyond the walls of campus to support programs internationally. But what may not be as well known about Mrs. Carter is she is a *career caregiver*.

Her passion and advocacy come from a personal place and a lifetime dedicated to understanding the challenges – emotional, physical and financial – that accompany caring for a loved one. Rosalynn was only 12 years old when her father was diagnosed with terminal leukemia, a battle he lost just three months later. As the eldest daughter, she helped care for her ailing father and after his death supported her mother, who had to go to work to support the family, by caring for her younger siblings.

She took up caregiving again for several relatives with cancer after she left the White House. She relates how all of President Carter's siblings succumbed to cancer and he also lost his mother to breast cancer. Rosalynn helped care for several of these in-laws and also cared for her mother for many years until she passed in 2000 at age 94. In 2002, she was called to care again for her younger brother who had a stroke. He was living all alone in Ohio so he moved closer to Rosalynn in Plains, Georgia, so she could care for him.

When I spoke to her, she said, "I have seen firsthand why it is important for families to have places to go to for help – it is so crucial." I also asked her if she had identified herself as a caregiver through the years and she laughed, "No, I didn't realize I was a caregiver until I got involved in this work."

Today she is a passionate advocate for caregivers taking care of themselves as much as they care for their loved one encouraging them to self-identify so they can find and accept help.

Career caregivers are at heightened risk of developing chronic illness themselves. According to a Commonwealth Fund report, caregivers are twice as likely as the general public to develop chronic illness earlier in life due to the ongoing stress they feel in their caregiving duties. In addition, the National Alliance for Caregiving found 23% of caregivers who have been providing care for 5 years or more report higher stress than caregivers who have been caring for a shorter amount of time.

In some families, the dynamic is one person is identified as the caregiver. Other family members default to this person because "she knows what she is doing – she has done it before," or "she has the time – I travel too much for work" or "I have kids and taking on caring for mom would be too much."

Spotlight on Stress
Caring for Multiple Loved Ones

Lost Generation

Children as Caregivers

It was Ernest Hemingway who originally coined the phrase *the lost generation* made famous in his novel *The Sun Also Rises*. Although some attribute the phrase to Hemingway's mentor Gertrude Stein, he wrote, "It is not about a generation being lost as it is 'the earth abideth' – the characters may have been battered but they were not lost."

When we think of caregiving and children, we think of the children *needing* the care not *providing* the care. Yet, a landmark study from the National Alliance for Caregiving showed 1.4 million children between the ages of 8 and 18 are caring for an ill parent, chronically ill or disabled sibling or grandparent.

> **1.4 million children between the ages of 8 and 18 are caring for an ill parent, chronically ill or disabled sibling or grandparent.**

Among this *lost generation* of young caregivers, 3 in 10 are ages 8 to 12; more than one-third are ages 12 to 15; and 3 in 10 are ages 16 to 18. Young caregivers typically live in lower income households where 70 percent are caring for a parent or grandparent – with two-thirds of these caregivers living in the same home as the one for whom they are providing care. In the 2010 U.S. Census Bureau data, 6.6 million children live in a household with a grandparent representing approximately 16 percent of all U.S. households. As our older population grows with aging baby boomers, this living situation may increase and thus create even more youthful caregivers.

The reasons for caregiving among these youth range from mental health issues to physical disabilities or ailments to chronic illness. However, the No. 1 reason – approximately 18 percent – that younger children become caregivers is because they care for a loved one with Alzheimer's disease.

While adults do have a choice on whether to become a caregiver (although as stated earlier 75 percent of adult caregivers say they felt they did not have a choice), young caregivers really have no choice. Psychologists call the phenomenon of children becoming caregivers *parentified* – a role reversal where the child becomes the parent, giving up nurturing to be the nurturer.

In countries such as the United Kingdom and Australia, they have identified young *carers* (their term for caregivers) and have created national support programs, but there is only one such organization in the U.S. and it currently operates on a regional basis.

Founded in 1998, the American Association of Caregiving Youth (AACY) was formed specifically to provide support for young caregivers. One of the first programs for the AACY is the Caregiving Youth Project providing in-school therapeutic support groups, tutoring, mentorship and extra-curricular activities that are both recreational, such as overnight camps, and educational, such as links to community resources and help with college and scholarship applications. The program operates in Palm Beach County, Florida for middle and high school age caregivers but AACY is reaching out to other school districts with plans to replicate the program in other communities across the U.S.

"Caregiving youth are the hidden providers of our health care delivery system," says Dr. Connie Siskowski, founder and president of the American Association of Caregiving Youth (AACY). "No one wanted to believe the statistics of children under age 18 providing the primary care for a loved one but it's real and it's a growing phenomenon with our rapidly aging population."

Siskowski sees the struggles these youth caregivers face. She says they struggle with stress over their role – at home they have to play an adult, but at school they have to revert back to being a child and this causes confusion and frustration for these kids. Often these child caregivers are sacrificing their own developmental needs which can result in their loss of autonomy, activities outside the home and the love and care they should receive from a parent.

These young caregivers are asked by mom or dad to care for an ailing or older grandparent in the home or to look after a sick parent or sibling, sacrificing their childhoods as they take on adult responsibilities. The caregiving tasks of children can range from household needs and chores to administering medications for a loved one or helping with their loved one's personal care such as bathing or dressing.

"Often the contributions these youth caregivers make are even overlooked by other family members, especially a parent who is overstressed themselves," says Siskowski. What adds to the dilemma according to Siskowski is, "The types of family health issues these youthful caregivers face are beyond the purview of the current school system."

Typically, these youth caregivers are not emotionally equipped to deal with this level of responsibility and it can affect other aspects of their lives. The Bill and Melinda Gates Foundation published a report, *Silent Epidemic – Perspectives of High School Dropouts,* showing 22 percent of children who drop out of school for personal reasons do so because they have taken on family caregiver responsibilities. Siskowski says while these youth caregivers should be concentrating on their school work and classroom interaction, instead they are worried about whether their grandmother took her medications on time. She says school problems often begin with these caregivers being late to school – for instance, they missed the bus because they had to feed their grandfather.

How children cope with these caregiver responsibilities can range from sadness to anxiety to resentment over being a member of *The Lost Boys (and girls)*. They are even more hidden and isolated from society than adult caregivers, and their peers and teachers often have no idea these children have a full-time job as caregiver.

TV actresses Madeline Stowe (*Revenge*) and Dianne Argon (*Glee*) both were young girls growing up in households where a father had multiple sclerosis. While Dianne declines to speak about this aspect of her childhood, it is only recently Madeleine has done interviews about the impact on her young life. Perhaps that is because Madeleine has had more time to reflect on her young caregiving experience whereas Dianne is still in her 20s and not too far removed from her family situation. You will also read in Marg Helgenberger's story the impact on a youth caregiver of caring for a mother and father simultaneously battling chronic illness. While Marg was not under age 18 at the time, she was just starting college, her brother who helped manage the caregiving was a teenager.

However, there can be some positive results to having children take on more of a role to help care for an aging or ailing loved one. That child can derive a sense of purpose, belonging and usefulness. Siskowski says youth caregivers also learn early about empathy, and they develop valuable skills in organization, time management and multi-tasking that serves them well as adults.

A lot depends on the family dynamic – ensuring one child is not more burdened by caregiving than other children in the home, that they have some balance between caregiving and interacting with their peers, and that they receive approval and support from the well-parent are essential.

Children deal with stress very differently from adults because they lack the coping skills most adults have developed. Depending upon the age and developmental stage of these youth, the stress of caregiving may cause tantrums, acting out, thumb sucking, drugs or alcohol abuse, anti-social behavior and teen pregnancy. In addition, the stress of caregiving may cause children to drop out of school all together.

One study showed many parents often underestimate the stress their child is feeling. This is not uncommon when a well-spouse is working thus, letting some of the in-home caregiving fall to the child. Children are unable to properly articulate their stress to the well-parent and the well-parent is often too exhausted or overwhelmed to appropriately identify the impact of stress on their caregiving child.

Stress on caregiving children also puts them at higher risk of depression than their non-caregiving peers. They suffer higher incidence of co-dependent relationships and can have difficulty maintaining relationships.

Spotlight on Stress
Children as Caregivers

Angels in America

Gay, Lesbian, Bisexual, Transgender Caregivers

The award-winning TV mini-series, *Angels in America*, was an adaptation of a powerful play about the Reagan-era epidemic of AIDS. The program focused on those affected and presented themes of love, loss, loneliness and finally acceptance.

Today, almost 10 years since the mini-series aired and nearly 30 years since the term AIDS entered the lexicon, lesbian, gay, bisexual and transgender (LGBT) caregivers are still an often overlooked segment of the entire caregiving population and yet, they may come into their caregiving role better prepared than most.

> **LGBT couples are now at an age where growing older is making them caregivers all over again – for aging parents and for each other.**

In the 1980s when the AIDS epidemic gripped the gay community, many gay couples and their circle of friends provided the care needed for the loved one dying an agonizing death. Having lived through the social stigma and discrimination of AIDS, these LGBT couples are now at an age where growing older is making them caregivers all over again – for aging parents and for each other.

In an American Society on Aging/MetLife Mature Market Institute study of gay baby boomers, *Still Out, Still Aging*, the report stated,

> "This is the cohort that advanced the U.S. gay rights movement and within one generation succeeded in changing social attitudes from seeing homosexuality as a psychiatric condition to winning same-sex marriage and acknowledgement of their civil rights in an increasing number of states."

Now the LGBT community is in a position to help change attitudes about caregiving as well.

The first national study of aging lesbian and gay baby boomers was conducted by the MetLife Mature Market Institute and the Lesbian and Gay Aging Issues Network and showed there is a higher incidence of caregiving among LGBT individuals (1 in 4) versus the general population (1 in 5) found in National Alliance for Caregiving studies. In addition, there is more gender parity among men and women when it comes to LGBT caregivers – equal numbers of men and women serving as caregivers as opposed to the almost twice as many women (66%) caring for a loved one than men (34%) in the general caregiving population studies.

And while LGBT caregivers are caring for a range of loved ones: (36% for aging parents and half that percentage for a partner), they have a higher incidence of caring for friends (14%) and non-relatives (12%) than the 11% of general population caregivers. This higher incidence of friend-caregiving is rare and you will read about a friend caring for a friend in the Alana Stewart and Farrah Fawcett story.

When it comes to being cared for, because older LGBTs are three-to-four times less likely to have children who will be caring for them as they age, who will be their caregiver becomes a huge issue for aging LGBTs.

"Baby boomers are the first generation to not have children who may be able to care for you," says John Feather, PhD and chief executive officer of Grantmakers in Aging. "If you are single, childless, or LGBT, odds are your caregiver will be a partner or a friend because you can't count on kids."

As with caregiving overall, not all LGBT caregivers are *one size fits all*. Catherine Thurston, senior director of programs for Services and Advocacy for LGBT Elders (SAGE), advises, "When it comes to the issues of caregiving, there is a difference for those LGBTs who are *first generation* – people in their 70s, 80s and 90s." She says these older LGBT caregivers often don't have the typical support network because they may still not be *out* so their level of isolation, especially through caregiving and after the loss of a partner, is profound.

According to the National Resource Center on LGBT Aging, twice as many LGBT caregivers are likely to live alone than the average caregiving population. In addition, they are more likely to be estranged or living apart from their biological family – either because of the conflicts with their family or just by sheer distance since many LGBTs have found more acceptance and social circles of support in urban areas. Bisexual caregivers also tend to not be as *out* as their gay, lesbian and transgender colleagues and are often more guarded and lack close friendships to support them through a caregiving journey according to the National Resource Center on LGBT Aging.

While isolation can be an issue for both caregivers and older seniors, according to a 2011 report, LGBT caregivers feel more isolated than general caregivers. We know isolation can lead to higher risk of depression. This is of concern for LGBT caregivers since SAGE reported the LGBT population is more likely to smoke and engage in heavy drinking than their heterosexual counterparts. We know in the caregiving population, 10 percent of those who felt overwhelmed and felt their health was declining because of caregiving turned to alcohol or prescription drugs to cope with stress and depression. This number could be even higher among LGBT caregivers.

However, the strength of the LGBT community lies in its *chosen family* defined as a close circle of friends. While no studies have explored in-depth the issue of caregiver isolation, many have reported caregivers feel all alone. As opposed to biological families, LGBT caregivers have created chosen families, or *logical families* according to Thurston, who help share the physical and emotional challenges of caregiving. These circles of care are a great example of how the general caregiving population can learn from LGBT caregivers. By creating a circle of care or chosen family, all caregivers can begin to alleviate the burn-out so common when caring for a loved one.

In addition, because biological family support is not always present, LGBT caregivers reach out more to neighbors, superintendents and others for help out of sheer necessity. This is a page out of the caregiving book that general caregivers should take – reaching out to those around you will ease the burden and daily tasks of caregiving that can cause burn-out and fatigue.

When it comes to health care and the medical community, a United Hospital Fund Next Steps in Care/SAGE guide found the challenges of social stigma and legal issues still exist for many LGBT caregivers. On the one hand only 22 percent said they were comfortable advising hospital or health care staff of their gay relationship to the patient.

In addition, in an article written for the American Society on Aging's newsletter, Robert Espinoza of SAGE, says "Researchers have also found severe health risks among LGBT older people that can aggravate social isolation. The 2011 study, *The Aging and Health Report: Disparities and Resilience among LGBT Older Adults* found, '…the stigma and discrimination many LGBT seniors have experienced across the lifespan continue into their later years…fearful of mistreatment by health care professionals and aging network providers, many LGBT elders delay seeking care until a crisis hits.'"

In contrast, LGBT caregivers have been proactive about discussing the legal necessities of caring for each other through end-of-life. The American Society on Aging/MetLife Mature Market Institute study found almost double the amount of LGBT boomers have made a Health Care Directive for medical decisions (34%) vs. general boomers (19%) – making LGBT couples ahead of the curve when it comes to having legal documentation in place for end-of-life wishes and having discussed it with their life partner. However, SAGE says when it comes to feeling secure about their long-term care, lesbians and bisexual females are in the same boat as heterosexual female caregivers who all feel they are less financially prepared for end- of-life and have a lower incidence of having a Living Will or long-term care insurance.

It becomes essential for LGBT caregivers to be clear about identifying you are the person authorized to make decisions and ensure you have the essential legal documentation confirming this – it will facilitate communication with health care professionals that can lead to improved or positive outcomes for your loved one. It will also go a long way to eliminate family strife when the loved one's desire about who is making decisions is clear.

In the end, Thurston says LGBT caregivers face the same issues, same challenges and same struggles as other caregivers. We will simply have more older Americans to care for and that leaves us all asking, "Who is going to take care of me?"

Aging alone and not having someone to care for you is a true concern for LGBTs. Catherine Thurston, senior director at SAGE, advises that ageism in the LGBT community still exists. If an older LGBT person loses a partner, they often find themselves very alone. This isolation can cause stress which is also related to older LGBTs not having the typical support network because they still may not be *out* publicly. This leads to higher levels of depression, stress and often misuse of alcohol to cope.

A study conducted by the University of California at San Francisco found gay men dealt with the stress of caregiving through greater or new-found spirituality. Much research shows we grow in our spirituality as we age which is also why many faith-based organizations are reaching out to the LGBT caregiver community to offer support.

Spotlight on Stress
LGBT Caregivers

It's A Small World After All

Multicultural Caregivers

I will never grow too old to take a ride through this wonderland of the world's diverse cultures and people at the *happiest place on earth*. In fact, we should gather the world's caregivers and take them to Disneyland just like they do the champions of the Super Bowl or the World Series – it would be hard not to forget your troubles for a few hours when you are in Walt's world.

When it comes to caregiving, it really is a small world. As stated earlier, caregiving crosses all cultural and ethnic boundaries – every community, country and culture has caregiving as part of its societal fabric.

According to the National Alliance for Caregiving (NAC) *Caregiving in the U.S.* study conducted in 2009, 13 percent of all caregivers are African-American, 12 percent are Hispanic, 2 percent are Asian American and 2 percent are listed as other. While the overwhelming majority of caregivers in the study were White (72%), the issues facing culturally diverse caregivers are important for employers, service organizations and policymakers to understand.

> **Caregiving crosses all cultural and ethnic boundaries – every community, country and culture has caregiving as part of its societal fabric.**

The study also took a more in-depth look at multicultural caregivers in comparison to the general caregiving statistics and showed Hispanic caregivers are more likely to be younger (age 43 on average) and are more likely to be Sandwich Generation (caring for children and older parents simultaneously). African American caregivers tend to be older than average caregivers (age 48 on average) and they are more likely to be single or never married. Asian American caregivers have almost an equal representation for men and women caregivers (compared to the 66% female and 34% male in the general caregiving statistics) and they are also more likely than any other group to have a college degree.

In many ways, there are lessons learned from multicultural caregivers. There tends to be more help from other family members in multicultural caregiving situations; this help relieves some of the burden on the primary caregiver. In Native American cultures, there is more intergenerational activity that can actually improve the health and wellness of older loved ones – especially the interplay between grandparents and grandchildren.

According to Pew Research Center, since the 1970s, the two largest immigration groups to the U.S. – Latin Americans and Asians – are more inclined to live in multi-generational households (18.8%) compared to native born Americans (14.2%). Having three generations under one roof paves the way for caregiving but also eliminates the issue of isolation, especially for older Americans whose physical and mental health are impacted from living alone and feeling isolated.

In a separate 2009 NAC study, *Hispanic Caregiving in the U.S.,* that focused on Hispanic caregivers only, 8 million Latinos are caring for a loved one and that represents 1 in 3 Hispanic households with a caregiver – higher than the 1 in 5 households of all caregivers. The study cited diabetes as the main reason for Hispanic caregivers to begin their caregiving journey, and 25 percent reported their loved one also had Alzheimer's disease.

Hispanics also represent a higher percentage of Sandwich Generation caregivers – more than half had a child under 18 at home while caring for an older relative. This is more than double the percentage for caregivers overall. The good news is there is more support through a circle of care for Hispanic caregivers – 82 percent reported getting help from other family members or friends in caring for a loved one compared to just six in 10 for caregivers overall.

In African American caregiving situations there is a higher incidence of spirituality and there is also more *kinship* caregiving. This is a term that means an aunt or grandparent actually becomes the guardian or caregiver to a child under 18 whose parent is not capable or competent to provide the nurturing a child needs. In addition, African Americans represent the highest percentage of single or never married caregivers (28%) – almost twice the percentage of caregivers overall, according to the Alzheimer's Association 2011 Facts and Figures report.

While you may not characterize kinship caregiving as *caregiving* – review the Lost Generation chapter which reveals how many children are caring for older loved ones especially if they live in the same household. While the situation may begin with a grandparent caring for a grandchild, the role reversal of caregiving is an increasing scenario in African American households where young grandchildren are caring for older grandparents.

Caregiving in Asian American families typically falls to the adult daughter or daughter-in-law. However, in one study, *Factors Affecting Elder Caregiving in Multigenerational Asian American Families,* researchers Suzy Weng and Peter Nguyen found second generation Asian American adult children may not share the same sacrificial philosophies around caregiving, and this "cultural dissonance between generations can result in adverse mental health outcomes for both the elders and their family members."

These diverse caregivers also experience some cultural differences when it comes to certain aspects of activities of daily living (ADLs). For instance, in the Hispanic caregiving study, some female focus group members expressed much distress and feelings of discomfort over having to bathe or help a father or father-in-law with toileting. Although essential, this was simply too delicate and embarrassing for both parties. They reported this is when their spouse – either the son or son-in-law – would get involved in caregiving.

There is also a language and cultural sensitivities issue. Many Asian American caregivers feel health care professionals and home and community based services are not equipped to deal with the sensitivities that come with their cultural backgrounds in caring for an elder. Among the Asian American population, there are nuances and differences between Chinese, Filipino, Vietnamese and Korean ethnic groups. These differences not only relate to language and communication but also to things like food and meals. An in-home health agency or meal delivery service that does not understand ethnic cooking can be upsetting for elders whose only comfort is their daily meals.

For Native Americans, respect of elders in a tribe and the caregiving journey toward spirituality and wisdom is something all caregivers can learn from. Native American cultures place much focus on younger generations listening to older ones – it is this communication rule that creates a stronger bond of trust and partnership between the caregiver and care recipient. The ultimate outcome of this discipline is a deeper *connection* between the two parties which tribal communities believe is essential to the healing process.

In tribal communities, the emphasis on spirituality is an essential part of healing that helps many Native American caregivers manage stress. John Lowe, a Cherokee and Assistant Professor at Florida Atlantic University and Christine E. Lynn, College of Nursing in Boca Raton, Florida, wrote "Spirituality is the basis of healing in Native American culture and is strongly connected to the continuation of traditional healing practices such as herbal medicine, ceremonies, and purification practices. It is the daily cultural practice that connects caregivers to the past, present, and future of their people."

Dr. Andrew Weil in his book, *Spontaneous Happiness*, recalls a conversation with Dr. Lewis Mehl-Madrona, a Native American psychiatrist:

> "In these ways of thinking of the mind and mental health, the *community* is the basic unit of study, not the individual…The idea is that we are formed by our relationships. It is not that our brain makes our relationships, but rather our relationships make our brains…Relationships with parents and caregivers actually create the brain… We are relational selves. We are not individual, autonomous units."

Culturally diverse groups of caregivers report less stress in their caring duties. More than one-third of Hispanic caregivers report less stress than non-ethnic caregivers in a National Alliance for Caregiving study.

In addition there is more emphasis on family and friend support in diverse cultures meaning more help for the caregiver. The National Academy on Aging Society reported, Hispanics and Asian Americans are most likely to receive help from their adult children and African Americans are most likely to receive help from a non-family member.

Spotlight on Stress
Multicultural Caregivers

Away From Her

Alzheimer's Caregivers

My fellow Americans,

I have recently been told that I am one of the millions of Americans who will be afflicted with Alzheimer's disease. Upon learning this news, Nancy and I had to decide whether as private citizens we would keep this a private matter or whether we would make this news known in a public way... In opening our hearts, we hope this might promote greater awareness of this condition ... Unfortunately, as Alzheimer's disease progresses, the family often bears a heavy burden. I only wish there was some way I could spare Nancy from this painful experience. When the time comes, I am confident that with your help she will face it with faith and courage.

– Ronald Reagan

The year was 1994. Up to that time, there was not a lot of awareness of Alzheimer's disease but since former President Ronald Reagan wrote this heartfelt letter to the American public, the spotlight on this disease has never dimmed but has only grown brighter. In recent years and months, celebrities such as the late film star Charlton Heston, the winningest coach in collegiate basketball Pat Summitt and country music great, Glen Campbell, have announced their Alzheimer's diagnosis.

According to the Alzheimer's Association 2012 Facts and Figures report, more than 5 million Americans and 36 million people worldwide are diagnosed with dementia and an additional 15 million Americans care for someone with dementia or Alzheimer's disease. In fact, every 68 seconds someone develops Alzheimer's-and it is now the sixth leading cause of death in the U.S. and the only cause of death in the Top 10 list that cannot be cured, prevented or slowed. Alzheimer's is the most common type of dementia, a disease of the brain that causes problems with memory, thinking and behavior.

President Reagan understood the difficult emotional toll it would take on his wife and as the disease progressed, he did not even recognize her. For family caregivers, Alzheimer's is known as *the long good-bye.* People with Alzheimer's – which is a progressive disease – typically live an average of eight years after diagnosis but some can live 4-20 years beyond the first signs or symptoms. The Alzheimer's Association has identified 10 Warning Signs of Alzheimer's – an educational effort to help people get an earlier diagnosis so they have more time to plan for their future care needs with their family.

> **Every 68 seconds someone develops Alzheimer's.**

Currently more than 50 percent of the people who have Alzheimer's or dementia are undiagnosed and five percent of those with early signs of the disease, known as early-onset or younger-onset are in their 40s and 50s representing approximately 200,000 Americans according to the Alzheimer's Association. Some of these early warning signs include:

- Memory loss – especially with recently learned information and not being able to recall the information later, occasionally forgetting names and appointments is normal, more frequent forgetfulness is not
- Misplacing things in unusual places such as putting car keys in the freezer
- Having trouble with simple words or replacing words with unusual options such as being unable to remember the name of an everyday item such as *toothbrush* and calling it instead *that thing I put in my mouth*
- Becoming lost in familiar surroundings such as your own neighborhood or not remembering how to get home

All the reasons for becoming a caregiver are important – Parkinson's disease, autism, multiple sclerosis, cancer, heart disease, ALS, Down Syndrome, PTSD, etc. – but I highlight Alzheimer's because it is truly becoming an epidemic for our society. While Alzheimer's is not a normal part of aging, statistics show 1 of every 2 Americans over age 85 will develop the disease. By 2050, more than 16 million Americans will suffer from this disease and the 17 billion hours caregivers currently provide to those with Alzheimer's will double.

In addition, research shows some of the risk factors for Alzheimer's might be similar for other diseases such as cardiovascular disease and diabetes including higher body mass index (BMI) and higher cholesterol. By maintaining good nutritional and exercise habits, caregivers can possibly prevent their risk for developing heart disease and Alzheimer's themselves. And as stated in the Bringing Up Baby chapter, almost 100 percent of children with Down syndrome who live to be age 40 or older will also have Alzheimer's.

Partially because Alzheimer's disease now costs the United States an estimated $200 billion a year, a first-ever National Alzheimer's Plan was established in 2011 with a goal of changing the trajectory of this disease that impacts so many families.

While other diseases are challenging, Alzheimer's actually robs the person of who they are. They can suffer progressive memory loss and fail to recognize spouses, children and other loved ones.

"One of the most difficult journeys for a caregiver to take is with a loved one with Alzheimer's," says Dr. Rosemary Laird, medical director at the Health First Aging Institute in Florida. "It is hard but essential to prepare yourself for the day your spouse or parent will not remember your birthday, your name and finally your face. We counsel that 'memory may fade but love never does' and that the brain no longer can grasp these details."

When it comes to dementia there are several different types including vascular dementia, the second most common form of the disease after Alzheimer's, which occurs after a stroke and affects more men than women. There is also dementia with Lewy body which can be found in Alzheimer's and even Parkinson's sufferers. According to the Alzheimer's Association, Lewy body symptoms can be similar to dementia or Alzheimer's in terms of cognitive impairment but may also include: excessive daytime drowsiness, visual hallucinations, movement symptoms including stiffness, shuffling walk, shakiness; lack of facial expression, and problems with balance and falls. In about 50 percent of cases, dementia with Lewy bodies is also associated with a condition called rapid eye movement (REM) sleep disorder.

Alzheimer's sufferers can also wander and get lost, something Sylvia Mackey lived with during her husband's diagnosis with frontotemporal dementia. All of these things change the person they are and are emotionally difficult for caregivers to understand and manage.

There is also a particularly unsettling symptom with some Alzheimer's patients called *sundowning*. Researchers still do not know the cause but they believe Alzheimer's and other forms of dementia disturb your inner clock and cause patients to have increased behavioral changes that begin at dusk and continue throughout the night.

This scenario was one of the heartwrenching moments in the touching love story, *The Notebook*, a great Nicholas Sparks novel and movie starring Rachel McAdams, Gena Rowlands, Ryan Gosling and James Garner. But while that scene was *reel* life, in *real* life, Joan Lunden deals with sundowners which affects her 94-year-old mother.

The recent film, *Away From Her*, starring a still-stunning looking Julie Christie, showcases the awful effects of Alzheimer's on a spouse and is played out on the big screen as her on-screen husband watches her fall in love with another man in a nursing home. She has forgotten who her husband is, creating for him a larger than life agony which many live with every day.

While these films seem like a dramatization for movie audiences, this same story played itself out in real life as former Supreme Court Justice, Sandra Day O'Connor, watched her husband John suffer with Alzheimer's disease. After she had to move him to live in a dementia care facility, John fell in love with another woman in the facility. The grace with which Her Honor accepted this situation is nothing less than *supreme* sacrifice for love.

It is often this lack of remembering loved ones that is the toughest issue Alzheimer's caregivers face. To have a loving spouse of more than 52 years who does not even recognize you for the last 10 years of your marriage – as was the case of Nancy Reagan – is devastating and can often impact the health and wellness of the caregiver.

While we know family conflicts can arise in caregiving, the story of the Reagans paints a different picture. What is perhaps most heartwarming was the strained relationship Nancy had with her stepchildren and with her own son and daughter, actually improved over the course of President Reagan's disease diagnosis and eventual decline.

As we know, it is not just the person diagnosed with the disease that lives with the disease – it is the whole family. As for the Reagans, their family grew closer during their Alzheimer's journey – one of the gifts that can come from caregiving. And although Alzheimer's robbed her beloved Ronnie of his memory of her, Nancy was never away from him.

When it comes to caregivers of those with Alzheimer's disease, the stress levels are higher than other caregivers. Sixty percent of Alzheimer's caregivers rate stress as high or very high and one-third of these caregivers suffer from depression according to the Alzheimer's Association. A recent UCLA study published in the *International Journal of Geriatric Psychiatry* stated it is closer to 50% of dementia caregivers who report depression.

The Shriver Report: A Women's Nation Takes on Alzheimer's found women are disproportionately impacted by this disease with more than 10 million women affected. Two-thirds of those with Alzheimer's disease are women and 60 percent of Alzheimer's caregivers are moms, daughters or sisters. The report found that due to the emotional stress and physical strain of caregiving, Alzheimer's and dementia spouses were six times more likely to develop dementia themselves.

Spotlight on Stress
Alzheimer's Caregivers

Rehearsals – Which Caregiving Responsibilities Will You Face?

All the real work is done in the rehearsal period.

– Donald Pleasence

Every star knows before you take the stage – whether you are acting, singing or dancing – you need to rehearse. No one would choose to walk into the spotlight cold with no preparation. Yet, this is what most caregivers do.

A crisis or event happens and all of a sudden you are expected to be an expert at health care, home care, special therapies and diets, medications, medical paperwork and insurance details, etc.

If you are getting married, you spend months or at least weeks planning all the wedding details. If you are about to be a new mom, you get nine months to educate yourself about the baby. When you become a caregiver, you may get a just a few minutes to get ready, set, go! And as opposed to weddings and babies, which are often seen as joyful events, caregiving typically is chaotic, stressful, emotional and a lot of other feelings that are not always happy and joyous. These are just some of the reasons why it is imperative you plan ahead for caregiving just as you would plan ahead for any other major life event.

Why plan for caregiving? Because it is going to happen so why take the ostrich-in-the-sand approach? Aging, and yes, death are inevitable. They may not be fun or happy thoughts but we must be thoughtful about these life events.

How do you rehearse for something you are not quite sure exactly what it will be? You may ask, "How can I plan ahead for a disaster I'm not even sure of – my loved one's heart attack? Cancer diagnosis? Early on-set Alzheimer's? All require different things so why bother – I'll deal with it when it happens."

When we think of caregiving, we often think of someone who is older – in their 80s or 90s. But caregiving is a role we can play at any time during our lives and our loved ones can be hit with a devastating diagnosis or accident in their 30s, 40s or 50s. Obviously, Tracy Pollan could not have planned ahead her young husband, Michael J. Fox would be diagnosed with Parkinson's disease at age 30. And Marg Helgenberger, a young college student, could never have dreamed her 45-year-old father would have devastating and debilitating multiple sclerosis.

Certainly you cannot predict the future, unless of course you are an ancient Mayan. However, you can still have the conversations and understand the details of your loved one's plans and wishes as he or she ages. This helps both of you be on the same page when the care needs to begin. There are some basics and fundamental information that will help you start to realize what caregiving is all about and how essential it is to have those caregiving conversations with your family sooner rather than later. When is the best time to have these conversations with your loved ones and other family? You will read in the C-A-R-E Conversation chapter there is no time like the present.

For now, I will call these care basics an important first step, otherwise known as the Caregiving Rehearsals plan. As you read through the Rehearsals chapters – remember this is a general guide. Each caregiving situation is unique. It is important to understand while caregiving is an international phenomenon, the help, resources and solutions you need are mostly local.

Dr. Rosemary Laird, medical director for Health First Aging Institute, told me, "There is a knowledge gap when it comes to caregiving. If we can get good information to caregivers on how to prepare to care, then we can help guide them on why finding time to care for themselves is as important as caring for their loved one."

If caregiving were a movie in which you are the star, this is the kind of good direction you would get from a Steven Spielberg or Francis Ford Coppola. "Ready and action!"

One Singular Sensation or A Chorus Line?

Solo act or team caregiving

When it comes to caregiving, there are two ways you can play your role: you can go it all alone or you can get support and help. I have spoken to hundreds of caregivers across the country and the one common sentiment I hear over and over is, "I feel all alone."

Caregiving can become an isolating event *if you let it*. Just think of Tom Hanks in *Castaway* – do you really want to be all alone on your caregiving island with no one to talk to but a soccer ball called Wilson? It is true some performers prefer to do solo acts. However, if you are a caregiver who believes no one else can provide the care your loved one needs then you have to know up-front you face possible burn-out and health risks as the physical and emotional toll of caregiving takes over.

Maybe your situation is one where there is no other family member who can provide you with assistance. In these instances, it is important to reach out to your spouse or partner, friends, a support group or a professional such as a therapist or geriatric care manager to help you shoulder the burden – if not physically and financially, then emotionally – while you are on your caregiving journey.

Most stage performers get an intermission and athletes get a break between innings, quarters or sets. If you are the only one providing care for your loved one, you have to get a break in between your caregiving duties. It is called *respite*. There are health care services that actually provide respite care workers, professionally trained or credentialed aides who can provide companionship and sometimes perform other small caregiving duties so you – the primary caregiver – can get a break. The largest national respite resources are the ARCH National Respite Network and Resource Center or the local Area Agencies on Aging located through the N4As and the elder care locator. You will read more about respite and getting a break in the Cocoon chapter.

Supporting Cast

If you have siblings, a spouse or partner, or other family members who can help you shoulder the burden of caregiving, it is important to know how to ask for and get their help. For instance, if you are caring for an older parent, you might be doing all the heavy lifting – literally – because you live close-by. Your sister, who lives in another state, does not have the proximity to give you a break physically but she can either provide financial support to get you more professional caregiving help or at the very least provide the emotional support so essential to keep a caregiver's fuel tank from hitting *empty*. A great example of this caregiving tag-team can be read in the story about Marg Helgenberger who supported her mother and brother in caring for her father while Marg was the long-distance caregiver providing the financial and emotional support.

You can and should also be able to turn to your spouse or partner when caregiving comes calling. You will read a great example of how a spouse can keep a caregiver from falling to pieces in the story of Jill Eikenberry and her life partner and husband Michael Tucker. Mike told me when Jill's mom, who has dementia, needed more care, his primary job was to take care of Jill.

Beyond your family and friends, a support group can become your life raft. These are other caregivers just like yourself who understand specifically what you are going through – whether it is caring for a spouse with cancer, caring for a child with autism or caring for a veteran with post-traumatic stress disorder (PTSD). In the story of Holly Robinson Peete, you will learn how a father's support group gave her husband Rodney the playbook he needed to understand his son's challenges with autism and how to create his new game plan on caregiving.

In addition to in-person support groups, many caregivers cannot find the time to get away to get this needed nurturing. This is when the wonder of the Internet comes into play. There are many online community support sites dedicated to caregivers. My recommendation is to first check with the association or organization that supports the condition or disease of your loved one – the Alzheimer's Association, Autism Speaks, National Multiple Sclerosis Society, Wounded Warriors Project, etc. These organizations typically have both in-person and online support groups you can join and then you are assured you are in the right place.

I spoke to one caregiver of a Vietnam veteran whose husband had cancer, which they think can be attributed to his exposure to Agent Orange. The social worker she spoke to sent her to a local support group for cancer caregivers. However, because this caregiver had the need to vent and talk about Vietnam as much as the cancer eating away at her husband, she didn't feel she got the support she needed. It is important to find the right group. I call it the *Band of Brothers* approach – you need to find those who have been in the same trenches you have. This becomes your troupe for support so you can get the critical circle of care you need. I have listed some of these great support groups in the LOST and Found chapter.

Caregiver Checklist

- ✓ Ensure you get a break – called respite – by asking for help.
- ✓ Find a support group, professional or someone who you can talk to lighten your emotional caregiving burden.

Martin Scorsese or Woody Allen?

Family drama or comedy

When it comes to caregiving, family dynamics dictate whether your journey will be a drama or a comedy. In other words, do you predict bloodshed like a Martin Scorsese film (like *Taxi Driver* or *Goodfellas*) or nostalgic comedy à la Woody Allen (like *Annie Hall* or *Midnight in Paris*)?

Somehow caregiving brings out the best and the worst in our families. It can be either like something out of *The Godfather* or *Meet the Fockers* (interestingly, Robert De Niro played the father role in both movies). What can be perplexing for many is how happy, congenial families become the Hatfields and McCoys over caregiving. It is amazing to watch siblings who have always gotten along fabulously; all of a sudden go at is like they are competitors in *Gladiator*, especially if mom or dad is incapacitated and cannot express his or her wishes for care. Sibling conflicts can flare up faster than hemorrhoids and feel just as painful. When families are facing a crisis with a loved one's illness, emotions are running high and the term *drama queen* does not even cover the confrontations I have witnessed.

> **Somehow caregiving brings out the best and the worst in our families.**

Then there is mom and dad. Ozzie and Harriet may be in denial about their increasing care needs as they get older. Your best efforts may be met with resistance like Archie Bunker rebuking any kindness or help from Meathead. Many parents do not like to discuss their long-term care but they also do not want to be a burden to their adult children. Unfortunately, these are two diametrically opposed concepts. If parents do not want to be a burden, they must *unburden* which means they have to spill it, sister (and mister).

If your caregiving situation involves caring for your spouse, such as in Sylvia Mackey's story, you might characterize it as *One Flew Over the Cuckoo's Nest* or *Romeo and Juliet*. Some spouses are in denial they need care. However, this approach gives you, the caregiving spouse, added burdens. The reality is life is not *normal* anymore and together you have to create a *new normal*.

If you find yourself caring for a child with special needs like Holly Robinson Peete – you may find yourself starring in *Kramer vs. Kramer*. Statistics show many parents of special needs children do not survive (the marriage not life). Happily Holly and husband Rodney are going strong as you will read in her story.

A lot depends on how your family has always acted with each other. You can rely on humor and strong family ties to get you through the bad times like *The Cosby Show,* or you may find your family lying, cheating and practically whacking each other (just think *The Sopranos*).

A lot of the drama scenarios can be avoided if older loved ones and their families get their paperwork in order AND have a conversation with everyone. For instance, a friend of mine received a call from Australian authorities that his parents had been killed in a freak sightseeing helicopter crash. As my friend sat with his brother and sister, these grieving adult children realized they had no idea whether their parents would want to be buried or cremated. Grief turned to animosity as these siblings fought over what their parents' wishes would have been. Since it was not included in the parents' legal documents, the kids were left to angrily debate when they should have been consoling each other.

Death is not easy. It is so much worse when everyone is fighting. Avoid the conflicts by having the conversation.

Caregiver Checklist

- ✓ Have the *talk* – start the C-A-R-E Conversation with your loved one, siblings, spouse or partner.
- ✓ If you find the conversation difficult to start, secure the help of a neutral party or a professional such as a geriatric care manager (GCM).

The Three Faces of Eve

From hospital to home to hospice - care transitions

In *The Three Faces of Eve*, Joanne Woodward won the Academy Award in 1957 for playing one woman who suffered from dissociative identity disorder (DID) – with three distinct personalities. The range of emotions caregivers go through particularly as you help a loved one transition from hospital to home to other housing or hospice can be confusing for caregivers. Each phase has different emotions associated with it and you may feel as if your personality changes to adapt to the latest crisis du jour.

When it comes to caregiving, your starring role can be short or it can be very long-lived. On average, the National Alliance for Caregiving states a caregiver's duration of care for one person is 4.6 years with 15 percent of all caregivers spending more than 10 years caring for a loved one. In the case of a child with special needs, your caregiving role may be the lifespan of that child. If you are caring for a parent or spouse with early on-set dementia or Alzheimer's, your loved one can be diagnosed in her 50s and live well into her 70s or 80s.

> **A caregiver's duration of care for one person is 4.6 years with 15 percent of all caregivers spending more than 10 years.**

What is important to understand about caregiving is there can be various stages where your caregiving responsibilities change over time. In addition, there are important knowledge factors when it comes to the transition of a loved one from hospital to home or to an assisted living or skilled nursing facility. The aging industry calls this *care transitions.*

The Wonder Years

Your caregiving role may begin innocently and easily. Perhaps mom or dad are just getting older and need more help mowing the lawn or shoveling snow in the driveway. Or, you offer to drive your parent to the doctor for an appointment or help manage the bills. While this just seems like something nice an adult child does for the parent who cared so lovingly for you, you have actually begun your caregiving journey.

In contrast to this smooth caregiving take-off, there is also the Apollo 13 caregiving situation – or in other words, "Houston, we have a problem." This is typically when a loved one has a medical crisis resulting in a hospitalization or a diagnosis of a devastating illness or disorder. You are thrown into your caregiving role, and if not prepared you are scrambling around not knowing where to start or who you can to turn to. This is the way most of us think of caregiving – crisis central. A colleague of mine, Candace Baldwin of the Village-to-Village Network calls this the "hair on fire caregivers." You are overwhelmed, under-informed and ill-equipped to deal with your new role.

Hospital discharge planners and social workers are usually the health care professionals physicians refer patients and their family caregiver to for next steps. However, these health care professionals often give caregivers a list of referral sources without making recommendations and leave you to navigate a complicated and complex health care system on your own. In the world of hospital jargon this is known as *treat and street.*

This situation is making more and more caregivers para-professionals without the skills and knowledge to back them up. Many studies have shown the lack of good care management in making the transition from hospital to home can result in adverse health effects and higher incidence of hospital re-admissions.

"Everyone is caught in this rushed process," says Carol Levine, director of the Families and Health Care Project at United Hospital Fund. "Discharge planners are under-resourced and are pressured by the hospital system to check patients out as quickly as possible. In addition, the physician at the hospital may be sending your loved one to a facility – either skilled nursing or assisted living – and has not discussed what this means or even whether this will work for the family."

This is why preparation is key. To help, United Hospital Fund has created checklists and other information to arm caregivers with knowledge about care transitions found on its Next Step in Care web site, a collaborative effort with the Centers for Medicare and Medicaid Services.

True Grit

As you enter the Caregiving Zone, not unlike the *Twilight Zone*, you realize the stamina, resilience, patience and intelligence it will take to make this caregiving journey – not unlike the pioneers seeking a better life out West. This is where your true grit emerges and you feel you have to be like John Wayne – riding tall in that saddle charging across the field, bullets whizzing by your head. However, being the hero every day is a tall order even for a rugged cowboy like the Duke.

In this stage of caregiving you are helping your loved one make decisions (or making the decisions for her) about senior living options, driving retirement and alternative transportation, senior nutrition, medication safety and administration, isolation and depression (both hers and yours). You may have to become Nurse Betty and Marcus Welby, M.D. all rolled into one.

Do you know how to put on a blood pressure cuff to get an accurate reading (many caregivers put it on upside down which results in an inaccurate reading)? Do you know about pressure sores and properly transferring someone from bed to wheelchair or wheelchair to shower without throwing your back out? Are you prepared to set up an IV pole at home or to manage oxygen tanks? Don't run but don't hide either – this could be your caregiving future.

"Care transitions are probably the biggest challenge caregivers face," according to Levine. In addition to lack of knowledge or good direction on how to care for your loved one at home, caregivers often become the only continuity point in their loved one's health care world.

Levine advises in years gone by, your loved one's primary care physician may have treated your parent or spouse in the hospital. That may no longer be the case. Now there is a *hospitalist* – an acute care specialist who sees your loved one only in the hospital setting, and does not have follow-up responsibilities for ongoing care. What this means is the opportunities for dropped balls and miscommunication are endless.

"The caregiver becomes the only continuity point in a patient's care," says Levine. This means you have to take a lot of notes, understand all the instructions and procedures, etc. so you can be the one to tell the primary care physician or facility staff what happened to your loved one in the hospital. Ideally, it would be safe to assume all these physicians and administrators are talking to each other but utopia is a fictional world. Your reality is more like *Alice in Wonderland* – you've fallen down the rabbit hole and now you must communicate with all these never-before seen characters. You can read more about health care literacy and communication with health care professionals in the chapter Lost In Translation.

Levine advises there are three new trends in care transitions caregivers should be aware of:

1. Understand the role of the hospitalist and the communication protocols with your loved one's primary care physician.

2. Know about observation status – This relates to Medicare reimbursements and can become a quagmire for caregivers. Essentially, if your loved one is not *formally admitted* to the hospital before tests are ordered, these services probably will not be covered under Medicare and will be considered a *fee for service*. This type of billing means higher costs to patients and possible financial burden for caregivers. Ensure you understand your loved one's official admission status any time she is hospitalized.

3. Realize discharge happens fast – If your loved one is hospitalized, she will most likely not be staying very long. The goal of the hospital is to discharge your loved one as quickly as possible. Levine also cautions often loved ones are discharged because they are stable "but stable does not mean healed or healthy."

Levine told me if "hospitals were hotels and you were treated this way, you would never go back to that hotel. We really should not accept this sub-standard service."

Until things change, understanding your lead role in care transitions becomes one of the most important things caregivers should learn to maintain your sanity.

Taps

If your loved one's condition is terminal or their age may mean your caregiving journey is entering its home stretch, there is another set of rules, regulations, responsibilities and requirements. By this third transition, hopefully you and your loved one have already had the conversation about end-of-life wishes. Beyond the legal documentation of Health Care Directives, Living Wills and funeral arrangements, there is the care of loved ones at end of their lives. At this caregiving stage, you have two options: palliative care and hospice.

Palliative (pronounced pal-lee-uh-tiv) care is part of the health care world few people know about. It is specialized medical care for people with serious or terminal illnesses such as cancer, chronic obstructive pulmonary disease (COPD), kidney failure, HIV/AIDS, etc. It is focused on providing patients with relief from the symptoms, pain, and stress of a serious illness, whatever the diagnosis.

Palliative care is a triumvirate of care between the patient, the health care professionals and the family – a team-oriented approach that addresses the medical, physical, social, emotional, and spiritual needs of the patient and provides emotional support to the family as well. Palliative care is provided by a team of doctors, nurses, and other specialists who work together with a patient's other doctors to provide an extra layer of support often called *comfort care*. It is appropriate at any age and at any stage in a serious illness and can be provided along with curative treatment. According to Doug Bates, palliative care social worker with the Motion Picture and Television Fund (MPTF), "Palliative care is about serious illness where someone may still seek clinical trials or treatments such as chemotherapy, whereas hospice is about terminal illness where the transition from cure to comfort for end-of-life happens."

The difference between palliative care and hospice is palliative care can be provided at any time after the diagnosis and can last years. Hospice provides end-of-life care that always includes palliative care. While many people think hospice care is only the last few days or weeks of a loved one's life, it can actually be provided for several months provided a physician continues to reauthorize your loved one's benefits for Medicare every six months.

"In order to qualify for hospice care and meet the criteria to receive the Medicare benefits, the physician has to sign on for six months or less for course of life for the patient," continues Bates. Some patients may exceed that timeframe but the physician has to continue to re-qualify the patient for the Medicare benefit. Bates says he even had one patient who remained on hospice care for almost five years. "As for palliative care, there is no set time and as our MPTF patients transition to hospice, the same palliative care team remains involved – they've developed this relationship with us already and since they are losing so much – loss of independence, loss of control issues, loss of health – we don't want them to suffer yet another loss by losing us as they transition from palliative care to hospice care."

You can read more about hospice and palliative care in the Curtain Call chapter.

"When it comes to palliative and hospice care, the whole family becomes the patient," says Bates. "And of course, 'family' is whomever the patient determines that to be – a friend, a partner, a spouse. Our role is to help normalize this process and that includes coaching the family caregiver through their feelings of hopelessness and powerlessness."

Caregiver Checklist

- ✓ Know the limitations of what a hospitalist can do for your loved one beyond a hospital setting.
- ✓ Ask a lot of questions of the hospitalist, case worker or social worker and discharge planner to find out everything you can about the transitions of care for your loved one. Use the Next Step in Care checklists for help with this.
- ✓ Ensure everyone on the care team for your loved one is talking to each other and keeping you in the loop.
- ✓ Don't wait to secure palliative care for your loved one if they are diagnosed with a serious or terminal illness.

Raiders of the Lost Ark

Elder Law attorneys, Medicare, Medicaid

Think of this step as if you are embarking on an adult scavenger hunt. You are Indiana Jones in *Raiders of the Lost Ark*, an intrepid archeologist searching for the truth and lost artifacts. You will have to do a little digging in order to uncover the secrets of your caregiving future. For instance, you will need to know where your parents' important paperwork is – things such as a Living Will or estate plan, an Advance Directive or Durable Power of Attorney (for both medical and financial decisions), DNR order (do not resuscitate, if they have one). You will also need to know where to find important information such as a driver's license, Social Security card, passport – all of which will be necessary if you need to have your loved one travel with you or step in as custodian of his well-being. As you learned in the stories about Jill Eikenberry and Michael Tucker, and Joan Lunden, if these items cannot be found or they are found but expired, your ability to help your loved one is jeopardized or at the very least delayed.

You will also need to know about their insurance, long-term-care plan, Medicare or Medicaid status and other health care coverage such as veteran's benefits. What is covered and what is not? Just know the basics for now. In the event of a crisis, you don't want to be searching in the dark, getting blindsided or making decisions that could cause a significant financial drain on your loved one or on you. It is also wise to know your loved one's doctors' names and contact information. If your loved one becomes incapacitated and cannot communicate, you do not want to spend endless hours searching for this vital information.

One of the reasons it is so critical to have the conversation with your older loved one and other family members earlier rather than later is to avoid court for conservatorship. In most cases, the spouse, meaning one of your parents or step-parents, will be the person who makes decisions for the parent who is incapacitated. However, if both parents are struggling, then it becomes essential to identify the person who is next in line to make decisions. It is much easier for families to know who will be making decisions for both the estate (assets) and the person (health care decisions). It is best to have your parent tell you his designate for these decisions when he is still healthy. This not only helps your parent but it takes a huge burden off of you when the time comes. There is no guesswork, no confusion among other family members and no anxiety over whether you are making the decisions your loved one would want.

Many people understand the need to have someone identified who can make financial decisions, but they don't often think about medical care, Medicare or Medicaid benefits and insurance issues. Since insurance policies deal with our health and long-term care issues, they are considered a financial matter. As a caregiver, the only legal way for you to make decisions affecting your loved one's medical decisions, is if you have power of attorney so you can receive and pay bills, view records, sort out coverage issues, and change policies on your loved one's behalf. You will probably need to give the insurance company proof of your status.

Without this legal paperwork you may have trouble helping your loved one as privacy issues are heavily guarded by most institutions under the regulations of HIPAA (Health Insurance Portability and Accountability Act). Without having power of attorney, HIPAA only allows a doctor to disclose medical information to you as a caregiver – whether you are a relative or friend – if the patient is present and does not object, and it is directly relevant to the patient's care. If the patient is unable to agree or object (for example, if he is unconscious) the doctor can choose to disclose information if the doctor feels it is in the patient's best interest. But the law does not require doctors to share medical information.

"HIPAA, while intending to protect privacy, has had some unintended consequences," says Carol Levine, director of the Families and Health Care Project at United Hospital Fund. "It has had a chilling effect on communication between physicians, patients and family caregivers, which can have an adverse outcome, since the caregiver is typically the only consistent factor in a loved one's care among various health care professionals and services."

Law and Order

When it comes to interpreting you or your loved one's rights, the aid of an Elder Law attorney can be essential. In the same way you would need a lawyer who specializes in a certain area – divorce, litigation, criminal defense – an Elder Law attorney understands the nuances of laws related to Medicare (federal laws), Medicaid (federal programs managed by individual states), Social Security and general aging issues that can be helpful in navigating a loved one's long-term care. It is important to note long-term care and other aging and legal issues vary state to state, making an Elder Law attorney your essential guide through these intricacies.

This is particularly important if your loved one has homes in two different states or travels frequently or if you are a long-distance caregiver and not as fluent in the state laws where your loved one lives. There is a national listing of these specialized lawyers you can find through the National Academy of Elder Law Attorneys (NAELA), which is the organization whose membership is dedicated to improving the quality of legal services provided to people as they age and people with special needs. You can also check with state bar associations which will have a listing of Elder Law attorneys.

"Approximately 40 percent of older Americans will end up in a long-term care facility and this becomes the single biggest cost to families helping a loved one who is over age 65," says Judd Matsunga, an Elder Law attorney in California. Yet Matsunga advises many of these seniors and their families don't have solid financial plans for their increasing longevity.

Matsunga says there are two huge issues he deals with when it comes to family caregivers seeking his counsel:

1. The caregiver has waited too long to get his advice. "So often adult children come to me two to three years too late when I could have saved them and their parent financially and protected their assets without sacrificing their quality of care or jeopardizing their benefits."

2. Parents often create long-term care or estate plans but do not communicate these wishes to all their family members. Once they are incapacitated, the sibling conflict begins. "Countless families are torn apart when a simple conversation would have resolved the problem before there was one," he says.

A good example of the value of an Elder Law attorney as your expert guide in understanding and interpreting certain restrictions and regulations that change annually when it comes to Medicare and Medicaid is called the *look back period*. This is a situation with Medicaid benefits and eligibility that currently states older adults cannot transfer certain assets to their adult children for a certain period of time prior to being eligible for Medicaid benefits (in most cases and states this period is approximately 5 years). This falls under the latest deficit reduction act (DRA) in most states. An older loved one can't simply give away all her assets and be eligible for Medicaid the next day. Here is an example from Judd Matsunga regarding what happens when a parent decides to transfer an asset to an adult child and encounters the latest DRA regulations in California:

> Your dad has passed away and your mom, who lives in California, decides to give you her Palm Springs vacation home since she won't be visiting the home alone any longer. The home's equity value is $460,000. To qualify for Medicaid benefits (called Medi-Cal in California) and receive nursing home care for your mom at a later date (which Genworth calculated to be approximately $7,800 per month on average for California facilities), she would have an ineligibility period of about 58 months before she could qualify for Medicaid benefits (home value divided by monthly nursing home costs). The clock starts ticking when your mom applies for Medicaid and *goes backwards* 58 months. If she gave you the home more than 5 years ago (60 months), no penalty period is imposed.

In many ways, an Elder Law attorney can serve not only as an expert guide on navigating the complicated system of protecting assets and securing benefits, but he/she can also be a mediator for family conflict as an objective, expert outside party.

Double Indemnity

Understanding your loved one's health care insurance can be confusing with so many nuances and codes that even Indiana Jones might have difficulty navigating this world. Today, according to the Kaiser Family Foundation, there are 50 million Americans who have Medicare benefits. Eligibility for Medicare depends on: age (must be 65 years old), certain disabilities (where you may qualify at any age), and end-stage renal disease (ESRD – which is permanent kidney failure requiring dialysis or transplant). Since Medicare benefits and policies change every year, it is important to know where to go online to stay on top of helping your loved one.

The best and first place to check is the Centers for Medicare & Medicaid Services (CMS) web site (medicare.gov). It is has a complete section dedicated to helping caregivers (medicare.gov/caregivers) understand benefits and eligibility issues. There are different types of Medicare plans (such as Medicare Supplement Plans, Medicare Private Fee for Service Plans, Medicare Special Needs Plans) and Medicare has different parts including:

1) Part A coverage is for inpatient hospital stays, care in a skilled nursing facility, hospice care, and some home health care;

2) Part B covers certain doctors' services, outpatient care, medical supplies, and preventive services;

3) Part C are Medicare Advantage Plans, a type of Medicare health plan offered by a private company that contracts with Medicare to provide you with all your Part A and Part B benefits;

4) Part D is an optional benefit to cover some costs for prescription drugs.

In addition to CMS, many private insurers offer guides to Medicare which help walk its members through information about Medicare benefits. Ask your loved one if she received this guide from her insurer or find it online at the individual insurance company web sites.

Medicaid is a jointly funded, Federal-State health insurance program for low-income and needy people. Eligibility rules are different in each state. In most states the benefits may cover children, the aged, blind, and/or disabled and other people who are eligible to receive federally assisted income maintenance payments.

Another resource for caregivers is the National Clearinghouse for Long Term Care operated by the Administration on Aging, which is part of the U.S. Department of Health and Human Services. The web site (longtermcare.gov) provides information about long-term care, the resources to help and what you can expect to pay and receive in benefits.

While the resources above will educate you about benefits and eligibility requirements for Medicare and Medicaid, there is a resource that can actually help you discover the Medicare benefits you may be overlooking. The Benefits Check Up web site, operated by the National Council on Aging (benefitscheckup.org), is a free service where anyone can uncover the programs and services that can help pay for prescription drugs, health care, utilities, and other basic needs. There are more than 2,000 federal, state and private benefits programs available to help but many people don't know these programs exist or how they can apply for them. Benefits Check Up asks a series of questions to help identify benefits that could save you money and help cover the costs of everyday expenses.

Network

In the 1976 film, *Network*, starring Peter Finch who won an Oscar® for this role, there is a defining scene where Finch's frustrated news anchorman character yells during a newscast, "I'm mad as hell and I'm just not going to take it anymore." I know many caregivers who want to yell the same thing when trying to navigate the fragmented health care and Medicare world.

There may be times when you feel like you are not getting all the facts you need to validate what you are being told with regards to your loved one's Medicare benefits. You can turn to the Medicare Rights Center – a national, nonprofit consumer service organization that counsels family caregivers about Medicare policies. These counselors can help you understand your loved one's rights and your rights as a caregiver when it comes to navigating the Medicare system. For instance, you have the right to talk to your loved one's doctors about her health, but you will be limited in what information you can get and what decisions you can make unless she has legally named you as her *proxy* or *agent* using a health care proxy document (also referred to as Medical Power of Attorney, Durable Power of Attorney for Health, or appointment of a health care agent).

If your loved one has named you as a health care proxy or agent, you will have the right to access almost any information and records she could. Your legal right goes into effect when your loved one cannot communicate her wishes because of temporary or permanent illness or injury.

In some states, if your loved one becomes unable to speak for herself (for example, if she is in a coma), decisions about her health may fall to doctors or hospital administrators rather than to you, her caregiver. And as discussed in the Trading Places chapter in the Casting Calls section, even in states where a family caregiver can make decisions, if you disagree with your siblings on the treatment, you may find yourself battling them in court over conservatorship for your loved one's care.

As mentioned earlier, if you do not have legal authorization, what you can find out will depend on the doctor. You do not have an automatic right to information about your loved one's health. While you can ask your loved one's doctor about some of these issues, you can also talk to your local pharmacist. Pharmacists can be helpful – particularly because so many questions do involve prescription drug benefits. You can also read about health advocates and government health insurance counselors who can help you navigate the world of health care insurance in the My Man Godfrey chapter.

Now that you have found all the vital information you need, how do you have the delicate conversation with your loved one about where this information can be found and how you might help her? Start with one of the stories in this book – relate what you read or perhaps you have a friend who encountered the same dilemma. Joan Lunden's story is a great start, because she says she wishes she would have had the family conversation around caregiving before the crisis happened. It would have saved her precious time; and eliminated her anxiety and frustration.

Tell your parent you want to be able to help when the time comes – ask the questions about legal and insurance paperwork. People of older generations feel this conversation is invading their privacy or is something they don't want to discuss for a variety of reasons. One of the things I have told caregivers is older parents may become paranoid you want your hands on their money or you are just a vulture waiting to pick over the bones. It is completely the opposite – it is the system that will feed off the bones of your loved one if you do not know everything and have the proper legal documentation and other paperwork in place.

Caregiving is a partnership – a sacred trust between care receiver and caregiver. Only by discussing how best to manage things – before a crisis occurs – can you be the best partner to your loved one. Remember, even Indiana Jones had help (from Marion and Sallah). Tell your loved one you are on this journey together.

Caregiver Checklist

- ✓ Know where your loved one's important information is stored – locations and account numbers, health care professionals' contact information as well.
- ✓ Ensure your loved one has at least a Living Will or trust in addition to Advance Directives or Durable Power of Attorney for both health care and financial decisions.
- ✓ Ensure your loved one has up-to-date identification documentation (driver's license or state ID card, passport, Social Security card).
- ✓ Investigate the help of an Elder Law attorney – it will probably save you time and money in the long run.
- ✓ Ensure your parents have identified the person (adult child or other person) they want to make decisions if they're both incapacitated. If your loved one is living alone, ensure you or a designate has the legal authority to access important information if a crisis strikes and she cannot communicate for herself.

The Money Pit

Costs and savings of caregiving

Cuba Gooding Jr. said it best in his Oscar-winning performance in *Jerry McGuire*, "Show me the money!" This section will show you where a lot of your money will go if you do not plan ahead and know as much as you can about your loved one's long-term care plans.

While these costs may change faster than I can update this book, this information will give you an idea of what the various prices and fees of caregiving are today. Again, every caregiving situation is unique and there are a lot of unknowns. Costs will vary state to state. Medicare will cover some but possibly not all of your loved one's health care costs which is the reason why many older Americans look to purchase Medicare supplement insurance plans. Medicaid will pay for all or most medical expenses but only after you have virtually nothing left in your piggy bank. Choosing a financial strategy is tricky business, because none of us knows what the future holds. Long-term care plans are not always the silver bullet in guaranteeing your safe financial future and reverse mortgages are still a question mark for many.

The best first step after you talk to your parent or other loved one for whom you are caregiving is to gather as much information as you can and then meet with your own financial planner. You may feel you have planned your own retirement future to be rock solid but with the possibility your parents or other loved one has not made the same solid plan for the future or has not been realistic about their life expectancy, you may find caregiving puts a crack in your future's nest egg.

When it comes to cold, hard cash and how caregiving may affect your pot of gold, here are some cold, hard facts about living longer you need to consider:

- Life expectancy in 1900 was age 47; in 2000 it jumped to age 78 (pretty good considering two thousand years ago the average Roman could expect to live to only age 22)
- The fastest growing segment of our population is people over age 80 – going from 10% today to 30% over the next 25 years
- If you reach age 65, you have a 20% chance of living to age 90
- 1 in 50 boomer women will live to age 100

The Women

One thing statistics tell us is women typically live longer than men – on average 3 to 4 years longer. In the recent U.S. census, there were twice as many women age 89 than men. This *female factor* can become frightening when it comes to finances. According to Cindy Hounsel, president of the Women's Institute for a Secure Retirement (WISER) a nonprofit organization based in Washington, D.C. that educates women on how to plan for a solid future, half of women age 65 will likely live beyond age 85, yet 92 percent of these older women do not have retirement plans to cover this 20-year period.

Some of this gap may be happening because women have often left the workforce for a period of time to raise children – thus, pressing *pause* on their potential 401(K) and Social Security earnings. According to *The Impact of Retirement Risk on Women* report conducted by the Society of Actuaries (SOA), by the age of 50, a woman's retirement plan should be well underway yet 4 out of 10 women over age 65 report relying solely on their Social Security income in their golden years.

"Women need to understand the full-blown drama of retirement," says Hounsel. "For most women, there is little room for error and being unprepared for nearly a third of their lives will have consequences."

Hounsel says the only way for caregivers and their moms to solve this dilemma is to take the mystery out of the future. There are online tools to help. AARP offers a Retirement Calculator and a Social Security Benefits Calculator on its web site, the U.S. Department of Labor site contains data and guidance on *Taking the Mystery Out of Retirement* and WISER offers checklists and other tools to help you make your financial future more secure.

How to Avoid the Caregiving Cost Drain

If you are caring for older parents, a sibling or another loved one and find yourself dipping into your own pocket to cover some of these costs – you are not alone. The National Alliance for Caregiving has conducted several studies over the last few years that uncovered unforeseen caregiving costs and issues. Here are some important things to know:

- More than half of all caregivers for someone over age 50 reported spending on average 10 percent of their annual income on care-related costs – this equates to $400 more than what they spent on health and entertainment costs *combined* – typically $5,531 based on a $46,000 salary.
- 63 percent of caregivers are saving less since the economic downturn.
- 65 percent of caregivers have difficulty paying for basic necessities like utilities and food and 64 percent are having a hard time paying other bills.
- 47 percent are using most or all of their savings to cover care costs and 4 out of 10 are borrowing money or increasing their debt to cover care costs.

On a positive note, another study conducted by Northwestern Mutual found while only 45 percent of respondents said they were not sure how to plan to address their own future long-term care needs, those who were caregivers were twice as likely as non-caregivers to have discussed long-term care plans with family and friends. But if you have not yet had the tough conversation about money with your loved ones, don't delay because caregiving could wind up bankrupting your own future. According to researchers at Harvard Law School and Harvard Medical School, "Nearly half of all Americans who file for bankruptcy do so because of medical expenses." The reality is the cost of caring for a loved one at home can make you go from *riches to rags* in no time.

Consider the average retirement savings for a couple over age 55 is $29,000. Depending on whether they have long-term care insurance and how much Medicare will cover, costs for assisted living or skilled nursing facilities and in-home care continue to rise. The annual

Genworth Cost of Care Survey found in 2012 a national average cost for a one-bedroom, single occupancy assisted living facility is $3,300 a month, and a private room in a 24/7 nursing home is $222 per day or a median annual cost of approximately $81,000 – about $15,000 more than you may have paid in 2007.

In addition, homemaker or personal care services you may secure for your loved one living at home average $18 per hour; licensed home health aides cost $19 per hour. Another Genworth study, *Beyond Dollars – The True Impact of Long-Term Caring*, found 42 percent of caregivers reported moving their older parent into their home for three years or more to care for them in order to help off-set some in-home care costs. Beyond housing and in-home care costs, there are costs associated with meal delivery, transportation, durable medical goods, home safety improvements, pet care and more.

And the ripple effects of caregiving are often felt beyond even the primary caregiver. This same Genworth study showed 36 percent of secondary caregivers – which can be a sibling of the primary caregiver, a sibling of the care recipient or even an independent adult child (such as an adult grandchild) – spent $2,600 on average (excluding facility care) and one-third lost 20 percent of their household income because they helped contribute to caregiving costs.

One way to ensure you and your loved one are getting the most out of available benefits is to use an online tool developed by the National Council on Aging called Benefits Check-up. You can find services to help pay for health care, medications, meals, utilities and more. It provides trusted information on federal, state and local programs and the benefits that may be covered for your loved one.

If you are working, another avenue to save costs is a flexible spending account (FSA) or a health savings account (HSA) through your employer benefits. Check with your human resources department to find out if your benefits include an FSA or HSA. It is possible if you are paying for your loved one's medications, dental and vision care and expenses, you may be able to apply these expenses to your FSA/HSA which means you could be paying for those services with pre-tax dollars – which can make these costs essentially tax-free. Typically your loved one has to be listed as a dependent on your FSA/HSA account to be able to do this.

In some cases you may even be able to have an Adult Day Care expense covered. In order to have Adult Day Care paid through a FSA/HSA however, both you and your spouse have to prove you are both working meaning no one in the home is able to watch your loved one during the day. Again check with your HR department for details.

Financial Gerontologists

Once you have discussed with your loved ones what their future financial picture looks like, it is time to talk to your own financial advisor. According to an AARP survey, 55 percent of Americans thought the government will pay for their long-term care. In fact, after a loved one is discharged from the hospital, some Medicare plans will typically only cover a partial amount up to 100 days in a rehabilitation nursing home facility. If a spouse needs to cover the ongoing costs for a nursing home, assisted living or in-home care, she can be brought to the brink of financial ruin if a plan wasn't in place ahead of time.

For instance, if your mom has to basically deplete her and your dad's savings in order to cover dad's care costs today; when her time comes she may be bankrupt which means the financial burden may fall to you, her potential caregiver. If you go bankrupt caring for mom, who will care for you and your spouse when your time comes? Your kids? This domino effect is what good financial planners, Elder Law attorneys and tax accountants can help you avoid if you sit down with all the facts and make a plan.

In 2012, Medicaid federal laws allowed the spouse of an ill loved one to retain $113,640 in assets so the loved one can still benefit from Medicaid. However, there are some instances when even these assets won't ensure the care of the well spouse when the time comes. In these circumstances, the well spouse, meaning the one who does not need the care, will seek spousal refusal. This law allows a spouse to refuse to cover the costs of care for a chronically ill spouse in order to protect the savings and assets for the future care of the well spouse.

Whether you turn to an Elder Law attorney (discussed in detail in the Raiders of the Lost Ark chapter) or a financial planner, you want to ensure they understand the intricacies of estate planning, but also Medicare/Medicaid rules and other legal elder care implications. A new crop of financial wizards are registered financial gerontologists (RFG). This special credential that financial planners, insurance brokers, CPAs and others earn helps them guide families through this elder care quagmire so no one need go bankrupt just because you hit the life lottery winning number of living longer.

According to Dr. Neal Cutler, one of the founders and current acting president of the American Institute of Financial Gerontology (AIFG), "Our goal is to ensure credentialed financial planners gain more insight and expertise into the aging of America – we don't train professionals on financial planning we train them to better serve their older clients through the understanding of aging and longevity issues."

The curriculum of AIFG is to help financial planners gain credentialed multidisciplinary expertise, building on relevant teachings from biology, psychology, sociology, and demography to understand the lifelong wealth span issues and aspirations of aging individuals and their families. For instance, a financial planner with RFG training will be better equipped to understand the costs associated with modifying your home or your parent's home to allow your parents to *age in place* (the aging industry euphemism for living in your home as long as possible). An RFG can also help you understand the costs and issues around driving and transportation needs, meal delivery, home health aide costs and even how to navigate some of the emotional minefields that can appear as you and your parents look towards the future of possibly being an 80, 90 or even 100-year-old.

To date only 300 financial planners hold an RFG certification but as needs of an aging population increase, hopefully more of our financial experts will up their game to keep us living as securely as long as possible.

"The idea that *lifespan* equals *wealth span* is one we feel empowers financial planners and their clients to collaborate on a financial future instead of just financial products," says Cutler.

Cindy Hounsel of WISER advises two things when it comes to considering your financial future as a caregiver:

1. Make sure you have an advisor that speaks *Venus* and not just *Mars*.
2. Approach your financial planning as you would your health planning.

She says many women who are not accustomed to having a seat at the table when it comes to finances, rely on their husband to handle everything with little or no input from them. This is a mistake. As a woman, you need to be as much in the know as possible since it is your future. When Cher divorced Sonny, she admitted she did not even know how to write a check since her husband had handled all the financial dealings for the couple.

When it comes to caregiving, husbands who work may not be as sensitive to the needs around caregiving. If your husband is handling the financial discussions with your planner, the caregiving for an older parent may never come up in conversation if you are not involved to ask those questions.

Hounsel also advises it is never too late to start a sound financial plan for your future just as it is never too late to start a healthier diet or begin a new exercise routine that puts you on a course for a healthier life. She says we are getting better at preventing chronic illness as we age, so we also need to get better at preventing poverty in our golden years.

The Taxman

There are some things to think about when it comes to caregiving and your taxes. For instance, if you can legitimately claim a parent or parents or other loved one with a disability or illness as your dependent, similar to a dependent child, you may be able to get a tax credit. You have to check with your accountant but even if your loved one does not live with you – he is still living in his home or even in assisted living – if you are helping to pay for that cost it might be considered as tax credit for you.

The ability to claim tax benefits all depends on your loved one's financial status. In many cases, annual income including their Social Security benefits must be below $3,600 annually. In addition, the tax credit may only apply if you are paying at least a minimum of 50 percent of a loved one's basic living expenses (meals, transportation, housing expenses, medications, incontinence products related to their chronic illness, etc.). You may also be able to write off certain itemized expenses such as gas costs for taking a loved one to and from doctor or medical appointments, or home safety improvements. Most of these expenses will need to meet tax eligibility and according to the 2012 tax code and rules they need to exceed more than 10 percent of your gross adjusted income. Again, check with your accountant on whether these costs may be eligible as a deduction for you.

There is also a tax benefit consideration even if multiple people are pitching in financially to care for a loved one. For instance, if you and your siblings collectively are covering at least 50 percent of the costs of care for your parents, once all eligibility requirements are met, one sibling may be able to claim the tax benefit. In this case, a Multiple Support Declaration needs to be filed with that year's tax return. There are many nuanced details to claiming tax benefits which is why it is always best to consult with your accountant or an Elder Law or tax attorney.

Your accountant should also stay on top of any legislative actions that may impact tax laws year to year. A study conducted by the National Alliance for Caregiving found higher household income caregivers (those making $100,000 or more annually) would like to see a tax credit for caring for a loved one while lower income household caregivers (those making less than $30,000 or less annually) prefer a voucher program where they could receive payment for the hours they spend caring for a loved one. To date, no legislation has been passed for either option but advocates continue to press Congress on addressing the needs of the nation's caregivers.

The Color of Money

One of the questions I get asked all the time when I speak to groups on caregiving is, "Can I get paid to care for my loved one?" The answer is: Maybe. The big caveat here is it all depends on Medicaid laws which vary state by state.

To date, there are 15 states that have embraced the Patient-Directed Services Program. This is a Medicaid waiver program whereby if your loved one qualifies for Medicaid benefits, you might be able to receive Medicaid payment for your loved one's personal care assistance. Modeled on the Medicaid Cash & Counseling Program that began in 1998, caregivers must qualify and then be overseen by a case worker who decides how many hours and what wage you will be paid. The National Resource Center for Patient-Directed Services (NRCPDS) offers a state-by-state map that displays the programs and waivers offered in each state to care for a loved one on Medicaid.

One caution: check with the local state Medicaid office or even better an Elder Law attorney on technicalities. Many ill or disabled loved ones, particularly older parents, want to compensate their adult child or other family caregiver for all the time spent caring for them. Particularly in cases where a caregiver has had to leave a job to care for a loved one – a situation a National Alliance for Caregiving study says almost 1 in 10 caregivers choose. Be aware if your loved one decides to start paying you cash for all the time you spend caregiving for them, it could jeopardize their Medicaid eligibility, particularly if you are paid more than the standard rate of a personal care assistant (typically below $10 per hour in most states).

Even if you can verify that it won't jeopardize your loved one's Medicaid benefits, it is wise to have a contract in place to help you and your loved one understand the services being delivered so expectations on both sides are met and future legal difficulties can be avoided which can cost you money. Also, remember any earnings must be reported to the IRS on both you and your loved one's tax returns. A great example of why having a written agreement in place with your loved one is so critical is found in the following *Mercury Journal Register* article written by Kathleen Martin, an Elder Law attorney in Pennsylvania. She wrote about a situation based on a 2011 legal case that emphasizes how important it is to have a written agreement in place with a loved one for which you are providing care – even if living in the same home:

"...case involves a son in New Jersey who provided nearly full-time care to his mother from 1994 to 2003, essentially abandoning his law practice. After the death of his mother, the son filed an inheritance tax return, claiming a deduction of $1.24 million as a debt that was owed by mother to son for care giving [sic] over the years. The son stated that his mother orally agreed to compensate him at her death. However, in the absence of a written agreement between mother and son, the court ruled that the estate was not entitled to the deduction."

Caregiver Checklist

- ✓ Educate yourself about the costs of caregiving and what financial plans your loved ones have to cover these costs should they live to be 80, 90 or even 100.
- ✓ Know the maximum benefit ceilings and eligibility for Medicare and Medicaid benefits.
- ✓ Always check with an Elder Law attorney before deciding to enact spousal refusal or other adjustments that can impact Medicare and Medicaid benefits and eligibility.
- ✓ Ask your accountant about tax credits of caring for a loved ones.
- ✓ Check with an Elder Law attorney or state Medicaid office on allowances and regulations about getting paid by your loved one to be their caregiver before any cash trades hands.
- ✓ Plan ahead for your own retirement and the possibility you may be dipping into your own pocket to help cover the cost of your loved one's care.
- ✓ Ask your financial planner and/or Elder Law attorney if she/he has an RFG certification or if she/he has had special training to understand the intricacies of Medicare or Medicaid financial issues and other aging-related knowledge.

Driving Miss Daisy

Senior driving safety, driving retirement and alternative transportation

One of the toughest issues you will face as a caregiver is when your loved one should no longer drive. Among aging experts, this is known as *driving retirement*. In the Oscar-winning 1989 film, *Driving Miss Daisy*, 80-year-old actress Jessica Tandy played Miss Daisy who resists her son's suggestion she have a chauffeur after she has an auto accident and cannot get insurance. What happens over a 25-year-period is a wonderful relationship develops between Miss Daisy and her driver, Hoke Colburn, played by the unforgettable Morgan Freeman. While this was just a movie, it is an example of what a person feels when told she/he can no longer drive: lost and frustrated. But there is hope (as Miss Daisy found).

This chapter will take you through the stages of one's driving career:

Stage 1 – Driving safety
Stage 2 – Driving retirement
Stage 3 – Alternative transportation

Route 66

Nat King Cole made this tune a hit in 1946 – the same year the first baby boomers were born. I am not suggesting you travel from Chicago to L.A., but the first step in assessing a loved one's driving ability is to take a ride with him. A quick trip to run an errand will give you the clues you need.

Today, 10 percent of all drivers are over age 70 – and by 2030 one in every five drivers will be over age 65. Among these older drivers; between 23-40 percent will have macular degeneration creating vision-related problems for driver safety according to the Macular Degeneration Partnership. The Automobile Club of America states men over age 70 outlive their safe driving ability by six years and for women it is 11 years. But those are just numbers. When it comes to driving, skills and judgment are more important than age.

What we do know is giving up the keys is equivalent to giving up your independence. However, the alternative is even more frightening. Take the 2003 tragic accident at the Farmer's Market in Santa Monica, California, when a confused 86-year-old driver accelerated rather than put on the brake and plowed through the crowd killing 10 people and injuring more than 50. The result was tragic and unavoidable deaths and the prosecution of a confused older man. In addition, the National Highway Traffic Safety Administration data shows 16 percent of traffic fatalities in the U.S. involved a 65-year-old or older driver. These are facts and the teachable moments we need to discuss with our parents and other older loved ones.

> **Men over age 70 outlive their safe driving ability by 6 years and for women it is 11 years.**

The good news is some older drivers are taking the keys out of their own hands – not entirely but cutting back to ensure their safety. A survey among older drivers conducted by the Massachusetts Institute of Technology (MIT) AgeLab and The Hartford Financial Services Group found two-thirds of the drivers self-regulated their activities in the car, restricting their driving for certain conditions. Time of day was a common factor, with some people choosing to stay home at night or dusk. Bad weather conditions and heavy traffic were other conditions. Over time, drivers developed conscious strategies to compensate for failing vision, slower reflexes and stiffer joints.

Following are several warning signs that are the most common cause for concern about your parent's driving ability. You want to look for patterns not just one incident. Keep in mind some of these issues are minor, others more serious.

1. They have become fearful, nervous or anxious about driving.
2. There are ongoing scrapes and dents to their car – and they confess they hit the mailbox or curb – again and again and again.
3. They have difficulty staying in lanes.
4. They have trouble following road signs or street markings.
5. They have a slower response time to basic driving skills like braking or accelerating.

If you've noticed the signs as well as taken a ride with your loved one, and felt like you were on Mr. Toad's Wild Ride at Disneyland, it's time to do two things: look into adjusting things in your loved one's car for better vision and mobility, and think about a driving assessment to determine your loved one's real driving performance.

The Adjustment Bureau

Sometimes a quick adjustment to seats or steering wheels can make a big difference. Remember, we shrink in size as we age. In fact, the *Harvard Health Letter* says after age 40 we lose ½ inch every decade – ultimately decreasing in size by about three inches in our *golden years*. In addition, arthritis or osteoporosis may make our driver's seat position, our flexibility and our reaction time different from 10-20 years ago. The MIT AgeLab recently conducted tests (one driving research program is actually called Miss Daisy) and found between the ages of 30 and 70 we lose 20-30 percent in our range of motion and develop poor neck rotation that can double the risk of an accident.

AARP, American Society on Aging, Auto Club of America and the American Occupational Therapy Association collaborated on a 15-minute, 12-point assessment for senior drivers at car dealerships, senior centers and other locations called CarFit to ensure drivers have the right car settings for their safe driving needs. Three out of 10 senior drivers who have taken the test had at least one problem – such as space between the steering wheel and chest or line of sight over the steering wheel – needing adjustment.

You can also work with an occupational therapist to assess your loved one's driving. These experts are called *driver rehabilitation specialists.* In the same way you would seek rehabilitation therapy for your loved one after an accident or surgery, these specialists assess your loved one's driving skills and prescribe a rehabilitation program or alternative transportation options. Your loved one's physician can refer you or the American Occupational Therapy Association will have these experts listed in your local area. Your loved one can also take an online driving assessment test from the Automobile Club of America called *Roadwise Review* or from AARP called the *Driver Safety Program.*

After adjusting the car to your loved one's new driving position and assessing his skills, it may be as simple as considering a newer model car that comes equipped with the latest driver safety technology.

Many auto makers such as Lexus, Prius, Lincoln, Mercedes Benz and BMW now include park assist and automatic brake features on cars intended to help drivers of all ages but definitely benefitting senior drivers who may have slower reaction times or decreased flexibility to perform certain car maneuvers. Ford, which has been a pioneer in senior driving features using its ThirdAge suit that simulates age limitations to help with car features development, has previewed a prototype car seat with built-in heart rate monitoring now being tested at a Ford research lab in Germany. Data from the seat could, for example, create a *driver workload estimate* to measure stressors that could affect safety. In addition, the OnStar feature on GM cars has addressed emergency safety issues for years and is compatible with 90 million vehicles on the road today.

In addition to driver assessment courses, there are also ways to hone driver skills from the safety of your loved one's living room chair – all he needs is a computer.

Posit Science® has a software product, Drivesharp, which is a suite of brain fitness exercises recommended by AAA Foundation for Traffic Safety. Numerous studies show that drivers who train for just 8-10 hours, process visual information faster, see more of the roadway, and react faster in situations where split seconds matter. In fact, reaction time improves by the equivalent of 22 additional feet in stopping distance at 55 mph. It has been embraced by several national auto insurers because it actually cuts crash risk in half for older drivers.

It is not a driver education or assessment, but rather a brain fitness software program that sharpens the brain. Studies show the benefits extend beyond driving to improvements in standard measures of quality of life, including functional independence, confidence, mood and overall health.

How to Set Your Car Mirrors for Best Visibility

According to Jim Snelling, former race car driver and founder of Advanced Driving Dynamics, a driver training school for teens and seniors, one of the easiest ways to improve driving performance and safety is a simple adjustment to your car's mirrors.

1. Start with the left outside mirror. Move it all the way to the left until it stops. Look in this mirror and find an object on the right hand side edge of the mirror.

2. Look in your rearview mirror on the inside of the car's front windshield. Adjust this mirror to find the same object you found in your left outside mirror. Adjust this inside windshield mirror to see the object on the left hand side of your inside mirror.

3. Now looking in your center inside windshield mirror, find an object at the outer right hand side of this mirror.

4. Looking at your right outside mirror, find the same object you just saw in the middle inside mirror and adjust the right outside mirror until the object is on the left edge of the right outside mirror.

Taxi Driver

If you believe having your loved one surrender his keys is best for everyone, be prepared to help with figuring out his transportation needs. A National Alliance for Caregiving study found 83 percent of caregivers provide transportation help to their loved one – either as the actual driver or coordinating the transportation services. And a report from AARP showed caregivers provide 1.4 billion trips a year for loved ones who no longer drive.

As a caregiver who may become your loved one's main source of transportation which means you may want to think about the type of car you own and whether it is *age friendly*. For instance, do you drive an SUV that your loved one will have to climb into or make a huge step up? Are the passenger seats at hip level making it easier to transfer someone from a wheelchair? Speaking of wheelchairs, will you need a van or larger vehicle to accommodate a wheelchair and ramp? Many automotive models are more conducive than others to your needs as a caregiver especially models from Toyota, Honda, Jeep and Hyundai. The National Mobility Equipment Dealers Association is a great resource for modifying your car for your loved one's mobility issues.

An option to becoming Robert DeNiro in *Taxi Driver* (without the crazy Mohawk and talking to yourself in the mirror), may be to explore some of the following services that offer alternative transportation for your loved one.

Companies such as SilverRide, offer much more than rides to and from the doctor or bridge club. Located in San Francisco but expanding to other cities, SilverRide bills itself as a lifestyle transportation service – offering companionship along with the ride. Drivers are also trained in Red Cross emergency techniques similar to EMTs giving you more peace of mind than calling a cab or putting your loved one on public transportation (which can be like a scene from *Throw Momma From the Train*). If your mom loves opera but has not been attending lately because she would have to go alone, SilverRide will find an opera buff/driver to pick her up, accompany her and bring her home safely.

"Driving isn't always about the driving it's about the experience of getting to a place you want to go," says Jeff Maltz, CEO of SilverRide. "Our service is about much more than just picking someone up and dropping them off. The passenger sits in the front seat, has a conversation with our driver, and maybe even attends an event or activity with the driver as companion. It's about much more than just getting around – it's about lifestyle and not giving up enjoying life because you can no longer drive."

There are also numerous organizations that offer low cost or no cost transportation. What you want to be careful about is whether the service is curb-to-curb (CTC), door-to-door or door-through-door (DTD). If your loved one needs a little help navigating the step into and out of the house, then you need the DTD service. Be aware some services will not agree to provide transportation to individuals with physical mobility issues, such as use of a wheelchair, because of the liability. While many of these services use the power of volunteers – the reality of volunteering can sometimes mean the service may not always be reliable.

Another service is Independent Transportation Network® (ITN) for older people who seek to replicate private auto ownership and mobility. Begun in Maine in 1995, ITN is staffed by paid and volunteer drivers. This service offers 24/7 transportation with some added extras like carrying packages, opening doors and offering a helping hand. The passenger or family caregiver is invoiced monthly and seniors can use their cars as trade-ins for the service. ITN Affiliates are located in several major cities: Los Angeles and San Diego, Calif.; Davenport, Iowa; Chicago, Ill.; Las Vegas, Nev.; St. Charles, Mo.; Lexington, Ky.; North Charleston, S.C.; Middleton and East Windsor, Conn.; Westbrook, Maine; Orlando and Sarasota, Fla., with planned expansion as senior transportation needs grow.

Other resources include the National Center for Senior Transportation (NCST) web site. Operated by Easter Seals in collaboration with the National Family Caregiver Support program through the Administration on Aging, there are tools and resources to help seniors and their caregivers with transportation needs in local communities, including rural areas. You can also check the Department of Transportation (DOT) web sites offering the latest in transportation alternatives for each state. In addition, some senior services agencies such as Right At Home and Home Instead will also help coordinate transportation services. While these agencies are not a taxi or limo service, they can help with incidental transportation such as trips to doctor appointments or physical therapy, some social activities such as faith services or special family events like birthdays and weddings, or running a simple errand such as picking up a prescription at the pharmacy or grocery shopping.

I have spoken to many caregivers who have had the driving conversation with their older loved one and afterwards sold the loved one's car and put the proceeds into an account to pay for these types of transportation services.

Going My Way

How do you start the conversation about driving retirement with your older loved one? It is not easy. One survey conducted by the National Safety Council and Caring.com showed this is the discussion we least want to have as we age. Thirty-six percent of survey respondents said "giving up the car keys" is their least favorite topic of conversation versus only 29 percent who said they did not want to discuss their funeral arrangements and 18 percent who did not want to talk about having to sell the family home. Basically, we would rather become homeless or contemplate death than have our car keys taken from us.

Several organizations have developed tips for caregivers on how to start this difficult conversation with your loved one. The Hartford has downloadable forms to help assess and address senior driving safety. One of the best tools Hartford offers is the *Conversation Inventory* which is a list of questions and things to consider when discussing driving issues with your older loved one. The Alzheimer's Association and AARP have developed several online videos on how to have these tough conversations. In the Alzheimer's Association videos various scenarios are depicted to give caregivers an idea of how to start the conversation that actually can help all caregivers, not just those who have a loved one with dementia. In one video, an older woman agrees with her family members to draw up a contract that she will give up the keys when a doctor or objective party deems it necessary.

In fact, a survey conducted by The Hartford showed 40 percent of older drivers prefer to hear about their driving issues from their doctor, while half want to hear it from a spouse. Caregivers should engage either one to help if they feel their loved one should stop driving. One-third of seniors say hearing about their driving from an adult child is also acceptable but the person they least want to address their driving issue is a law enforcement officer. But waiting for that to happen may take time. Unless your loved one is in an accident or stopped by a police officer for a driving infraction, most states don't have requirements that older drivers renew their license with an actual driving test.

If it falls to you to start the conversation, consider beginning with asking your loved one how he feels about his driving skills. This may be a frightening or maddening topic for him. He will think you are trying to take away his independence. Remind him you are his *co-rider* in this situation – together you have to figure out how to keep everyone safe and able to get around. Say things such as, "Let's explore how to keep you and others safe but still get you to places you want to go." It's about *prevention* and *protection* – for your loved one and others on the road who could be injured or killed. Remind him of the statistics – the National Highway Traffic Safety Administration says:

- People age 75 years or older have more fatal crashes of any age group except teens (ages 16-20).
- Older drivers over age 75 have a 37 percent higher crash rate than other age groups.
- Just giving up nighttime driving or driving far distances may not be enough - most fatal accidents involving senior drivers occur during the day and actually close to their home.

If he is still resistant, one avenue is to talk about senior driving in a similar way we deal with health issues. As we age, things change; we cannot control it but we can manage it. In the same way your loved one has annual health check-ups, or tests such as a prostate exam, he should consider an annual driving exam. Tests can be administered by a driving school instructor, a driving rehabilitation specialist or in a driving simulator. The agreement between you and your loved one should be if the test shows he should no longer drive, he has to agree to discuss alternative transportation plans, just as he would discuss medical solutions for an exam that showed a health problem.

Keep in mind the loss of a driver's license is a reminder to your loved one of his loss of many things in his life: possible memory loss, loss of physical strength and ability, loss of feeling relevant in a fast-paced world, and especially loss of independence. Not being able to get around makes your loved one vulnerable and unhappy. It also is a loss of identity. Our driver's license is typically our main source of ID. When your loved one decides to give up his license, it is important to take him to the DMV to replace his license with an ID card. This is a critical and symbolic gesture in the transition from driver's seat to passenger seat. In the end, your loved one can still get around, be independent and be safe at the same time. The focus of your conversation needs to shift from *loss* to *assurance*. Your goal together is not to stop your loved one from getting around, it's to come up with alternative plans to make getting around safe for everyone.

Most of all, be sensitive to what your loved one is facing. Think of yourself having to hand over those car keys. One way to really put yourself in your loved one's position is to download the Driver Seat Game app by Liberty Mutual for your smartphone. This iTunes app is billed as the world's first senior driving simulator mobile app game. It's important when faced with this difficult conversation about driving retirement to you know what it feels like to be an 80- or 90-year-old driver.

One user of the app posted this comment, "I want to thank you for making such a great game; it's nice to know what's it like to be in someone else's shoes."

By getting a virtual glimpse of your driving future as you age, it will give you more sensitivity when the time comes to have that conversation with your loved one.

Caregiver Checklist

- ✓ Understand warning signs your loved one should no longer drive.
- ✓ Check into services to help you assess your loved one's driving safety – CarFit, driving schools and driving simulators. You can also get an assessment from an occupational therapist which can be prescribed by a doctor.
- ✓ Before you have the *driving retirement* conversation, have alternative transportation plans scoped out.
- ✓ Think about who is best to talk to your loved one about driving retirement – your other parent, doctor or you. And don't delay the conversation – it can be a matter of life and death.

Cocoon

*Home safety modifications, home care services,
respite care, senior living options*

Remember the great 1985 movie by Ron Howard starring some of the most memorable actors from the '40s, '50s and '60s like Don Ameche, Wilford Brimley, Hume Cronyn, Maureen Stapleton, Jessica Tandy and Gwen Verdon? These septuagenarians live in an assisted living facility but take a swim in a magical pool created by aliens and infused with everlasting youth juice. Suddenly these seniors act and feel like teenagers.

In today's world, where and how you will live out your golden years is one of the most important decisions and conversations caregivers and their loved ones can have. A survey by AARP showed more than 80 percent of older Americans prefer to stay living in their homes as long as possible rather than contemplating a move to a retirement community or the *dreaded* nursing home. Another poll conducted by *Parade* magazine and Research America showed 58 percent of Americans want to reach age 85 and 26 percent want to live to be 95.

> **80 percent of older Americans prefer to stay living in their homes as long as possible**

What all these statistics tell us is that we're living longer and we want to stay in our homes but the questions become:

Is this practical for all involved?
Can I afford it?
What are my options if I have to consider moving?

What it really comes down to are three options for your loved one: remain in their current home, move them into your home or find them a new *home*:

1. The first option is to help a loved one stay in her home as long as possible called *aging in place* requiring some modification to make the home safe as she ages.

2. The second option is to have her come live with you but this has be part of a larger family discussion.

3. If option 1 and 2 are not possible, the third option is to have a conversation about alternative senior housing – of which there are many choices depending on the level of care your loved one needs.

The goal is to find the choice which is *just right* not just for the present but for a lifetime to minimize frequent moves as the care needs of your loved one changes over time.

When it comes to the conversation with your loved one about where he/she will live as they age, there are a few questions that need to be asked and answered to make the best choices for everyone:

1. Does she need minimum assistance? (grocery shopping, mowing the lawn or raking the leaves, etc.) – *can she still live in her home?*

2. Does he need moderate care? (transportation, paying bills, help with bathing or cooking) – *can he live in his home with some help or live in your home?*

3. Does she need maximum care? (she needs help with bathing, feeding, dressing, toileting, etc.) – *can she live in your home with full-time help or need to consider alternative living arrangements for constant care?*

4. Is he a safety hazard? (with some dementia patients they can wander or become violent posing anxiety and danger for a family or professional caregiver or others which may require more institutional or special care facilities.) – *does he need specially trained professionals who know how to manage these types of patients?*

Once you have answered these questions, following are the options for where mom or dad will live.

Option 1: There's No Place Like Home

As Dorothy expressed in the *Wizard of Oz*, staying in (or in Dorothy's case returning to) our own homes is a wish most of us share. This idea of living at home as long as possible is coined by experts as *aging in place* and a cottage industry has grown up to support this dream.

Typically, aging in place services requires home safety modifications such as adding grab bars to showers and baths, eliminating throw rugs or carpets that can cause falls by being caught on walkers or wheelchairs, widening doorways to accommodate wheelchair access and perhaps pulling off an *Upstairs, Downstairs* – moving a master bedroom from the second or third floor to a main floor.

A wonderful nonprofit organization with chapters in many cities across the U.S. that helps with small home modifications is called Rebuilding Together. For more than 30 years, Rebuilding Together has used volunteer help (both non-professionals and skilled tradesmen) and donated supplies, to help lower income seniors and people with disabilities, such as many of our veterans population, to ensure their homes are safe and livable for a lifetime. There is no cost to your loved one and the peace of mind you receive as their caregiver is priceless.

While the Rebuilding Together option is cost-efficient and easy (if you qualify for its low-income requirements), it is also more of a bandage addressing only those immediate, small modification needs than the sometimes more comprehensive changes that have to be made to your older loved one's home.

There are experts who can help caregivers – called CAPS which stands for Certified Aging in Place Specialists. These CAPS experts have obtained certification to help them understand aging issues and how they apply to home building and modification. A CAPS expert may be an actual contractor or a professional geriatric care manager. The important note here is you do not want to simply engage a handyman who does not have the expertise to identify and understand the specific needs of your loved one as she ages. If you think about it, we don't have to wait until mom and dad are more frail or infirm to make these changes to their home. In fact, most of the following safety modifications are good for all of us to make in our homes today. This idea of *home for a lifetime* is what experts call the concept of *universal design* – to ensure something works for any age from 18 to 80. To find a CAPS expert, the National Association of Homebuilders has a directory of these specialists on its web site which is listed in the Resources section.

In an interview Sharon Dworkin-Bell, senior vice president of 50-plus housing at the National Association of Home Builders, did with United Features Syndicate, she said, "Universal design isn't just about older people with chronic conditions, it is for everybody and all circumstances, whether you are pushing a wheelchair or a stroller."

Since we know there is no place like home, I contacted the great *wizard of oz* when it comes to home modification, Louis Tenenbaum, one of the nation's most respected CAPS experts and the founder of the Aging in Place Institute. Tenenbaum took me through a litany of home safety modifications that are actually beneficial for any age. (read the sidebar on the Universal Design Home Tour). According to Tenenbaum, "The reality is many of these modifications we should be making to our homes now – whatever our age – because they make the home safer and that is good for everyone."

A 2011 Hartford Insurance survey conducted in collaboration with MIT AgeLab showed 96 percent of baby boomers are aware of changes they should make to their home for safety but only 26 percent have actually made any of these changes.

The key things to consider when modifying the home are what I call the three S's:

1. **Safety from falls.** As we age, falling becomes a serious health hazard and for those with certain chronic illnesses, such as multiple sclerosis or Parkinson's disease, balance can be a challenge making falling more possible. According to the Centers for Disease Control and Prevention (CDC), 2 million seniors are treated in emergency rooms every year for falls at home and falls are the leading cause of injury death among those age 65+. One general tip is to remove any rugs that can catch canes or wheelchairs and can easily trip your loved one. (You will read more about fall risk and solutions below).

2. **Stretch and strain reduction**. Whether in a wheelchair or just having trouble bending or reaching as we age (weak knees, arthritis) – every day tools for living such as bathroom or kitchen items and things such as clothes need to be within easy reach – with most items stored at waist level.

3. **Strength challenges**. As we age our strength levels change. Tenenbaum advises it is typically easier for us to pull than to push as we get older. Therefore, modifications that accommodate this *pull* rather than *push* action are another key to making your house your home for a lifetime.

The Village People

Another version of aging in place is called the Village Movement. This grass roots effort takes the desire to remain in your home as long as possible and makes a collective out of it. Villages, which can be a few blocks in urban or suburban areas or a 20-mile radius in rural towns, are formed by local residents who create a nonprofit organization that provides services and programs the members choose. The pilgrims of this movement, not surprisingly, were located in Boston, Massachusetts in 2002 in the Beacon Hill area of the city. By 2012, more than 89 villages exist across the country with 125 more in development – all based on similar principles and all connected to each other through the Village-to-Village Network (VtV).

These Villages are usually spontaneously created by and for residents age 50 and over. Each member pays an annual fee that can range from $50 to $1,500 although the average is $435 with all Villages offering some type of discount or scholarships for lower-income residents. Most Villages have between 150-200 members and the average age for a Village member is a 74-year-old woman who is known as a *tweener* – a middle income person not eligible for Medicaid programs but not sitting on the long-term care goldmine she might need for nursing home or assisted living care. Does your loved one need a prescription picked up from the pharmacy? Does he/she need grab bars installed in the shower? Does your mom need some extra exercise, such as tai chi, that is conducive to healthy senior living? The Village will find it and coordinate it for your loved one.

The programs and services are managed by a concierge-type staff or volunteers and customized by the membership. Typical offerings include a variety of social and cultural activities, in addition to services needed as we age such as help with the household – everything from computer/tech experts to dog walkers to plumbers, discounted nutrition and exercise programs and access to geriatric care managers and transportation services. The VtV network has a web site with a national map of current and future Village locations and helps identify group discounts on products and services for Village members through more than 200 organizations across the country.

Candace Baldwin who oversees the VtV Network for NCB Capital Impact says, "Baby boomers are really driving the Village Movement in two ways – first, they are purchasing the membership for their aging parents which gives them peace of mind; and second, they believe this is the model they want for their future housing as they grow older and they are starting that conversation in their own neighborhoods."

Mr. Rogers Neighborhood

Similar to the Village Movement, Naturally Occurring Retirement Communities (NORCs) are associated with the NORC Aging in Place Initiative which is a program of The Jewish Federations of North America (JFNA). The 157 Federations comprise a community-based network of 1,300 health and social services providers that provide humanitarian assistance to millions of people nationally who want to age-in-place.

Typically located in lower-income areas, NORCs allow seniors to stay in their own homes and access local services, volunteer programs, and social activities through a concierge-like service. A NORC may be a small, single urban high-rise or spread out over a larger suburban area. The Motion Picture and Television Fund (MPTF) identified several NORCs of its members in Southern California. These retired Hollywood industry veterans – the cameramen, make-up artists, screenwriters – who comprise the majority of membership in MPTF are found clustered in several communities including Toluca Lake, a suburb near Glendale, California where Bob Hope once lived.

Independent Living

Independent living is a general term for any housing arrangement designed exclusively for older adults, typically age 55+. In general, the housing accommodations may be more compact (e.g., single apartment/condo complex or confined community), and includes outside maintenance and sometimes transportation services and organized recreational activities.

Someone To Watch Over Me

One of the key considerations when helping an older loved one to age in place is the type and cost of in-home care and services that may be needed. According to the Kaiser Family Foundation, more than 10 million Americans — mostly people 65 or older — need long-term services and support to help them with daily activities. These in-home care services vary from small tasks such as grocery shopping or housekeeping to 24/7 nursing care including administering medications. The good news is as opposed to volunteer friends and family, if someone gets sick or an emergency comes up and that friend or family member cannot come through for you, professional home care services will always fulfill their duty.

Services such as HomeInstead, LivHome, Right at Home, SeniorHelpers, CareLinx and Care connect caregivers and their loved one to various personal care services. There are also regional services such as Best of Care, a Boston-area home health services agency, and local city or county agencies that can be found through the Area Agencies on Aging Elder Care Locator.

Often, you may not know what level of care worker you need. If you are looking for light housekeeping and companionship you may need a personal care aide or home health aide (HHA). Note there is a difference. Personal care aides have typically completed a certified nursing assistant (CNA) training program (you find CNAs in skilled nursing or assisted living settings) but not the home health component. Home health aides are allowed to check pulse and temperature and administer prescribed medications but cannot change dressings, catheters or assist with medical equipment such as breathing devices. They can also help with bathing, feeding, dressing and transferring a loved one from bed to bath to wheelchair. For more skilled nursing help, where your loved one needs help with injections, changing open-wound bandages or dealing with pressure sores, you need a more skilled nurse such as a Licensed Registered Nurse (LRN).

When it comes to hiring in-home care, the Visiting Nurses Association of America has a great list of questions to ask in an interview situation with service providers. You should also write a job description with the *dos and don'ts* of what you and your loved one need. Include your expectations, always check references, ask to see background checks for verification of criminal or other history, check to see if they have a Facebook page – you will be amazed at how put together someone can be in an interview and then you view their Facebook page and there they are – half naked, chugging a beer bong or perhaps some other behavior which may concern you.

Your goal is to attempt to find an in-home care worker or team you can form a relationship with and who becomes a consistent, comforting presence for your loved one. A revolving door of help can be confusing and add more stress for both you and your loved one. A great example of how an in-home care team becomes like family can be found in the story of Jill Eikenberry and Michael Tucker. Remember hiring in-home care for your older loved one is the same as hiring a nanny or anyone else who comes into your home and is there to watch over your most precious thing in life – your loved one.

A lot of family caregivers want to know if they can get paid to care for their loved one. You will find more information about this in The Money Pit chapter. There are regulations about payment but you can become trained under a Medicare waiver program to provide personal care assistance to your loved one. You can find more information about this at the National Resource Center for Patient-Directed Services (NRCPDS). You can also find valuable help, assistance and training information through the Administration on Aging's National Family Caregiver Support Program.

Grey Gardens

One area of concern about in-home care is finding low-cost help from online help listings such as Craig's List or from what is known as the *gray market* services. These are care workers who are found through *word-of-mouth*. A friend may have a good experience from a gray market worker who has a cousin looking for similar work. But beware – these gray market and Craig's List workers are often not credentialed, trained, bonded or insured and certainly Medicare will not cover the cost of these workers.

But beyond cost it is the jeopardy you may be putting your loved one in to save a little money or expedite a search for a match for your loved one's needs. While some agencies may have restrictions on the minimum number of hours you need to hire in-home care helpers (in some instances it can be a minimum of 8 hours, although the online service CareLinx has no minimum hours for its help), gray market or Craig's List workers in my opinion may not be the way to go.

In April 2011 the California Senate Office of Oversight and Outcomes issued a report indicating California is one of the few states that does not require background screenings for in-home care workers and it was highlighted there was a "significant incidence" of these workers who had criminal records. You run the risk of elder abuse – everything from physical violence, sexual assault, neglect and abandonment of your loved one – which according to a National Elder Abuse Incidence Study conducted for the Administration on Aging happened to more than 500,000 older Americans. You also risk identity theft for your loved one, stolen goods, driving cars not authorized to drive and other bad news situations because the in-home care worker has access to your loved one's home and belongings. The rewards of having in-home help at a low cost are not worth the risk. You can read more about gray market services in the My Man Godfrey chapter.

Only You

You may have professional in-home help, friends or family who help you out or you may be doing all the caregiving duties for your loved one at home yourself. Regardless, if you are the primary caregiver for a loved one, you still need to get periodic breaks called *respite*. The Administration on Aging (AoA) has funded programs through its National Family Caregiver Support Program in 24 states which have established locators for respite care service providers and provide information on how to pay for these services. You can access this information through the ARCH National Respite and Resource Center. They have an online locator for services in your community and a great *ABCs of Respite Care* downloadable brochure that gives you a complete overview of the various ways you can receive respite care for your loved one.

Respite can be provided in your loved one's home or can be a service that gives you a break where you can take your loved one to a location where they can be watched over such as provided in Adult Day Care Centers. You can even find respite services in case of an emergency where you need someone to sit with your loved one while you handle the emergency. Following is a quick rundown of the various respite care services you can find:

Adult Day Care – These centers may require reservations while others offer *drop in* supervision and socialization for loved ones who need monitoring. Caregivers can leave their loved one in professional care during the day and loved ones will typically receive a meal or snack in addition to the opportunity to engage in a variety of activities. A great option for caregivers who need to work, run errands or just need a break for an hour or a day to find some *Me Time*.

Residential Facility Respite – More assisted living facilities are setting aside beds or facilities where caregivers can bring a loved one for a few hours, a weekend or even an extended stay. This gives a caregiver an opportunity to take a business trip or even a family vacation and know their loved one will be looked after in a trusted facility.

Respite Camps - This is not a new concept but an exceptional way for children with special needs, people with disabilities or caregivers of loved ones to get a break, interact and socialize with others and experience a different side of life from the focus on their constant health care needs. Examples of some of the best camps can be found in the Planes, Trains and Automobiles chapter.

Respitality – An innovative concept where participating hotels provide you as the caregiver (and your family) with a room, dining and even entertainment while a local respite service provides the companionship care to your loved one in their home or another location such as an assisted living facility. This model was created by the United Cerebral Palsy of America.

Sitter Companions – Either a volunteer from a local organization such as the Junior League, the Jaycees or a faith-based organization, there may be some training for the sitter and the respite is provided on a volunteer basis.

Home Alone

When it comes to having your loved one stay in their home, two main safety issues arise for caregivers: risk of falls which can lead to serious injury or even death, and isolation which can lead to depression and other health risks. Caregivers need to be in tune with these issues, know the warning signs and understand the solutions to address them.

Falling Down

One of the key problems of aging, and especially living in our homes sometimes alone as we get older, is the risk of falls. The Centers for Disease Control and Prevention (CDC) says more than 2 million seniors are treated in Emergency Rooms from falls each year and every 29 minutes an older American dies from a fall at home. Falls can be caused by many things: balance problems caused by certain medications (always ask your loved one's physician if prescribed medications have balance implications); issues with multiple sclerosis, ALS or Parkinson's disease which affect balance; osteoperosis which causes bones to become weak and thin and not able to sustain the body in a fall; Alzheimer's and dementia which can impair judgment and can distort physical limitations for a loved one; inner ear and hearing problems; diabetes which can cause neuropathy that affects feeling in hands and feet; and hypotension (low blood pressure). The MetLife Mature Market Institute and the National Alliance for Caregiving created a publication free to caregivers called *The Essentials: Falls and Fall Prevention* that offers a number of tips of how caregivers can help loved ones avoid *taking a trip* they definitely don't want.

Former First Lady Nancy Reagan has had some recent falls that are impacting her health and ability to stay engaged in the activities she loves. In 2008, she suffered a fall and was hospitalized for a few days and then a few months later fell again and broke her pelvis. She did not realize she had the break until persistent pain finally caused her to see a doctor where the fracture was discovered. Then in 2012 she fell again and broke several ribs missing an event at her beloved Reagan Presidential Library.

There are several things you can do to help prevent your loved one from falling at home:

1. Vitamin D – according to the U.S. Preventive Services Task Force, its report found taking 800 IUs of Vitamin D daily will reduce your fall risk by 17 percent. You can also get Vitamin D through nutritious eating such as Omega 3 fatty acids found in salmon or walnuts or drinking nutrient-rich milk, and even 10 minutes of sunshine a day will help build strong bones to help reduce falls.

2. Clear the clutter - remove piles of newspapers, magazines or other obstructions from hallways to keep pathways in the home clear.

3. Vision - Ensure your loved one's vision is good and keep eyeglass prescriptions up-to-date. Eye issues such as glaucoma or cataracts can make a loved one more at risk for falls.

4. Embrace technology - Devices such as Personal Emergency Response Systems (PERS) found in watches and cell phones can help alert you automatically when a loved one has fallen and cannot get up.

5. Core strength – helps your loved one build strength through exercise like tai chi or a senior exercise program such as Silvers Sneakers or Silvers & Fit offered at many fitness clubs nationwide.

One unique program was developed by a two-woman team – a former Broadway dancer and an occupational therapist – specifically to help older Americans understand how to use dance techniques and tips to avoid falling. The Fall Stop Move Strong class is provided in New York City but a DVD is available for anyone to follow at home. The program provides exercise benefits but also awareness of the environment such as managing hazards like uneven sidewalks, icy crosswalks or getting into and out of cars or cabs. The program, which offers three levels of training classes and has a 12-week course for each level, is part of a study being conducted by the Martha Stewart Center for Living at The Mt. Sinai Hospital in New York City.

"I got to a point in my dance career where I wanted to use my skills to do some good and found senior mobility issues could benefit tremendously from dance technique," says Celeste Carlucci, one of the two creators of the program. "We call this 'joyful exercise' because many older participants are hesitant at first to take the class but then they flourish and actually form friendships with other class members in addition to improving their core strength."

During the month of September, the National Council on Aging celebrates its Falls Free program (typically tied into the first day of fall) where it works with thousands of senior centers across the country to offer free seminars, testing and other activities and education for older Americans and caregivers on how to avoid *falling down*.

Dark Shadows

When it comes to living at home, many older Americans find isolation to be a huge issue that not only impacts their emotional wellness but ultimately can impact their physical wellness. Just because a senior lives alone or is naturally reclusive does not necessarily mean he is lonely or risking his health because of isolation. Instead, *senior isolation* occurs when an older adult feels he has no place to turn to for help or for social support.

For the 40 percent of people over age 65 who live alone, a major health concern is isolation leading to a risk of depression. More than 6 million seniors suffer from depression and older white males have the highest suicide incidence among any age group according to the National Alliance on Mental Illness (NAMI). Retirement, death or severe illness (such as Alzheimer's disease) of a spouse, significant health problems, reduced income, adult children who move away, death of a friend, or the sense of becoming irrelevant or undervalued – all can create situations where one pulls away from social interaction. These are all issues to be watched carefully particularly if your loved one is living alone at home.

Again, Martha Stewart is helping to redesign healthy aging when it comes to isolation. The Martha Stewart Center for Living at The Mount Sinai Hospital in New York City has clinical experts who help caregivers better understand issues such as isolation and how we treat our senior population – infusing respect and social connectivity for improved health outcomes. Martha, the ultimate home makeover expert, was a caregiver for her mother who lived into her 90s, and is dedicated to creatively making our lives fulfilling as we age and in making our caregiving role easier.

The Universal Design Home Tour

Going room by room with Louis Tenebaum, one of the nation's top CAPS experts, here are things you need to know to make your loved one's home and your own home safer, more *livable* and your future dream house for a lifetime:

Entry to the home

- Remove steps and make a gradual grade up to your doorway that is slip-resistant. If there is too much rise for a sloped entry, consider adding a mechanical lift or ramp to achieve a no step entry.
- Ensure the porch or entry to your home has a protective cover so if it is raining or snowing you are shielded as you open the door. It may also be easier to make your no step entry to the home at the side or back door or through the garage instead of the front door.
- Add good lighting near the keyhole where many porches have poor lighting. Also, ensure you have good light inside the entry. It is also a good idea to add high contrast or lighted house numbers on the home and the street to make it easier for emergency responders to find your house.
- Create a package shelf near the door – a convenient place to set your handbag or a grocery bag so you can easily find your keys to open the door.

Hallways

- Add *On/Off* switches at both ends of a hallway, near the top and bottom of stairs, and right outside major rooms leading into a hallway (such as a bedroom). Many homes have switches only at one end of the hallway.
- Change doors – moving doors within a hallway may create the space needed for maneuvering a wheelchair, walker or other device in hallways.

Kitchen

When it comes to the kitchen – the key words are "within easy reach."

- Lower the counters - most typical kitchen counters are 36 inches high. Lower counters and knee spaces allow you to sit as you chop or mix food (this height level applies to pull out cutting boards as well).
- Additional outlets and switches - these are typically located on the backsplash of counters making them hard to reach. Move these to the ends of counters or just below the counter or inside a lower cabinet for easier access. Also, do not forget to move the switch for the garbage disposal as well.
- Appliances such as ovens should be at lower levels (instead of the higher stacked wall ovens) and have side doors instead of a heavy door which makes it a burn hazard to lean over to get food out. Stoves should have controls on the front of the stove instead of the top or back, again making them hard to reach. Refrigerator doors can be heavy – side-by-side door models are best.
- Store everyday items on middle shelves for easy accessibility. Also invest in sliding shelves for pantries, storage space and even in the refrigerator.

Stairs

- While an elevator may be a little pricey for your budget if your loved one has a multi-story home, an electric stair chair lift may be a reasonable alternative if your loved one has bad knees or a heart condition. Be aware the lifts may drop your loved one on the edge of the top step where falls can happen more easily. Straight run lifts may cost less (typically $2,700 - $3,200). Stairs with bends and curves and landings require custom track (typically $6,000 - $9,000).
- If your loved one doesn't yet need a lift, ensure there are hand rails on both sides of the stairwell.
- Consider marking (in a fashionable way with designer paint or different wood stains) the rise from the tread so it is easy to see the steps.
- The other option is to move your loved one's master bedroom and bathroom to the ground floor to avoid the fall risk associated with stairs.

Bathroom

- Remove all towel bars – they are all too flimsy to hold your weight if you grab for them when falling or off-balance. Instead replace the towel bars with professionally installed grab bars – both for the towels and inside tubs and showers. Add vertical grab bars to help get in and out of the tub as well as horizontal bars. There are really stylish heavy-duty bars from Great Grabz that I like.
- Change the shower to a curbless or no-step shower. Also, add a shower stool if it is easier for your loved one to sit in the shower. Change the showerhead and controls so they can be accessed at waist or sitting level. A handheld model is best.
- A major consideration is having enough room in the bathroom if two people need to be in there at one time. Whether you are helping your loved one or you have a home health aide or personal care assistant that helps with bathing and toileting, you need room for this multi-person activity. Also consider a seat adjuster for the toilet to help easily transfer a loved one who is in a wheelchair.
- One of the most important bathroom modifications is to ensure the door swings *out* not *in*. If your loved one falls in the bathroom with the door shut, even if help arrives, they may be blocking the door making it harder to get to them.

Bedroom

Many people have higher beds that almost require a step to get into; this will not work as you get older.

- Purchase a lower-height bed or thinner mattress; in fact, it would be ideal for lifting in and out of bed to have one at wheelchair height. Also consider installing a trapeze pull above the bed so it is easier to get out of bed (here is the *pull* rather than *push* concept).
- Keep every day clothing and shoe items at waist level to avoid bending down for shoes or reaching high above on shelves for them.
- If you are having electrical work done, such as changes to the outlets in the kitchen or adding light switches in hallways, ensure you add more outlets to the bedroom and main living space to accommodate medical equipment or technology assistive devices which need an outlet.

> **Garage or Laundry Room**
> - Front loading washers and dryers are great investments just remember to plan for enough space so they are not stacked on top of each other. Front controls are best as well.
> - Remember good lighting for the garage – most garages have low lighting that needs to be improved.
> - Ensure you have enough room to get a wheelchair in and out of the car or van. And again, add a ramp so wheelchairs, walkers and canes do not get caught on the bottom lip of a side garage door.
>
> As Louis told me, "We need to think of our lives and our homes as more of a movie than a snapshot – we want to see the whole picture as we age, not just what our needs are today in freeze frame."

Option 2: Golden Girls

This hilarious 1980s-90s TV sitcom showcased two things which are becoming more reality than fiction in our lives:

1. Women are living longer – typically 3-4 years longer than their male counterparts.
2. Many baby boomer and younger generations are looking at mom, dad or even grandparents becoming roommates.

A National Alliance for Caregiving study on caregivers and the economic downturn showed there was a 21 percent increase in co-residency of caregivers and their older loved ones.

Bill Cosby famously said, "Human beings are the only creatures on earth that allow their children to come back home."

There is a twist on that thought today where it is our older parent who may be moving in with us revisiting a trend from days long gone in multigenerational housing. The U.S. Census Bureau reported from 2008 to 2010 there was a 15 percent increase in multigenerational homes – more than 4 million U.S. households currently have three generations living under one roof.

A variety of options are springing up to have mom move in with you or at least be closer. There are temporary garage converter experts such as Next Door Garage Apartments that take a 2-car garage and make it into a cozy, comfortable living environment for your loved one with a bed, bath and kitchenette. With the help of the local Habitat for Humanity volunteer force, the installation takes about 10 days. In addition there are pre-fab installations – either temporary or permanent – that can fit in your backyard if you have space to allow a 300-square foot or 14-foot x 44-foot modular design. Other options known as *granny pods* such as MedCottage™ from N2Care, Care Cottage from Nationwide Homes and PALS (Practical Assisted Living Solutions) from the Rockfall Company all offer a variety of ways to keep mom close and cared for but give you both the privacy and independence you want.

Before you take the plunge of moving mom or dad into your home, garage or backyard, HomeInstead, an international organization that provides personal care services in the home recommends the following things to ask yourself about co-habitating with your older loved one:

1. **Health concerns** – depending on whether your loved one is just recuperating from a surgery or broken hip or has a diagnosis of dementia means different things in terms of home care. Consult with your loved one's physician to find out the details of what the care will entail and possibly cost.

2. **Emotional concerns** – acknowledge this will be an adjustment for both you and your loved one. If your loved one needs someone to help with bathing them, dressing them, feeding them, it can be hard for both parent and adult child to switch roles. It can also mean a loss of independence on both sides. Ensure you talk these things through.

3. **Physical concerns** – does your loved one need to be transferred from bed to wheelchair or wheelchair to shower? If so, can you do the lifting alone or do you need help?

4. **Financial concerns** – will you need to cut back on hours at work to become the caregiver or will you need to hire home health aides to be with your loved one while you are at work?

5. **Physical space** – does your loved one need a special hospital bed, oxygen or IV poles or wheelchair accessibility? Also, you may have to make modifications to your home such as a special commode seat adjuster or rails on front or back steps. If you have stairs and your loved one has difficulty navigating them, you will have to consider first floor accommodations.

6. **Family dynamics** –if you still have children at home, will there be too much commotion or hub bub for your loved one who needs more peace and quiet? Will both you and your loved one still be able to have some privacy? What if you need an overnight nurse – is there room?

Option 3: Sunset Daze

This reality TV show about frisky seniors living in a retirement community in Surprise, Arizona (think *Jersey Shore* for the over-65 crowd), is a Viagra-induced view of what senior living communities are all about. Below you will find a tamer version of what is available when it comes to senior living options.

What is changing is moving from your home as you age used to mean two words: nursing home. Now the options are almost unlimited with a range of opportunities for what is best for your loved one. There really is a home for everyone.

According to Larry Minnix, CEO of LeadingAge, an association of 6,000 not-for-profit organizations dedicated to older Americans, "Home is going to be however we define it. What is important is there are more choices and more value today than ever before."

Minnix believes while most Americans are pinching pennies in our current economy there is value to be found in our senior housing choices. One trend he does see is our health care will be delivered to us rather than our current model where we have to go where the health care services are found.

"Health care will be like the home entertainment evolution – delivered to our doors, delivered in our homes," continues Minnix. He believes this trend is being driven by the migration of the baby boomers desire to move from an institutional setting for their care to a more patient-centric care model – wherever we wish to live.

Adult Family Homes

Also called Board-and-Care, Adult Family Homes (AFH) are residential homes licensed to care for up to six elder residents or couples. All adult family homes provide housing and meals (room and board) and assume general responsibilities for the safety and care of the residents.

Assisted Living

As the name implies, assisted living facilities (AL) are designed to assist individuals who may need help with some day-to-day tasks, but do not need the extensive nursing care provided by skilled nursing facilities or nursing homes. This allows older Americans to remain relatively independent but have the reliability of professional care when needed. Most ALs are set up as small, efficiency apartments and are staffed with nursing assistants and aides who are able to help with bathing, dressing and grooming. In some states medication administration is also a benefit for residents in an assisted living facility. Most facilities also offer dining programs and structured social events. Assisted living facilities may also be a good choice for couples who want to remain together but simply cannot care for each other at home without help because of health limitations.

What you may not know is there are some requirements necessary to live in an assisted living facility. Some people believe a common myth that wheelchair-bound loved ones cannot choose assisted living. This is not necessarily true. While rules and regulations can vary from state to state and even county by county, mobility independence is encouraged among residents of most assisted living facilities and wheelchairs are not always prohibited. However, residents must be able to transfer (move from bed/chair to wheelchair, etc.) with the assistance of one other person. Those who require the assistance of two people or who cannot bear any weight may require more assistance and thus, their care exceeds the licensure of assisted living facilities.

Similarly, residents who experience urinary incontinence are usually accepted as long as their condition can be managed with a toileting schedule, incontinence products and reminders on a consistent basis.

According to the Alzheimer's Association 60 percent of nursing home residents have a diagnosis of dementia or Alzheimer's. However, there are Assisted Living facilities that specialize in the care of Alzheimer's and dementia care patients. They are called memory care facilities or sometimes special care units (SCUs) and can be a great choice for individuals with memory impairment who need some supervision without fully having to relinquish independence.

One model for memory care is Silverado Senior Living with communities in several states. While the specialized assisted living for those with Alzheimer's and dementia is the foundation of the operation, there is also hospice care and at home care services as well. The Silverado model is based on the philosophy of founders, Loren Shook and Steve Winner, who co-authored the book, *The Silverado Story* and believe caring for someone with Alzheimer's or dementia means instilling trust, choice and love in everything they do. While the Silverado services may be expensive for some on limited incomes (Silverado is known as the Ritz Carlton of Memory Care), its model and services have been selected by organizations such as the NFL as part of its 88 Plan for long-term-care for its retired players (which you will read more about in Sylvia Mackey's story).

There are also group home facilities for aging adults with autism, Down syndrome and other special needs. Caregivers should note many of these homes are similar to the assisted living facilities above with typically four to eight residents maximum per home. Because the availability is limited, many states have wait lists for group home admission. In addition, parents of special needs adults need to consider that currently many group homes accept many different disorders and you may have a mix of residents with autism, mental health or other issues. This can be difficult for caregivers who have a high functioning adult child who needs minimal supervision and care. Many attorneys are now specializing in estate plans for caregivers of special needs adult children to ensure their future housing needs are met in the best possible way if the parents are gone and no other family member can assume their care.

Continuing Care Retirement Community

Continuing Care Retirement Communities (CCRCs) are facilities that include independent living, assisted living and nursing home care in one location, enabling seniors to stay in the same general area as their housing needs change over time. CCRCs are typically the most expensive alternative housing option and it is important to know costs include contracts for entrance fees and monthly service charges. There may also be additional fees when your loved one moves from one accommodation to another even when it is on the same campus.

One advantage is the blend of different types of senior living. Couples who need different levels of care can live on the same campus or even together, something other alternative housing options do not often offer. Couples who are split up can experience anxiety and depression that can affect their health.

Eden Alternative

Literally breathing new life into what we think of as *nursing homes* the Eden Alternative is a not-for-profit organization with 300 registered homes in the U.S., Canada, Europe and Australia. The focus on both health and wellness within the environment, or *habitat a*s they call it, is as important as the care provided.

In these beautiful facilities you will find plants, pets and grandchildren playing. Residents and their families are encouraged to work with facility administrators to develop new ideas that will enhance the loved one's daily living. The culture of collaboration and connectivity among residents helps to eliminate the isolation and loneliness typically associated with growing older and with being in an *institution.* In fact, the Eden Alternative strives to *de-institutionalize* its facilities to make these living arrangements an attractive alternative to living at home alone.

For those who do want to stay in their homes, there is also the Eden at Home initiative which takes the principles of creating a nurturing, caring environment and ensuring the loved one's home, community and life are infused with connecting our elders to people and services that feed their bodies and their souls.

The Green House Project

Similar to the Eden Alternative, the Green House Project caters to the lifestyle of our loved ones instead of just addressing their health needs. These facilities replace what we know as institutional settings like a skilled nursing facility (SNF) by creating an intimate living environment that is warm (features similar to your own home), smart (utilizing the latest technology) and green (dedicated to environmentally friendly design and operations) while delivering a level of care similar to a nursing home setting.

Started in 2004, there are more than 134 Green Houses operating in 32 different states with another 250 in development worldwide. Each facility has only six to 10 residents per home and each person is provided with a private room and bathroom that can be decorated to each resident's liking – making it as much like home as possible. The professional health care workers are mostly certified nursing assistants (CNAs) called *shahbaz* who are self-directed and have a less than half the lowest turnover rate of nursing home care workers. These shahbaz (a name based on a fable where shahbaz means a royal falcon that protects and cares for people – a title both the professionals and the residents embrace as part of this unique culture) blend health care needs administering medications and checking on vital statistics with personal care such as cooking and housekeeping for all residents. Each resident receives four hours of care a day with 24/7 shahbaz on site at all times for any emergencies.

Each Green House is customized to its residents' needs with most having an open living and dining area, to encourage the socialization that is critical to our health and wellness as we age. The Green House Project was created by Dr. William Thomas, the same innovator who created the Eden Alternative with funding from the Robert Wood Johnson Foundation and planning and development managed by NCB Capital Impact.

"The biggest benefit of the Green House concept is this becomes your home for life," says Robert Jenkins, director of The Green House Project for NCB Capital Impact. "If and when your health and personal needs increase or change, you do not have to leave the facility, we can accommodate these care transitions for our residents so they can remain in the Green House through palliative and even hospice care."

Nursing Home/Nursing Care and Rehabilitation

Also called Skilled Nursing Facilities (SNFs), a nursing home is usually the highest level of care for older adults and those with disabilities or disorders that can be found outside of a hospital setting. Nursing Home care typically provides two types of care: short-term care for those who need rehabilitation but will eventually return to their own home; and long-term care for those with chronic illness or aging issues which require round-the-clock professional care. Many facilities provide similar services to those found at other retirement living options, but nursing homes differ from other senior housing by also providing a high level of medical care and skilled nursing care. Doctors supervise each resident's care, and a nurse or other licensed professional is always on the premises. Some skilled nursing care facilities also provide occupational or physical therapy, as required by residents. Most residents spend a majority of time in a wheelchair or their bed and have limited mobility.

The Goldilocks Syndrome

In many caregiving situations, the choices and evaluation of alternative living for a loved one are not always clear. Many caregivers I have talked to, and as you will read in the stories of Joan Lunden and Jill Eikenberry and Michael Tucker, find they are operating in a crisis and making decisions on the fly which may not always be well-informed. Many caregivers and their loved ones wind up *testing* different facilities and find that multiple moves are necessary because the facility does not offer the right level of care (as Jill Eikenberry and Michael Tucker found), or perhaps the facility looks beautiful and offers wonderful amenities but your mom is just not the person she used to be and all this activity is disturbing rather than delightful (as in Joan Lunden's story).

While your loved one's care needs may change over time, multiple moves to different facilities, particularly in a short span of time, can be detrimental to her health. Finding a location that can provide the care needed and is adaptable to those needs over time is the best option. But that requires planning ahead, discussing the options with your loved one, and understanding the costs involved with the various options.

"There is no right way or wrong way when considering a move for your parent," says Dr. Rosemary Laird, medical director of the Health First Aging Institute in Florida. "However, if your parent is living alone, there are safety and health concerns and having them closer so you can be their advocate on health care issues can make a big difference."

Dr. Laird advises if you are one of the 7-8 million long-distance caregivers, ensure you have a health care advocate who can be there in person with your loved one. You can read more about this in the My Man Godfrey chapter. You will also find online resources and other services can help you find the best facility for your loved one but Dr. Laird recommends looking at a loved one's current and future care needs to minimize the moves you may have to help your loved one make.

A pitfall for many caregivers when reviewing alternative living facilities is putting our own lifestyle preferences in place of our loved one's needs. We see a beautiful dining room, maybe a gorgeous view, beautiful architectural or design appointments, and great social or lifestyle activities such as free transportation to malls or church. Instead we should be asking more questions about staffing (how often do nurses or health care workers check on loved ones and what is the professional to residents ratio?) If your loved one's mobility becomes an issue is this still the right home? Is there a therapy pool on-site? A nonprofit organization called HelpGuide provides a full listing of questions to ask on your visit to a senior living facility.

It is hard to know a loved one's prognosis over time but Dr. Laird says knowledge about care transitions will help you make better decisions – both health- and wealth-wise – in the long run when it comes to where our older loved one will live out their lives.

Beth Kallmyer with the Alzheimer's Association says, "Always visit a facility at different times and on different days. You should evaluate how the staff treats residents when you are not on a tour and also how the facility looks and feels at different times."

If your parent has Alzheimer's or another dementia, she cautions a move can engender anger or fear in your parent. Your mom may be trying to tap into her memory for her environment and she may be frustrated or scared over not being able to find a bathroom or bedroom because she is in a new place. Eventually your loved one will likely settle in but it may take time so be patient.

And don't be uncomfortable or shy about asking facilities for their ratings and any fines or violations they may have received. Some web sites, such as Caring.com, CareScout.com and SnapforSeniors.com offer ratings from actual users or caregivers that can be helpful. Official ratings by a regulatory organization are difficult if not impossible to find. The Centers for Medicare and Medicaid Services (CMS) offers some ratings on its web site but several experts I talked to said the information is not a complete enough picture to base your choice – it should be considered but don't neglect researching other sources or using the help of an expert. In the end, if you have done your homework and feel you have asked a lot of questions, sought referrals from actual residents or caregivers and had some input or guidance from an expert such as a GCM, you will at least feel confident you did everything within your power to make the best choice for your loved one.

Witness for the Prosecution

If you ever witness an issue or your loved one complains about the care received in these facilities or living environments, there is recourse for caregivers to get help. Residents of nursing homes, board and care homes and assisted living facilities have access to a Long Term Care Ombudsman program.

Operated by the U.S. Administration on Aging, the LTC Ombudsman program provides advocates to work with residents and caregivers on complaints and who also advise on improvements to be made to LTC facilities and operations. The network has 8,700 volunteers certified to handle complaints and more than 1,300 paid staff. Nationally, in 2008 the ombudsman program investigated over 271,000 complaints made by 182,506 individuals and provided information on long-term care to another 327,000 people.

Follow the Yellow Brick Road

Wherever we choose to live, cost issues will drive a lot of decisions. Lea Pipes, vice president of community services for the Motion Picture and Television Fund (MPTF) says, "The factors driving housing choices are family, financial status, available resources and safety." It is this infrastructure that Pipes says caregivers have to discuss with their loved ones to make the best decisions about where our loved ones will live as they age. She believes too many caregivers are acting "impulsively – they aren't thinking this through in a methodical way, it is all coming as a surprise." And while she sees the surveys and reports that say most older Americans want to age at home, she says, "Care at home is not cheap."

One trend MPTF is seeing is a lot of older adults who are upside down in their home mortgages and an increase in home foreclosures – especially in depressed housing markets like those in California. This is exacerbating the senior living choice question and she says MPTF is conducting a lot of counseling with family caregivers because their parents aren't financially prepared for their long-term care needs.

When it comes to housing for your loved one, we all have different definitions of what makes a house a *home*. In the end, we can't just click our heels like Dorothy and have it all solved. We have to plot a plan and have the conversation with family so our yellow brick road of caregiving is a smooth and safe journey.

Caregiver Checklist

- ✓ Ensure you have the C-A-R-E Conversation with your loved one about where they may want to live out their *golden years* – discuss all three options (their home, your home or alternative living) so everyone has a chance to voice their opinions.
- ✓ Secure a CAPS expert to help you modify your loved one's home so they can *age in place*.
- ✓ Understand your options when it comes to securing in-home care.
- ✓ Write up a job description for the in-home care you need – use this to interview and select your best candidate.
- ✓ Think about securing an expert in senior housing and in-home care services – either through a senior care service or a geriatric care manager (GCM) to help you know all your housing options and to avoid the Goldilocks Syndrome.
- ✓ Always visit a senior living facility at different times of day when helping a loved one make a decision about a move.
- ✓ Understand two big aging issues: Falls and Isolation and what you can do to help prevent both.

My Man Godfrey

Caregiving information, online matchmakers, telemedicine, advocates/navigators and professional geriatric care managers

Wouldn't it be nice to have someone you trusted who you can reach day or night to help you keep your loved one healthy, happy and safe? The beautiful comedienne Carole Lombard had that luxury in her on-screen butler played by William Powell in the 1930s screwball comedy, *My Man Godfrey*. In nicer hotels, there is a concierge to find you a great restaurant and get you reservations or secure you theater tickets; in some apartment buildings or townhomes there is a concierge who can find you a plumber or a taxi to the airport. And as you read in the Cocoon chapter, the Village Movement has a concierge service for its residents.

When it comes to caregiving a *concierge* would be a dream come true. As you will read, in the world of caregiving there are some online sites that offer information and tools, some services that match you with in-person professionals, some services that can cut through the maze of insurance and red tape of Medicare/Medicaid, and some services that provide in-person experts in elder care who come close to this idea of a caregiving concierge. But don't confuse these services with the latest trend in medical concierge services like the TV series, *Royal Pains,* where a doctor makes house calls to the rich and famous in the Hamptons.

While a concierge service typically connotes a *high-end* option, you will see with many of the following services, some are free and some come with a fee. All are dedicated to helping you navigate a complicated, fragmented health care world, and many use online services to get you answers faster. These caregiving concierge-style services typically fall into two categories: online help and live help either telephonically or in-person.

I have grouped these services into the following categories starting with the basic online self-help (free of cost) all the way to the most valuable (and costly) – an in-person professional geriatric care manager (GCM):

1. Online information sites – great content, data, tools, resource links and *how-to* information.
2. Telemedicine – this is what I call *virtual docs*.
3. Online sites that actually match you to in-person help and other services – I call these *caregiving matchmakers*.
4. Expert navigators and advocates – this new breed of services help you navigate the hospital environment, help with insurance paperwork, etc.
5. Geriatric care managers – the best of the best – trained professionals who can guide you to the best decisions for your loved one and can serve as your caregiving coach.

The Social Network – *Online Information*

Ever since Google, caregivers can let their finger do the clicking (with a mouse rather than let your fingers do the walking through the Yellow Pages). While Pew Research found 88 percent of those with access to the Internet looked up health information and 67 percent said they looked up the information for someone other than themselves, we know going online is the way to go when searching for caregiving and related information.

However, if you put the following terms into your Google search bar, you get more than 6 million results for *caregiving*, 28 million for *caregiver*, 8 million for *aging loved one* and 146 million for *special needs child*. If you try to search what you need via the Internet, be prepared to be sitting at your computer about as long as Robinson Crusoe spent on the island. The key is to be specific in your search – do not type in words like *Alzheimer's* instead type in *Alzheimer's early warning signs* or *Alzheimer's medications* or *Alzheimer's living facilities*, etc.

One of the biggest complaints caregivers have is they do not have time to sit at a computer all day or all night searching for information that can help and then wonder if the data they found is:

1. Accurate and the most-up-to-date.
2. The best choice for their loved one.
3. Going to be useful based on their specific needs and situation.

To get the peace of mind and confidence in decision-making, you need to find a geriatric care manager which you will read more about later in this chapter. However, when it comes to online information, here are the sites I find to be the most helpful. Keep in mind these are sites that offer full-spectrum caregiving information – the home and community based resources, valuable tools for caregiving and the psychological/social aspect of caregiving. You will read more about the medical/disease/disorder online services and sites later in this chapter under Close Encounters of a Third Kind.

While there are many sites that may have a fact sheet or a page dedicated to caregiving information, the sites I listed here (alphabetically) have robust, comprehensive information, tools and resources to help caregivers:

AARP Caregiver Resource Center (aarp.org) – Comprehensive content and videos on various topics to help explain things visually. Tools include a long-term care calculator, state-by-state listing of advance directives, a care provider locator, *AARP Caregiving Advice and Help from Genworth,* and *Many Strong*, a free online service to help you coordinate care for a loved one. AARP also offers periodic webcasts on different topics where anyone can join the conversation whether it's about senior driving issues, housing options, etc.

Administration on Aging - Aging and Disability Resource Centers (aoa.gov) - The Aging and Disability Resource Center Program (ADRC), a collaborative effort of AoA and the Centers for Medicare & Medicaid Services (CMS), is designed to streamline access to long-term care. ADRCs target services to the elderly and individuals with physical disabilities, serious mental illness, and/or developmental/intellectual disabilities. The ultimate goal of the ADRCs is to serve all individuals with long-term care needs regardless of their age or disability. The ADRCs provide information and assistance for those needing public and private resources for long-term care.

Alzheimers.gov (alzheimers.gov) – Launched in 2012 by the U.S. Department of Health and Human Services, the site is part of the overall National Alzheimer's Plan dedicated to finding a cure and helping caregivers manage their loved one's dementia care. A great source of information but mostly focused on government agencies and help with paying for services; should be seen as complementary to the alz.org site by the Alzheimer's Association.

Alzheimer's Association Alzheimer's and Dementia Caregiver Center (alz.org/care) – Specific to dementia care but one of the most comprehensive sites for caregivers, it offers checklists, videos, links to support groups either online (ALZConnected.org) or in local communities, guidance on financial and legal planning, disaster planning, traveling and more. There is also a Community Resource Finder, which links you to local resources and options such as dementia care facilities, specialized care at home and adult day centers; an online Care Team Calendar, where you can coordinate offers from family and friends to help you care for your loved one; and an online assessment program, Alzheimer's Navigator, which provides customized action plans for care management. You can also purchase location management services such as Alzheimer's Association Comfort Zone® and MedicAlert® + Alzheimer's Association Safe Return®. And there is great information on caregiver health such as the Caregiver Stress Test, Caregiver Notebook and more. The Alzheimer's Association also offers a toll-free, 24/7 helpline for caregivers (1-800-272-3900).

Ask Medicare (medicare.gov/caregivers) – Operated by the Centers for Medicare and Medicaid Services (CMS), this is the *go to* site for caregivers on how to navigate this government agency and the Medicare/Medicaid benefits provided for your loved one. The site includes videos that take you through the steps of planning for hospital discharges, care transitions and more.

Caregiver Briefcase (apa.org) – Created by the American Psychological Association to aid professionals and family members in understanding the caregiving challenges for someone with mental health issues. While much of the information was developed to help the professional psychiatric and psychology field professionals become more sensitized to caregiving issues, the information is valuable for family members to help them understand how professional therapists can assist them in caring for a loved one with a mental illness or disorder.

Caring (caring.com) - This is the highest traffic online site dedicated just for caregivers, with a lot of great articles and information such as state-by-state senior driving laws and Medicare information. The site also has tools such as the Alzheimer's Steps and Stages for care transitions planning and *what to expect* information for dementia caregivers, and a *senior care finder* of more than 100,000 resources for in-home help, housing options and Elder Law attorneys – all with ratings by other caregivers who have used the services. They also offer toll-free telephonic service to talk to a Caring Advisor who is a non-commissioned customer service professional who can help caregivers understand different care options available.

Caring from a Distance (cfad.org) – The only online site dedicated to the 7-8 million long-distance caregivers and the special issues they face. The site is operated by the national nonprofit organization by the same name. The site has downloadable brochures, resource links and information on how to make care decisions; and a searchable resource directory for the Washington, D.C. metro area of 3,000 services available to help in that area, with links to directories in 17 other states.

CareLike, formerly known as Snap for Seniors (carelike.com) – This site has more than 250,000 profiles of various senior living options from assisted living facilities to skilled nursing facilities (nursing home). An affiliate of HealthLink Dimensions, the site also lists end-of-life resources, medical facilities such as for diabetes care, medical equipment, Elder Law attorneys and other resources.

Center for Disease Control and Prevention (CDC) (cdc.gov) – The Family Health page of this extensive web site about national health issues, contains comprehensive resources and related links for caregivers of special needs children.

Elder Care Locator (eldercare.gov) – This site is a public service of the U.S. Administration on Aging and operated by the National Association of Area Agencies on Aging (N4As). Caregivers can put in their zip code, and find a variety of services in their local state or county. The services listed are mostly government agencies or nonprofit organizations, and do not include available private sector services. The site offers fact sheets and links to other government agencies that may be helpful to caregivers. There is also a toll-free number for caregivers to call to chat live with an information specialist who can help find resources locally at 1-800-677-1116.

Family Caregiving 101 (familycaregiving101.org) – This site offers some basic tools and information about caring for a loved one while balancing caring for themselves. Created by the National Family Caregivers Association (NFCA) and the National Alliance for Caregiving (NAC), the site includes checklists and information about how to get started as a caregiver.

Family Care Navigator (caregiver.org) – This site offers a nationwide map where you can click state-by-state to find both public (including government-run and nonprofit organizations) and private services resources to help you care for your loved one. Operated by the Family Caregiver Alliance and its National Center on Caregiving, there is also a Frequently Asked Questions (FAQ) section with many answers to specific caregiving issues.

National Clearinghouse for Long Term Care Information (longtermcare.gov) – This site provides information to educate you about long-term care services, resources and options. Operated by the U.S. Department of Health and Human Services.

National Resource Directory (nationalresourcedirectory.gov) – This site offers the most comprehensive directory of federal, state and local resources to help wounded veterans and their caregivers. The site was developed as a partnership between the U.S. Departments of Defense (DoD), Labor and Veteran's Affairs.

National Resource Center for LGBT Aging (lgbtagingcenter.org) – This site is the clearinghouse for all services, information and links to other resources for Lesbian, Gay, Bisexual and Transgender caregivers and is operated by SAGE (Service and Advocacy for Gay, Lesbian, Bisexual and Transgender Elders).

Next Step in Care (nextstepincare.org) – Operated by the United Hospital Fund and created in collaboration with more than 40 other organizations including the CMS, the site offers checklists and guidelines on how to manage care transitions – from hospital to home or facility.

Veteran's Administration (caregiver.va.gov) – This site offers questions to ask your veterans' health care provider, a *MyMedicationList* to help caregivers keep track of medications and instructions, a *Caregiver Tool Box* with helpful checklists and tools to keep you connected to other caregivers of veterans. The site plans to update the links to Veterans Services Organizations (VSOs) many of which offer help to individual veterans of specific veterans groups such as the Vietnam Veterans of America, Wounded Warrior Project, National Family Military Association and others. There is also a toll-free caregiver of veteran's number to talk to a live operator about veteran's services and benefits at 1-855-260-3274.

In addition to the sites listed above, there are many online destinations that offer a range of services helpful to caregivers. I would begin with the disease or disorder for your loved one which may then link you to other great resources:

- Disease or disorder-related nonprofit organizations, from Autism Speaks to the MS Society, have comprehensive sites rich in information about individual conditions and help educate caregivers.

- Support groups – Often found through the disease organizations or through referrals from hospital social workers or geriatric care managers.
- Regional agencies such as Network of Care focus in California, Colorado, Ohio and Texas. Some of these sites can be found through the ElderCare Locator, others through geriatric care managers.

Matchmaker, Make Me a Match – *Online Services*

When it comes to home care services or finding alternative living options – whether assisted living, nursing home or in-home care services (see the Cocoon chapter for more details) – it is hard to know if your choices are the best if you are doing an online Google search. There are services available that actually can provide matchmaker services for you and your loved one. Similar to relationship matchmaking services, you create a profile with specific details about what you and your loved one are looking for, view the options matched to your profile, coordinate a meeting or tour of the facility and hopefully fall in love.

Keep in mind these types of services make their money in one of two ways: either you will pay a fee for their service or they are paid by the facility or service providers to make referrals. I am not making an argument one way is better than another and of course your other option is to seek services on your own. Each option has advantages and disadvantages and you must weigh cost versus value. I advise some professional guidance is always helpful so I do recommend you do not do it all on your own. Remember to ask a lot of questions, ensure you get referrals from others who have used the service or facility so you have covered all the bases for making the most informed choice.

Following is a rundown of these different senior care services:

A Place for Mom – This service site allows you to put in your zip code and the type of senior living facility you are seeking to receive your matches. You can compare amenities and costs; and if you aren't sure which type of facility you need, there is a toll-free number you can call to talk to a senior living advisor. The advisor can then meet you to tour the facilities you want to see in person. The cost to caregivers is free since the list of 18,000 facilities pay to be listed as part of this service. Joan Lunden serves as their celebrity spokesperson after she used the service to find a facility for her mom.

Care – This site offers a wide spectrum of in-home and facility care options for families including child care, senior care and pet care. It also offers services to employers and military/government organizations needing back-up care for its caregiving employees. You are asked to post a job description and provide a few details (such as your cost range), search for free and pay the health care worker or facility directly. Care conducts background checks and provides telephonic advisors for additional help.

CareLinx – Offers an efficient and cost-effective way to find a personal care aide, also known as a personal care assistant. The matches are limited to personal care services such as meal preparation, transportation, medication reminders and companionship, also known as respite care. They do not provide skilled nursing care.

Caregivers create a free profile for the care needed for their loved one, view online videos of the personal care worker selections, conduct a video chat interview with the home health aide or arrange to interview him/her in person and negotiate the fee. CareLinx manages the scheduling, billing and other necessary administrative tasks to make this a fully integrated service. And since the health care service is provided through an online *virtual* agency rather than a *bricks and mortar* location such as other health service agencies, ultimately the caregiver saves money because there are limited overhead costs.

Sherwin Sheik, CEO and founder of CareLinx, created the service after experiencing his family's struggle with in-home care for his sister who has multiple sclerosis and his uncle who had ALS. He says, "Traditional home health agencies have a minimum number of hours or limited weekend services available. We have no set minimums. We fill the gap for families who are disenfranchised and need to match their loved one's needs with the family budget."

Sheik advises that a recent client was a caregiver in Phoenix who needed to find in-home care for her father in Los Angeles after his hospital discharge. She used CareLinx and will ultimately save about $10,000 over the next 12 months for the care service versus using a traditional agency.

CareScout - This is the same service that administers the AARP Caregiving Help and Advice from Genworth. Both an online and offline service, the database of local senior housing and home health care service options includes 90,000 entries across the country which caregivers can search free of charge.

For a membership fee (or included in AARP membership where caregivers can access the information using a loved one's AARP member ID), caregivers can receive the *SmartMatch* service, which matches your loved one's care needs to specific providers in your loved one's area. CareScout has created an extensively detailed database with care provider answers to more than

80 questions about its service including holiday and weekend rates and split shift offerings. CareScout uses this information to create its own rating system that caregivers can review. In addition, the services are also rated by the caregivers or loved ones receiving the care provided, so you get a second rating from actual users to help you make an informed decision.

CareScout also offers Care Advocates – its own network of professionals across the country who can conduct assessments and help caregivers put together a care plan for their loved one based on a variety of needs. Bob Bua, president of CareScout, a Genworth company, says, "I like to say we're *old-fashioned* because we offer both the convenience and information at your fingertips of online caregiving services but we also offer the in-person, high-touch service so many caregivers need for peace of mind."

Caregiving SVU (Special Victims Unit)

One caution I have for caregivers is to beware of finding in-home care services known as the *gray market* that can sometimes be found from personal services listings found online and in local community newspapers. While at first blush these listings may be attractive because you can save money, in the long run you are risking your loved one's health, safety and well-being to pinch a few pennies. The *risk versus reward* is simply not there and the problems than can arise from an uncredentialed, non-licensed and perhaps not even background-checked health care worker can include identify theft, stealing from your loved one, elder abuse, elder neglect and enough problems to fill Pandora's box. Remember, you are hiring someone to come into your home or your loved one's home and take care of one of your most precious things in life – your loved one.

In a 2011 *Los Angeles Times* article, one woman described following a home health aide she found from an online personal health care worker listing for her mom who was wheelchair-bound. The home health care worker told the caregiver she was taking her mom to the park every day. But a friend had a chillingly different story. The friend said she had seen the mom sitting for more than two hours in a hot car in front of a home in her neighborhood. The next day, the caregiver quietly followed the home health worker as she clumsily and without care tossed her mom into the car, drove a few blocks and parked in front of a house and went in leaving her mom in the hot car as her friend had said. When the caregiver rang the doorbell, a half-dressed man answered the door with the scantily clad home health worker standing in the background. Buyer beware.

You can read more about these gray market services in the Cocoon chapter under the section Grey Gardens.

Close Encounters of the Third Kind – *Telemedicine*

Navigating the health care world on behalf of your loved one is like entering an alien world. As I tell you in the chapter Lost in Translation, everyone seems to be speaking a foreign language and you may be confused about whether to trust just one source such as your loved one's health care professional. The following listing of online tools and consultation services can help you as a family caregiver to navigate the intricacies of the complicated, fragmented world of health care. It can also ensure you – the caregiver who has no time to get to your own doctor appointments – don't neglect your own medical health needs.

While these tools and services should never replace the advice of your love one's health care professional, such as a primary care physician, I think of them similar to how I use WebMD or Medline Plus (the library of health information from the National Institutes of Health). When I have an ailment or odd feeling, I immediately look up my symptoms on WebMD. I read everything I can and then I take this information with me to my doctor visit. Nine times out of 10, I have, with the help of WebMD, correctly identified my problem. While I would never skip the actual doctor appointment, it is nice to know reliable information can now be found on the Internet from certain trusted sources.

Online caregiving sources, such as WebMD and Medline Plus, help educate you and steer you in the right direction to ask those health care professionals more intelligent questions and give you better peace of mind when helping to make health care decisions with your loved one. These resources are supplemental to meeting face-to-face with your loved one's doctor and should never replace long-standing physician-patient relationships.

Another category of online resources and services falls into the growing sector called *telemedicine* or as I call it *virtual doctors* or *docs in a box*. Essentially telemedicine is exactly how it sounds – professional medical advice and services delivered via phone, video chat or email to bridge the distance when the patient and health care professional cannot be in the same room. According to the American Medical Association, 70 percent of doctor and ER visits are informational, and do not require face-to-face interaction.

Quickly becoming part of mainstream health care delivery, telemedicine is actually not a new concept. In the 1960s, NASA used telemetry to monitor the daily health of its astronauts during the space missions. A decade later, satellite technology allowed physicians to conduct consultations with residents in rural communities in Alaska and Arizona. In today's fast-paced world, telemedicine allows patients and family caregivers to ensure their health care needs are being met even if they cannot always get to the doctor's office.

Telemedicine should not be confused with telehealth which refers to clinical and non-clinical health information, administrative services and research information. Telemedicine is a consult with a clinical health care professional who can diagnose and write prescriptions. There are also nurse help lines, many provided through insurance plans, but telemedicine connects you with physicians who have more medical training in diagnosing conditions so weigh your options accordingly.

One caveat I have for some of the following resources is most do not accept personal insurance or Medicare reimbursement. While costs for the consult can vary, the cost is completely the responsibility of the person requesting the consult. In some instances, these telemedicine consults may be covered by an employer health benefit plan but be sure to check with your HR department before using these services if cost is an issue for you.

Following are some of my recommended online telemedicine resources that may be useful for non-emergency health care services:

My Consult – This online medical service connects you to top specialists in various disciplines including nutritionists and dieticians to give both your loved one and you a valuable second opinion when assessing health care advice. This service is offered by the prestigious Cleveland Clinic which was rated #4 in 2010 among all hospitals in the United States by the *U.S. News & World Report*. Essentially, this is a sophisticated, web-based extension of Cleveland Clinic's 90-plus-year role as one of America's most respected referral institutions.

The MyConsult program gives patients secure, online access to Cleveland Clinic's physician specialists for over 1,100 diagnoses. Getting a second opinion from Cleveland Clinic enables you to make the most informed decision about your health care or the health of your loved one. As cautioned, the cost of each consultation is a little steep (can be upwards of $565 depending on your condition) and it does not accept personal insurance or Medicare reimbursement.

MDLiveCare – An on-demand 24/7 network of health care professionals provides you access to board certified and licensed therapists and nutritionists. The virtual doctor visits are conducted via phone, video chat such as Skype or email and all are through secure networks to ensure the privacy and security of your health care information under HIPAA (Health Insurance Portability and Accountability Act) regulations.

You pay a fee per online consultation which can last up to one hour (about $40 per consult if you are a $10 per month subscriber; non-members pay $60 per consult). You can synchronize PHRs (personal health records) online via GoogleHealth or Microsoft's Health Vault.

AmeriDoc - Similar in service offerings to MDLiveCare, AmeriDoc physicians are required to undergo a formal review process every six months and are regularly assessed on patient feedback, a formal rating system, patient outcomes track records, and peer reviews from fellow network physicians. This site also provides patient advocacy services to communicate with doctors and health insurers and solve disputes or billing questions (you will read more about this type of service later in this chapter). Costs vary depending on type of consult or service after you sign on as a member.

RingaDoc - Similar to MDLiveCare in its medical consultation services, this network of physicians is part of Global Medical Networks and is the only service boasting doctors who are both English and Spanish speaking. Each doctor consultation is approximately $40 or there are annual membership programs providing a discount on the individual consultation cost.

Other players in this telemedicine sector include Zipnosis (whose CEO is the same person who started MinuteClinics, bought by CVS Pharmacy), Teledoc, AmericanWell and many more.

While no studies I could find prove telemedicine is as successful or better than in-person physician visits, it is wise to look to telemedicine consultations for simple routine issues – sinus or bladder infections, skin rashes, upper respiratory illness, sniffles or a cough – for yourself or your loved one.

The Avengers

Sometimes when wading through mounds of paperwork and insurance forms, you need a *superhero* on your side. Welcome to a whole new world of service providers cropping up to help you do just that.

Patient Advocate – These are professional services offered free of charge through a treating hospital or senior living facility that can solve every-day non-medical and non-health care-related problems for your loved one, such as getting a special lunch or getting an in-room TV fixed. Some define patient advocates as the liaison between patients and their health care providers, and sometimes get involved in navigating financial aid for patients and families. They help when your loved one is receiving treatment or living in a facility, thus you only receive this service while your loved one is *under their roof.*

The Patient Advocate Foundation (PAF) is a national nonprofit organization that provides patients and caregivers with arbitration, mediation and negotiation to settle issues with access to care, medical debt and job retention related to your loved one's illness or condition. The site also offers downloadable brochures, Web chats and Webinars on these topics. In addition, there are professional case management services for Americans with chronic, life threatening and debilitating illnesses to serve as active liaisons between the patient and their insurer, employer and/or creditors to resolve issues related to their diagnosis with assistance by doctors and health care attorneys.

Patient Navigators - (Also called Health Navigators or Health Advocates) – These services typically include caregiver education about the disease or disorder, advocacy in managing the maze of administrative paperwork and interfacing with insurance claims and provider billing departments. Some services also include complementary medicine, typically defined as nutritional counseling, meditation techniques and alternative therapies that complement traditional medicine. These services are paid for by the patient or caregiver and operate on hourly fees or service subscription packages.

One new entry in this category is CarePlanners started by Alan Blaustein, a successful entrepreneur who faced the frustrating and fragmented world of health care as he successfully battled cancer; and his long-time friend, Dr. Nancy Snyderman, chief medical editor for NBC News and caregiver to her older parents. CarePlanners manages health information and care coordination for the patient working with the member's health care providers and family caregivers. They also handle complicated billing, claims and insurance issues.

One example is a 94-year-old member, Charlotte Stern, who has spinal stenosis needing frequent spinal cord steroid injections. When the tragic outbreak of fungal meningitis causing more than 14 deaths occurred in 2012 because of problems with the compounding site providing the medication, CarePlanners immediately sprang into action. They confirmed Charlotte's steroid injections were not from the contaminated Massachusetts compounding company and contacted Charlotte's son to assure him his mother's injections were fine. "CarePlanners is a real gift to families," says Charlotte. "My son was frantic when this news broke, but CarePlanners called and took the weight off his mind without him even having to ask for their help."

Health Advocates – This service category varies but most are organizations that require membership fees. They become your *go to* source for help answering questions about a diagnosis, treatment, costs, insurance claims, etc. They will interface on issues with your health care insurance, Medicare and other health care professionals particularly on billing issues and insurance payments. This category provides peace of mind but at a cost to the caregiver or loved one.

Government Health Insurance Counselors – Typically offered through the State Health Insurance Assistance Program (SHIP), which was formerly known as the Information Counseling and Assistance (ICA) Grants Program. The SHIP offices are located in each state's capitol city, and offer free state-wide counseling services that help seniors and their caregivers understand Medicare and Medicaid benefits. Anyone can call these offices to ask questions of a volunteer advisor.

The SHIPs were created to ensure seniors and people with disabilities receive the counseling they need to take full advantage of their federal and state benefits under Medicare/Medicaid. They can answer questions about insurance options, medical bills and appeals, and Medicare. All states have a toll-free number to call and some states also offer face-to-face counseling by appointment. In some instances, you will see SHIP used interchangeably with other designations such as SHINE (Serving the Health Information Needs of Elders), HICAP (Health Insurance Counseling and Advocacy Program) and SHIBA (Statewide Health Insurance Benefits Advisor).

Even James Bond Needed **M**

In the James Bond movie franchise, Bond is the suave, shaken-but-never-stirred spy but it is **M** who is at the helm of the fictional Secret Intelligence Service known as MI6, who keeps Bond on track and often saves his life. **M** directs his missions and advises him on when danger lies ahead. (My favorite **M** is Judi Dench – magnificent in her cool, controlling style).

In your life as a caregiver, your **M** just may be a geriatric care manager (GCM). A professional GCM is trained in social work or some level of nursing care with additional, specialized credentials in elder care. GCMs will conduct an assessment of your loved one, her living environment and your caregiving role. From the assessment, they prepare a care plan, discuss it with the family, and if needed, help coordinate local home and community based services or make referrals. They can also typically help mediate family conflict related to caregiving situations and help coach you on how to have those tough conversations with your loved one.

What makes a GCM your special weapon in caregiving is their training in all aspects of elder care – not just the health aspect of getting older but the social, psychological and home and community based services aspects of aging – so their expertise goes beyond what a doctor or family therapist may be able to provide.

"GCMs are great resources for caregivers because they are integration specialists," says David Solie, author of *How to Say It to Seniors*. "Our health care system, and particularly elder care resources, is so fragmented, a GCM can help you map out a plan and understand all the moving parts." Solie also feels they are a caregiver's best resource when it comes to coaching caregivers on conversations which you will read more about in the C-A-R-E Conversations chapter.

Many GCMs can be contracted directly through the local Eldercare Locator listings of the Area Agencies on Aging or through the GCM professional organization, the National Association of Professional Geriatric Care Managers (NAPGCM). You can also find national agencies with local GCM services such as SeniorBridge, which in addition to its GCM network provides live-in home care, telecare delivered through remote monitoring (read more about this in The Jetsons chapter) and private daily nursing services.

Nora Jean Levin, executive director for the nonprofit organization Caring From a Distance says, "The only drawback about GCMs is not enough caregivers and people in general know about them."

If you are an employed caregiver you may want to also check with the HR department of your employer to see if your benefits package includes an Employee Assistance Program (EAP) or work-life benefit that may offer access to a GCM. For instance, UnitedHealthcare has a program called Solutions for Caregivers, which provides the services of a GCM to more than 500,000 employees nationwide through their employer benefit services. Genworth Financial also provides employer services, where participating employers can offer their workforce Care Advocates, Genworth's national network of professionals, part its CareScout division.

"We are definitely on the verge of senior living options and home based services taking the Angie's List approach but you can't get the personalized approach from the Internet," says Larry Minnix, CEO of LeadingAge. "In the same way we do banking online but when it comes to the personalized expertise needed to create an estate plan we sit down face-to-face with a financial planner, [working with a GCM or other professional] this will be the trend in aging." Minnix adds there really is no replacement for professional help such as a geriatric care manager because "you can't diagnose through the Yellow Pages."

Caregiver Checklist

- ✓ Know the *matchmaker* services that exist to help you in your search for in-home care or alternative housing for your loved one.
- ✓ Understand the benefits and limitations in using telemedicine to ensure you are getting to your doctor when certain serious health issues arise for both you and your loved one.
- ✓ Know the services to help you navigate hospital, medical insurance, Medicare/Medicaid and other complicated but important paperwork and issues.
- ✓ Consider the expert help of a geriatric care manager (GCM) who can save you time, money and give you peace of mind.
- ✓ Check with your employer to see if you have access to GCM help through a work-life or EAP benefit.

Lost in Translation

Health care literacy and expert support

One of the biggest challenges facing family caregivers is health care literacy. According to the Agency for Healthcare Research and Quality (AHRQ), 1 of every 10 adult Americans lacks the skills needed to manage their own health. Health care literacy is the ability to obtain and use health information, make informed choices and appropriate decisions, weigh the risks and benefits of different treatments, manage costs, understand insurance coverage and fill out complex medical forms.

A survey by Kelton Research and eHealthInsurance.com found:

- 43% could not explain what *deductible* meant
- 41% were unable to define *premium*
- Only 25% knew how to explain *coinsurance*
- 19% could not define the following common insurance terms: *out-of-pocket, open enrollment, PPO, HMO* and *HSA*
- More survey participants were able to state how much their monthly cell phone bill was versus knowing the monthly cost of their health care insurance premium

Caregivers are not dumb – quite the contrary. They are like foreign exchange students, who must first learn and understand the language and culture of health care. Then you will have no trouble speaking and reading this *new language.*

Part of the problem resides in our health care system. Sara Honn Qualls, professor of psychology at the University of Colorado at Colorado Springs says, "Unfortunately our health care system is very oriented toward the patient rather than the family context of a patient."

Dr. Qualls says even though the family caregiver may be the one needing to understand the results of tests, the prescribed therapies, the insurance implications, the next steps, two barriers emerge:

1. Privacy issues where the health care professional is held to privacy regulations under HIPAA. Once the patient has identified you as the caregiver the doctor is free to share this information with you. It is also important to be in the room with your loved one and their doctor to hear the same thing your loved one is being told. Until that is made clear, the caregiver is in this "awkward insider/outsider role" which makes it difficult for caregivers to get good information and just the facts.

2. Often health care professionals use technical jargon or reports are written with data a layman cannot understand. "For instance, if you have a neuro-psychological test report, it is written for other neuro-psychologists," says Qualls. "The information may be helpful but the caregiver does not understand it."

However, there is hope. If Rex Harrison could teach the *Cockney guttersnipe,* Audrey Hepburn, to speak like English royalty, well, by George, you too can become proficient at health care-speak.

Health care literacy has nothing to do with how many years of schooling you have had or your reading level. It has nothing to do with intelligence level but more to do with understanding prescription medication instructions, filling out insurance form claims, understanding a doctor's directions and providing consent for certain procedures. The reality of health care literacy is this: the less you know or understand, the more costs you or your loved one will incur and the more at risk your loved one's health is – it's elementary my dear Watson.

If all this sounds silly, consider this: a Georgetown University study found among adults who stayed overnight in a hospital in 1994, those with low health care literacy averaged six percent more hospital visits, and stayed in the hospital nearly two days longer than adults with higher health literacy skills.

What is your health care IQ and how you can you improve your score? Here are the basics:

- Visual literacy (understanding graphs and charts)
- Computer literate (understanding how to search the Internet and fill out online forms)
- Numeric and computational literacy (understanding how to calculate or reason with numbers)
- Verbal skills (not just the ability to speak but to speak up, ask questions and continue to probe until you understand and feel you have all the information you need)
- Listening skills (it is not just a matter of speaking up but also of listening carefully)
- Strong decision-making skills

Given this criteria, certain populations including those older Americans who are not computer-savvy, low-income individuals and minority or non-English speaking groups are more at risk for health care illiteracy. According to a study by the U.S. Department of Education 36 percent of adults have only basic or below-basic skills for dealing with health material and the Institute of Medicine reported that almost 90 million Americans lack basic health literacy and may be considered limited English proficient (LEP).

There is a safety risk when it comes to health care literacy. According to the National Patient Safety Foundation communication breakdowns are the leading source of medical errors and the health care literacy of patients and caregivers are critical to preventing these errors. Patients and caregivers have to be their own heath care advocates and need to ask these three essential questions of their health care professional in every health care interaction:

1. What is the main problem?
2. What do I need to do to help my loved one?
3. Why is it important to do this?

Improving your health care literacy IQ score includes educating yourself and having the health care industry meet you half way. There is a movement among health care professionals to create more *consumer-friendly* language in medical and health literature and to adopt this language in conversations with patients and caregivers. Many brochures and online data now contain icons to make it easier to interpret how the data provided relates to the different areas of health care. Think of it like *The Da Vinci Code* – icons and symbols are becoming the key to understanding our health care information.

While some health care professionals are making an effort to use simple words – the average American who has at least a high school education actually reads at a 7th or 8th grade level. It is up to you to ask a lot of questions. Many doctors use complicated medical terminology because that is how they were educated but these words are going to fly over your head because you did not go to medical school (or watch every TV episode of *ER* or *Grey's Anatomy*).

Caregiving's *60 Minutes*

Don't be intimidated to ask about anything you don't understand clearly. And remember to always be a *journalist*. As you will read in the stories of Joan Lunden and Alana Stewart, you want to have your notebook or your tape recorder, have your questions ready and be ready to ask a lot more, take a lot of notes and then you will have this information for future reference.

Any conversation requires effort on behalf of two people: caregivers need to hone their health care literacy comprehension and health care professionals need to learn how to communicate simply and effectively. The web site, Next Steps in Care, offers numerous fact sheets and questions to ask of health care professionals especially for the critical transitions from hospital to home with your loved one. The information was created by the United Hospital Fund in collaboration with 30-40 partner organizations including the Centers for Medicare and Medicaid Services (CMS).

"Caregivers are often the continuity factor in their loved one's care," says Carol Levine, director of the Families and Health Care Project at United Hospital Fund. She advises patients treated in a hospital setting are seen by a hospitalist who only looks after their acute care needs but does not have ongoing interaction with your loved one. In addition, hospital dispatch planners and social workers may provide the caregiver with a list of resources, medications to be taken, or the facility where a loved one is being transferred – all without much conversation taking place.

The hope is the hospitalist, your loved one's primary care physician, the social worker or case manager involved and perhaps the facility administrator are all talking to each other. The reality is typically it is the caregiver who is managing this *care coordination* ensuring all these different health care professionals have shared instructions and had discussions about your loved one. This requires caregivers understand the details of care and how to interpret them. You can read more about the transitions from hospital to home or skilled nursing or assisted living facilities in the Rehearsals chapter called Three Faces of Eve.

One way to maintain good records for your loved one (and for all your family members and yourself) is electronic health records (EHRs). Sometimes EHR is used interchangeably with EPR (electronic patient record) and EMR (electronic medical record). However, the U.S. Department of Health and Human Services (HHS) says these are distinctly different. EMRs and EPRs are used mostly by hospitals and health care providers and EHRs contain holistic health information not just medical information. The EHR may include a range of data, including medical history, medication and allergies, immunization status, laboratory test results, radiology images, vital signs, personal statistics like age and weight, etc. Although not yet experiencing widespread adoption, EHRs allow a caregiver to keep all records at your fingertips any time day or night. Many health care insurance providers keep some patient or member data electronically but a caregiver may not have access to this information unless your loved one has specifically designated you as someone who can access this information. You can also create and maintain your own records using online resources such as Google Health and Microsoft Health Vault.

Find Your Professor Higgins

There is also professional help in understanding the technicalities of health care information. Credentialed health care interpreters, health navigators, patient advocates and health advocates are available to help patients and caregivers understand complicated health care information. You will read more about this new group of professionals in the chapter My Man Godfrey.

One of the ways to stay health care literate is to keep up with trends in how the names of some functions or services will evolve. Many in the health care world see terminology changing in how we describe certain services or professional designations. Much of this change will be driven by the baby boom generation, many of which are not in *age denial* but definitely in *age defiance*. In years past, boomers have ushered in terminology such as all-natural, organics, disposable income, family values, self-expression, the good life.

Larry Minnix, CEO of LeadingAge, an association that supports older Americans, says baby boomers will change the health care terminology of today to fit their age defiance posture.

"The language of health care will change, a social worker will become a concierge, a therapist will become a health coach, a nurse aid will become a companion and today's senior citizen van will be a limo." Staying up to speed will require caregivers to get engaged and embrace the *lifelong learning* of caring for a loved one.

In the end, being a caregiver means being the best advocate for your loved one in discussions and dialogues with the health care world. The American Medical Association stated, "poor health literacy is a stronger predictor of a person's health than age, income, employment status, education level, and race." It is time for caregivers to learn the lingo and be heard.

Caregiver Checklist

- ✓ Find resources that can improve your health care literacy such as information from sources such as Next Step in Care or securing the help of a health or patient navigator.
- ✓ Become a journalist – ask a lot of questions, write down or tape record discussions with doctors and other health care professionals.
- ✓ Think about creating an electronic health record (EHR) to help you maintain your loved one's health history.
- ✓ A geriatric care manager (GCM) can help you understand and navigate health care options you don't understand.

Drugstore Cowboy

Medication safety and adherence

A business colleague recently told me a story about her 80-year-old parents. As they got ready to go to their favorite Italian restaurant, her mom asked her dad if he had taken his Lipitor medication (for managing cholesterol). Grumbling, he made his way to the bathroom, grabbed the pill bottle, swallowed the pill and they set off for their favorite fettuccini Alfredo dinner. Half way through their meal, her dad did a face plant into his pasta. Her mother thought he had a sudden heart attack and as she called the waiter to help and found they couldn't revive him, she thought her husband was dead. As the EMTs lifted him into the ambulance, he groggily came alive. My business associate got a call from her shaken mom who was at the ER. The doctors discovered he had taken his wife's Lunesta sleeping pills instead of the Lipitor for his cholesterol.

This could have been a scene out of an *I Love Lucy* skit – and the thankfully happy outcome still makes my colleague and I chuckle. However, taking the wrong medication is no laughing matter.

According to the *Journal of the American Medical Association*, more than 106,000 Americans die every year from adverse drug reactions – three times higher than deaths from automobile accidents. In addition, the CDC and FDA reported 177,000 seniors are hospitalized because they had taken their medications incorrectly. In fact, half of all prescriptions are taken incorrectly and this has now become the fourth leading cause of death in the U.S. In addition to all your other responsibilities and concerns as a caregiver, medication adherence and safety is another thing you can add to the list. However, unless you are there to administer the right prescription, in the right dosage at the right time, what is a caregiver to do?

"The two most important things for a caregiver who has a loved one coming home after being hospitalized is to have a medication management checklist and to remind themselves to keep it up to date," says Carol Levine, director of the Families and Health Care Project for the United Hospital Fund (UHF).

The UHF has a Medication Management Form downloadable in four languages from the Next Step in Care web site – a campaign UHF and the Centers for Medicare and Medicaid Services (CMS) collaborated on to help caregivers with the care transitions discussed in the Three Faces of Eve chapter. The Next Step in Care web site provides caregivers with valuable, important information on a variety of topics focused on transitioning loved ones from hospital to home. Podcasts, videos and checklists with questions to ask are invaluable to caregivers who have loved ones who are *treated and streeted* in hospital jargon. In other words, they discharge your loved one and you are on your own.

Something To Talk About

Another way to help manage your loved one's medication adherence is to take advantage of the latest tech gadgets for this purpose. In the old days (which in technology terms means 18 months ago), we used pill boxes that had the day of the week printed on them. Now we are well into the digital age and there is an endless supply of tech gadgets, products and services that can help caregivers help their loved one take the correct medication at the right time.

Among U.S. adults aged 65 and up, 40 percent take five to nine medications and 18 percent take 10 or more, according to a study published in the *New England Journal of Medicine*. With poor eyesight and possible forgetfulness, it's easy to understand why medication mix-ups can do more harm than good. While you should talk to your loved one's physician about their medication list and possibly *Just Say No* to some of the drugs if possible, for the prescriptions that do need to be managed there is help.

Tech to the rescue. A pill bottle cap from Vitality™, called GlowCap™, uses an embedded wireless GPS chip that provides an audible reminder. The GlowCap fits most prescription bottles and comes with a home hub device that illuminates and plays a ringtone when it's time to take the medication. Your loved one will get a reminder call from the service if the bottle is not opened two hours after a scheduled dose. The system also provides a weekly email to family caregivers or your loved one's physician with a medication adherence report and contacts the pharmacy for automatic refills. A clinical study by Partner Healthcare's Center for Connected Health found users of the GlowCaps had a 27 percent increase in their medication adherence.

While GlowCaps *talk to you* another device called Tabsafe® does everything except take the medication for you. This product cuts back on the caregiver needing to say to their loved one several times a day, "Did you take your meds?" The caregiver or health care professional receives this information remotely. In addition, Tabsafe allows the doctor or pharmacist remote control of the device so changes to the dispensing of medications can be managed as instructed by a pharmacist or doctor. The only drawback for many caregivers is cost. The device runs more than $1,000 with a monthly service fee. Some Medicaid programs in certain states will reimburse the cost and private insurers are evaluating reimbursement. However, Tabsafe estimates this cost outweighs the repeat hospital admissions from seniors not taking meds correctly. According to a study published in the *New England Journal of Medicine*, 66 percent of older adults over age 80 were hospitalized because of unintentional drug overdoses.

The future of medications becomes even more James Bond-ish with a prototype product from Accenture. They have developed a medicine cabinet with a built-in mirror with a camera and online computer with face recognition software. When you look in the mirror, you are greeted by name and the mirror will tell you if you are taking the right medication and automatically order refills. This completely changes the idea of "Mirror, mirror on the wall…"

Several other products that include a medication safety reminder communication function are also available. Some of these devices offer multi-function services including Presto℠, Celery®, Ceiva®, Independa™ and the Great Call® cellular service with the Jitterbug® phone. You will read more about these devices in the chapter called The Jetsons. Lastly, there are the low-tech products such as vibrating bracelets, watches and necklaces that remind your older loved one or child with diabetes it is time to take a medication or to test blood sugar.

"When it comes to technology to help ensure you or your loved one are taking your medications properly, the options are growing for caregivers," says Peter Radsliff, CEO of Presto and co-founder of AgeTek Alliance, a consortium of companies dedicated to aging technology development.

Love and Other Drugs

"A big issue for caregivers is re-admission of a loved one to the hospital because of drug interactions or medications not being taken properly," says Carol Levine of United Hospital Fund. She says often miscommunication is a culprit. When a physician or nurse talks to your loved one but not to you about medications – and you are going to be the one administering or helping administer the drugs – there is a gap in communication.

According to Levine, the reality is we are an over-medicated society. "In my experience, doctors are great at adding medications but not so great at taking them off the list," says Levine. She adds often your loved one may ask about a new medication and a doctor may prescribe it because it won't do any harm and actually may help. The issue according to Levine is the entire list of medications should be reviewed each time a new drug is being added to ensure it doesn't duplicate other medications and also to cut any unnecessary drugs off the list to make adherence more manageable.

One area that is particularly dangerous but seemingly safe is over-the-counter (OTC) drugs. Sometimes caregivers or loved ones believe because it is OTC it won't do any harm. Wrong. Not only are drug interactions an issue but dosages on the packaging may not be appropriate for your older loved one. Levine warns many medications are tested on people far younger than your parent or older spouse, and tolerance and the effect of a medication changes as we age.

Often we believe our doctors or even nurses are the best health care professionals to talk to about medications. However, many caregivers are finding pharmacists have more time to explain medications to a you, can walk you through any drug interactions especially with OTC drugs, and can review a complete medication list and make a recommendation with changes that can then be discussed with your loved one's physician. It is also helpful to have all your loved one's medications filled at one pharmacy chain so the pharmacist and the chain's computerized systems can help monitor drug interactions.

Lastly, Levine says medication names can be a hang-up for both caregivers and their loved ones. "The names used for brand drugs are typically easy to remember and have a *catchy* ring to them but generics are long, complicated, non-user-friendly names that anyone without a medical degree can't understand or remember."

This is just another reason to write it down or keep a medication list in an electronic health record (EHR) for easy reference. It is also wise to have this list handy at all times, such as keeping an electronic copy where you can access it with your smartphone or a printed copy in your wallet. This helps when you have to answer questions in an emergency for health care professionals or emergency technicians.

Altered States

One of my favorite refrigerator magnets is by the artist Anne Taintor who uses a vintage 1950s era advertising shot of a happy-looking housewife with the caption, "Medicated and Motivated." While we can laugh at the fact there seems to be a pill for everything these days, there is not a pill yet to relieve you of the stress and worry of being a caregiver. In fact, you may have a very different relationship with prescription or other drugs than your loved one. Theirs is need, yours may be dependency.

As I have discussed throughout the Casting Calls chapters, stress is a caregiver's biggest enemy. Each caregiver copes with stress in different ways but a National Alliance for Caregiving study showed 10 percent of caregivers whose health had declined were misusing or abusing alcohol or prescription drugs to cope with caregiving. In addition, Paul Lehrer, PhD, author of *Principles and Practice of Stress Management*, wrote that tranquilizers, antidepressants, sleeping pills and antianxiety medications exceed 33 percent of annual U.S. prescriptions. The use of prescription drugs to deal with caregiver stress, depression, insomnia and other issues are far more prevalent than most people realize.

Often caregivers feel undervalued, isolated from other family and friends, and overwhelmed. The sobering reality is they turn to drugs to cope. It can start as a glass of wine to de-compress from a stressful day, one glass becomes two and suddenly they cannot get through the day without their bottle of merlot. Or, they find themselves *Sleepless in Seattle* – insomnia is a huge problem for caregivers but taking a sleep aid can become addictive.

Another pitfall for caregivers is falling back into bad habits. Caregivers who had given up cigarettes years before, find themselves returning to these nicotine sticks to calm frayed nerves or take the edge off. What you are taking off is years of your life by jeopardizing your own health while caring for your loved one.

The best way to avoid this slippery slope of health risks and addiction is to ensure you have a support network you can talk to about your stress and challenges in caregiving. Being able to let off steam can provide amazing relief for the chaos of caregiving. In the chapter, LOST and Found, I will give you some great tips on how to find support online and at home.

Caregiver Checklist

- ✓ Have an updated list of your loved one's medications (names, why prescribed, dosages and frequency).
- ✓ Always ask your loved one's physician if newly prescribed medications are necessary and review the entire list of drugs your loved one is taking with their doctor.
- ✓ Check out the latest technology products that can help you and your loved ones ensure they are in medication compliance.
- ✓ Be aware if you are misusing prescription medications or other drugs to cope with the stress of caregiving and find help to avoid this *slippery slope*.

Breakfast At Tiffanys

Nutrition and meals for your loved one and for you

One of the most iconic images from film is Audrey Hepburn, elegant and slim in her little black dress and sunglasses pulling up in a taxi to Tiffanys on Fifth Avenue in Manhattan. As dawn breaks, she eats her Danish and drinks her coffee at her favorite place in the world. I can hear the lilting Henry Mancini theme song, *Moon River*, in my head as I write this.

Breakfast of any type is something many of our older citizens either miss or mismanage. It may surprise you to know more than 6 million Americans over the age of 60 suffer from malnutrition and hunger according to the Meals on Wheels Association of America (MOWAA). Good nutrition is something many of us struggle to maintain but when you are caring for an older loved one it is easy to overlook the fact she may not be eating properly or enough.

Some warning signs when it comes to your older loved one's appetite:

1. **I have trouble chewing** – Your loved one's dentures may not fit properly or she may need important dental work. You can also suggest she try eating softer foods.

2. **Food does not taste good anymore** - As we age our sense of smell and taste can change. Foods can taste flavorless or medications may leave an aftertaste in the mouth or depress our appetites. You may want to also check the refrigerator and cupboard to see if there are expired foods your loved one may not realize.
3. **I cannot get out to go shopping** – Your loved one may be fearful of driving or has trouble carrying groceries.
4. **It's too much trouble to cook for just one person** – Perhaps arthritis is prohibiting your loved one from handling pots and pans or she is depressed from being alone and chooses to not eat rather than cook.
5. **I'm just not hungry** - Your loved one may be suffering from indigestion, gas, stomach pain or has recently become lactose intolerant.

As we age our nutritional needs change. According to the National Institute on Aging, eating more fiber after age 50 can prevent stomach and intestinal problems such as constipation. Fiber can also help lower cholesterol and regulate blood sugar. Make sure you add fiber slowly into your loved one's diet to avoid gas (and it is not a bad idea to grab some high-fiber snacks for yourself).

Soul Food

Over the last 10 years, there has been a 79 percent increase in hunger among people age 50 plus according to an AARP Foundation report. Several others studies show seniors are often choosing between a hot meal or paying utilities or health care costs. If you are caring for a parent or other older loved one, hunger and malnutrition are cause for concern, especially if he or she is housebound.

Meals On Wheels president and CEO, Enid Borden, calls these older and disabled Americans "the hidden hungry." She says, "They are literally hidden from society and because we do not see them at food banks – they are behind closed doors because of mobility issues – a nutritiously delivered *meal*, not just food, can mean the difference between life and death."

The Meals On Wheels Association of America is comprised of 5,000 local groups that deliver nutritious meals across the country – even in hard-to-reach rural areas. "We deliver 1 million meals every day through the efforts of our 2.5 million volunteers," says Borden. However, Meals On Wheels delivers much more than just a nutritious meal.

Beyond the benefits to your loved one of a home-delivered, nutritious meal, services such as Meals on Wheels bring socialization as well. One of the biggest concerns caregivers may have about their loved one – whether it is an older parent or perhaps a disabled sibling – is isolation. This can be a problem for a loved one living alone at home because she recently lost a spouse or partner. When a housebound person does not have someone to talk to, does not attend church or synagogue or is not seeing friends regularly, this can lead to isolation and ultimately depression and other health issues.

Seeing a young volunteer regularly who delivers meals and checks in on your loved one can have positive impact for both generations – it is about food and friendship. The older loved one gets to look forward to a visit. The young volunteer gains newfound respect for the vulnerabilities of aging and feels uplifted in the gifts she brings. Ultimately, you, the caregiver, gain peace of mind not only that your loved one has a regular nutritious meal but also that she is having interaction and conversation to keep her spirits up. This is particularly important for the 7-8 million caregivers who may live long-distance from their loved one – sometimes hours or even a plane ride away.

Caroline Sorensen, a high school student in New York who volunteers with Meals On Wheels, recently told me, "I love knowing I made someone's day easier and happier." She has been a teen volunteer for Meals On Wheels through her school for the last four years. Borden believes meal delivery is nourishment for the soul – for the meal recipient and the volunteer.

The Breakfast Club

When it comes to children with autism and other chronic illnesses such as celiac disease (autoimmune disease triggered by the food component gluten that causes abdominal pain) and multiple sclerosis (an autoimmune disease attacking the central nervous system), there has been a lot of attention on gluten-free diets.

According to the Mayo Clinic, a gluten-free diet eliminates the protein gluten found in grains such as wheat, barley and rye. This also includes avoiding foods or beverages made with these grains such as bulgur, most pastas, soy sauce, french fries, cookies, matzo balls, potato chips, some salad dressings, soups and vegetables with certain sauces. A gluten-free diet can improve cholesterol levels, boost energy and promote digestive health.

You will read in Holly Robinson Peete's story she believes a gluten-free diet helped her son R.J. who is living with autism. In addition to gluten-free, some parents of children with autism believe in casein-free diets that eliminate milk by-products from the diet.

For those suffering from multiple sclerosis or looking for alternative medicine treatments for cancer, a recent trend is an alkaline diet. Over-acidity in the body can result in a host of chronic illnesses. By balancing the acidity in your system for proper cell function, you can reduce inflammation, boost the immune system and prevent premature aging. Alkaline diets involve eating certain fresh citrus and other low-sugar fruits, vegetables, nuts, and legumes. The diet recommends avoiding grains, dairy, meat, sugar, alcohol, caffeine, and fungi.

Guess Who's Coming to Dinner?

In addition to Meals On Wheels there are meal delivery services that can cater to the special dietary needs of diabetics, heart patients, those needing gluten-free meals, seniors, etc. Two of my favorites are:

1. **Mom's Meals** – This family-owned business delivers great tasting, high quality, fresh and nutritious meals throughout the United States. Everything is shipped fresh in a patent pending package and you can specify food for diabetics, gluten-free, vegetarian, low carb or heart healthy meals. Average cost per meal is $5.99 plus shipping and handling. Mom's Meals is dedicated to the senior nutrition and meal delivery market and currently works with numerous Area Agencies on Aging and providers across the United States as an approved home delivered meal provider (you can use a Medicaid waiver for this service).
2. **Dinewise** – Gourmet food meals ordered online. The home-delivered frozen meals are offered as part of a package where you choose several meals at the same time with average meal cost between $13 - $17 plus shipping and handling. Customers can order for their loved one and for themselves or for entire family meals.

Caregiver Happy Meals

It is not just our older Americans, people with chronic diseases or children with special needs who need to focus on good nutritional habits. Caregivers are at great risk of gaining or losing weight because they become overwhelmed with their caregiving responsibilities. In fact, almost 4 out of 10 caregivers reported weight management as an issue in a National Alliance for Caregiving survey.

Stress, which is a caregiver's No. 1 complaint, can cause caregivers to forget to eat or turn to bad habits such as downing an entire box of Oreos or hoovering half a pizza while standing up in the kitchen at 10 p.m. when you finally get a break.

Caregivers often have no time to focus on sound nutritional habits and choose instead a steady diet of fast food burgers, fries and tacos. You have only to watch the documentary *Supersize Me* to know where this path leads.

What should you eat and how do you manage this when you have no time? First of all, *super foods* will make you a caregiving superhero by increasing your energy level, helping you stay focused and alert and increasing your physical and emotional stamina. We know every body is different. Some of us have special nutritional needs to manage conditions such as diabetes, high blood pressure or arthritis. In many cases, weight gain can be attributed to a thyroid condition.

If you have not joined a weight loss center such as Weight Watchers or Jenny Craig but you experience rapid weight loss, this can be an indication of illness. And not getting enough calcium can make you more at risk for osteoporosis which can put you at risk for falls and bone fractures later in life.

Before you start any new diet, you should have a wellness exam by your doctor and talk to her about any fluctuations in weight. Always explain your role as caregiver so your physician understands the whole picture of what may be impacting your diet and body. She may feel you need a nutritionist's help since your time is limited to focus on proper nutrition. Your doctor, a nutritionist or a counselor such as those found at weight loss centers can be invaluable sources to help you stay in super caregiving shape.

You will read more about how stress affects cortisol levels in our bodies causing weight gain and you will review a list of super foods and other nutritional tips for caregivers in the Backdraft chapter.

Julie and Julia

Having the C-A-R-E Conversation with your loved one around nutrition and meals is not always easy. Again, it is important to emphasize maintaining proper nutrition helps both of you – it will keep her body as strong as possible, give her energy to do the things she wants, improve her mood, help with her risk of falls and all of this helps you as her primary caregiver. Read the C-A-R-E Conversation chapter for my tips on how to start this conversation with your loved one.

Caregiver Checklist

- ✓ Know the warning signs of why your loved one may not be eating enough.
- ✓ Understand your meal delivery options.
- ✓ Educate yourself about various diets to address different disorders (such as autism) or chronic illness (such as multiple sclerosis) and healthy senior nutrition.
- ✓ Maintain your own healthy diet to ensure you have the energy to continue to be a caregiver.

Nine to Five

Working caregivers and employer support

When it comes to working, caregivers are already putting in as many hours as any part-time or full-time job. According to the National Alliance for Caregiving (NAC), 1 in 4 caregivers spend 20 hours a week caring for a loved one while 13 percent spend more than 40 hours a week. Add to these statistics that 73 percent of caregivers actually DO hold a part- or full-time job and you have one very over-worked group of Americans.

According to the Bureau of Labor Statistics, today more than 51 percent of the workforce is age 40 or older – approximately 69 million workers – a 33 percent increase since 1980. By 2020, 1 in every 5 employees will be over the age of 55. In fact, every nine seconds a baby boomer turns age 63, and given the economic downturn and lost retirement savings, this means fewer boomers will be leaving their jobs. In addition, almost half of all U.S. employees are women, and 17 percent of all full- or part-time employees are also caregiving according to a Gallup/ReACT survey. These numbers will only grow as our population ages, and we have more parents to care for than children. When you add all these statistics together, you have a lethal caregiving cocktail that would knock any *Mad Men* character on his tush.

As our workforce, and population in general, gets grayer, Corporate America is facing a workplace crisis. What is alarming is the *silver tsunami* is approaching, the warning bells are going off but U.S. businesses are ignoring the signs. It is not unlike New Orleans when the category 4 hurricane, Katrina, approached the city and many officials knew the levees may not hold.

"One of the challenges for employers is those companies that do offer some services to support employees have these programs coordinated through human resource departments where the personnel are not trained on aging issues," says Gail Hunt, president/CEO of the NAC. "The lack of training and knowledge creates a gap in understanding the need and communicating the support available to its employee base who is caregiving."

According to the Society of Human Resource Management, over a decade ago 24 percent of U.S. companies offered its employees some type of elder care or caregiving assistance through an Employee Assistance Program (EAP) or work-life benefits. Some of the services employers have included: online and telephonic support for research and referral to elder care services such as transportation, Adult Day Care services, meal delivery or home health aides; on-site support groups; flex time; educational training such as *Powerful Tools for Caregivers*, a six-week comprehensive course for long-term care solutions and how to manage caregiver stress; in-person geriatric care management services and back-up respite care.

In the same way companies recognized working mothers needed more support on the job when women began joining the workforce in record numbers in the '70s and '80s, companies were beginning to recognize the growing need to support workers who were supporting their older parents. Yet today, with the biggest age wave our nation has ever faced approaching fast, less than half of these same employers – about 11 percent – maintain any type of support for these hardworking caregiving employees. There has been much discussion around why employers have cut back on caregiving services in recent years, not the least of which point to the continuing sluggish economy and intense pressure on companies to trim costs where they can.

While the demographic and caregiving statistics point to these employee benefits as essential, the reality is utilization of caregiving benefits remains below 2-4 percent on average and thus, are difficult to justify as continued benefits by most human resources departments. The utilization problem may not point to a lack of need or interest from employees but rather lack of good internal communication these services exist, lack of self-identification among caregivers and concern by working caregivers the stigma of being identified as a caregiver may make them a target for a lay-off, if they are perceived as being less productive.

Productivity and Preventing Chronic Illness

For years, the argument to maintain caregiver support in the workplace has focused on employee productivity and impact to the bottom line. With many working caregivers also put in 20-40 hours a week providing care to a loved one, studies show U.S. business suffers from a $33 billion annual loss due to the productivity issues of caregiving employees. These workers have to leave work early or come in late, take time at work to conduct research or make phone calls on behalf of their loved one. But the real news is in the health care costs of caregiving employees.

A study conducted by the MetLife Mature Market Institute and NAC showed because of the health impacts of caregiving that typically arise from chronic stress, depression and burn-out, caregiving employees cost employers on average 8 percent more than their non-caregiving employee colleagues in terms of their health care coverage costs. The MetLife/NAC studies make an argument that caregiver services provided through employers may improve productivity as well as improve overall workforce health and wellness and ultimately save employee costs for U.S. businesses.

In this tough job market, caregiving employees are definitely feeling the need to *stay in the closet* when it comes to their caregiving responsibilities. Another NAC study showed since the economic downturn, 50 percent of caregiving employees were less inclined to ask their boss for time away from work to care for their older loved one. In addition, according to the *The Shriver Report: A Woman's Nation Takes on Alzheimer's*, 46 percent of female respondents wanted time off for caregiving but could not get it.

Sacrificing the Future to Care Today

While many families are still struggling in this economy, a working caregiver may be the one keeping food on the table. For those working caregivers who feel the need to leave the workplace, this may jeopardize their own retirement savings. In the same MetLife/NAC study on working caregiver health care costs, caregivers who left their jobs to continue to care for a loved one suffered greatly – lost individual wages and benefits, such as Social Security, averaging from $283,716 to $324,044 for a typical caregiver.

All of this would seem to spell doom for working caregivers, especially Boomer women. Since women represent 50 percent of the workforce and are 66 percent of the nation's caregivers, women are at a particular disadvantage. However, numerous studies show flexible workplace policies – similar to those to support working moms – help caregiving employees achieve a better work-life balance, enhance employee productivity, reduce absenteeism and improve employee wellness. Employers benefit from reduced employee health care costs, and these programs can aid recruitment and retention efforts. Caregiving advocates believe the positive results borne out over past decades for employers that adopted child care services and flex time for working moms will yield the same positive results if implemented for working caregivers.

The American Psychological Association (APA), which polls Americans each year on stress impacts in its *Stress in America*™ surveys, found 36 percent of Americans experience chronic work stress. Based on this fact, the APA began working with companies to find ways to de-stress employees without the use of prescription drugs. For example, one company working with the APA, is holding a meditation class.

Many industries and our entire health care system would be seriously impacted if caregivers had to give up their jobs to care for older loved ones or decided they cannot juggle a career and caregiving. Today, caregivers are the lynchpin in a fragile health care system – they provide 80 percent of the long-term care to keep an older loved one living at home as independently as possible. In addition, caregivers make or influence 79 percent of all care-related purchases in an $800 billion annual market – everything from health care insurance and prescription drugs to durable medical equipment, home health aides and home safety improvements, etc. Losing the caregivers on either side of the corporate divide spells disaster.

The solutions are clear and both employer and caregiving employee have a role in making caregiving a life event that does not have to become a life-threatening event. Here are my recommendations and some solutions for each group's role:

Employers – U.S. companies need to view its workforce as one of its greatest assets. By acknowledging the realities of an aging workforce and supporting working caregivers, companies will enhance their bottom lines. Some areas employers can address are the training of supervisors and HR departments on caregiving discrimination issues, such as demoting, not promoting or laying off employees who have acknowledged their caregiving role and responsibilities to their manager. Some of these workplace issues are addressed by the U.S. Equal Employment Opportunity Commission *Best Practices for Workers with Caregiving Responsibilities Report*.

In addition, holding health fairs, educational events and webinars and encouraging workplace support groups give employees tools and support for their caregiving role. And allowing for more telecommuting, which can help long-distance caregivers who want to move closer to older parents without losing their job, or a simple flex time policy would help working caregivers remain productive and valuable outside of the confines of a *Dilbert* 9 to 5, five-day a week, cubicle work environment. Employers will do well to sympathize rather than stigmatize caregiving employees.

Caregivers – Individual responsibility in a caregiving situation requires balancing self-care while caring for a loved one. Sometimes this is easier said than done. Employees should start by asking about the services their employer may provide to get the help they need.

Employees should also familiarize themselves with The Family Medical Leave Act (FMLA). This program provides 12 weeks of unpaid time off in a 12-month work period and 26 weeks for caregivers of military service men and women (exceptions are California, Connecticut, Hawaii, Maine, Minnesota, New Jersey, Oregon, Rhode Island, Vermont, Washington, Wisconsin and the District of Columbia, which do provide some pay over that period) with job protection when caring for an ill or injured parent or spouse. However, if you are a lesbian, gay, bisexual or transgender (LGBT) caregiver, you may face ongoing inequality as compared to heterosexual, married couples when it comes to FMLA. On a national level FMLA does not recognize LGBT couples; however some states (such as California, Maine and Oregon) as well as some employers make different allowances for FMLA.

In the end, if you do not maintain your own health and wellness, statistics show you can become too fatigued or ill to care for your loved one – and then who will provide that care?

Caregiver Checklist

- ✓ Know the services and benefits your employer may provide through an EAP or work-life program to help you in your caregiving journey.
- ✓ Know your rights and benefits under FMLA.
- ✓ Find support – through respite care, Adult Day Care, or create an online community for volunteer help of family and friends – to help you carry the load at home, at work and as a caregiver.

The Jetsons

Aging and technology

Who can forget the 1960s TV cartoon, *The Jetsons* – the space age equivalent to *The Flintstones*? The cartoon originally aired for two seasons, but was rebooted in the 1980s and can still be seen on cable channels, The Cartoon Network and Boomerang. *The Jetsons* is an obvious choice for a chapter on aging and technology – the cartoon supposedly took place in 2062 where robotic contraptions, holograms and innovative inventions made life easier. What you will see as you read this chapter is technology is going to make our lives easier: keep us safe, keep us connected (including grandparents with grandkids), keep us healthy and keep us feeling relevant as we age. This is great news for older Americans and great news for caregivers.

"This is an exciting era to be in your 70s, 80s, 90s or even reaching age 100," says Jeff Cole as we discussed what tech can do to help caregivers. Cole is executive director for the USC Center for the Digital Future, and he travels the world advising companies and heads of state on technology advances for our rapidly aging global societies. "Technology can help people avoid isolation, maintain family relationships, feel confident loved ones who live near or far are doing all right, and connect us to each other and the world."

Whether it's a wristwatch that can make a call to you if your loved one has fallen, an Apple® iPad® app that helps your non-verbal autistic child take control and communicate, an ink jet printer or medicine cabinet that can remind you or your spouse to take your medication at the right time in the right dosage, a walking shoe with a built-in GPS that advises you if your loved one with Alzheimer's has wandered too far from home, or finally a robot that can help you transfer a loved one from bed to bath to wheelchair. This technology is not the future – it's here today.

One of the driving factors in how fast this technology will become available to all families is cost. We know prices for gadgets and other tech products start on the high end for early adopters and gradually decrease as the masses make them more popular. When it comes to aging technology, a report from the AARP Foundation examined the attitudes toward technology of people age 65 and older as well as their family caregiver. The study found both groups have a willingness to try technology such as home security services, sensors to detect falls and devices to regulate temperature, lights and appliances. But cost remains a factor, with 75 percent of caregivers and 80 percent of those over 65 not willing to fork out more than $50 per month for the service.

Eric Dishman, an Intel Fellow and general manager of the Intel Health, Strategy and Solutions Group, believes technology and who pays for it will fall into two main categories: those products we purchase as consumers that aid things such as safety and communication and those services and devices that fall into a medical bucket we have come to expect will be covered by our health insurance plans.

From Green to Gray

But regardless of who pays, Dishman believes the baby boomer generation who are caregivers today and will need care in the future will "transform health care and take caregiving from a silent majority to a vocal, mobilized effort." Dishman, who has been a global leader, guru and advocate for technology that will help us live independently in our homes longer, calls this the tipping point of a new evolution. "Just as we had the environmental and global warming movement with green technology, we now have a global aging movement where 'gray technology' will help caregivers." The shift will happen when more caregivers start demanding tech tools to help them in their role.

"We're still an ageist society," says Dishman. "We've improved, but by and large we're still a youth-obsessed culture and high tech in particular is a youth-fueled industry." He also points out the gender gap for caregiving tech development. "Most start-up companies that are creating innovative technology are dominated by male engineers who are not on the frontlines of caregiving every day like the women in the workplace and in the home."

Dishman related a story to me about a meeting he had many years ago to secure funding for Intel caregiving technology development – concepts which were very innovative for that time.

After the presentation, he said the lead executive, a man, responded that no one was going to be really interested in these concepts. Dishman asked him right in the middle of the meeting to call his wife. He said after he explained the technology to her if she didn't like it, Dishman would stop asking for funding. Astonished, Dishman says to the executive's credit he did just that, he called his wife right then and there. As Dishman explained to the executive's wife what he wanted to do, she had Dishman put her husband back on the phone and told her husband this was the first time in his 25-year career at Intel he would actually develop something she needed. She was caring for her mother-in-law at the time. Dishman got his funding.

"This is an illustrative story that shows it's not malice, it was just that the caregiving his wife was doing was completely invisible to him," says Dishman. "He is at work all day and he doesn't see that she's at work all day with a caregiving job. It took that jarring of his consciousness to say 'Wait a minute, if my wife is going through this maybe millions of other people are as well.'"

In fact, what I found fascinating is many of these tech pioneers have either been or are caregivers or are dealing with aging challenges themselves. Eric Dishman was a 16-year-old caregiver for a grandmother who had Alzheimer's; Martin Cooper, the global telecommunications innovator and undisputed creator of the cell phone at Motorola wanted his mother and anyone else with special needs to have a better phone so he gave input to his wife Arlene Harris, also a telecommunications pioneer, who created the Jitterbug®; Peter Radsliff, who heads up Presto℠ and is co-founder of the AgeTek Alliance helped care for an aging father; Tim Rowe, head of Vitality™, created the GlowCaps™ pill bottle caps because he wanted a better way to remind himself to take his cholesterol medication; Susan Ayers Walker, managing partner of SmartSilvers Alliance cares for a husband with a chronic illness. The personal caregiving stories abound and it is this personal experience that is driving the technology breakthroughs we see.

Caregiving Tech

Laurie Orlov, market research analyst who offers comprehensive insights and updates on her Aging in Place Technology Watch blog identifies four categories for technology to help caregivers:

1. Home Safety and Security
2. Health and Wellness
3. Communication and Engagement
4. Contribution and Learning

Orlov predicts the aging tech marketplace, which today is a $2 billion industry, will grow to be a $20 billion industry by 2020. A 2010 report by Berg Insight, which offers premier business intelligence to the telecommunication industry, reported the home monitoring and safety industry is $9.88 billion and growing nine percent every year. According to other studies, 79 percent of these purchases will be made by a family caregiver.

One of the drawbacks of writing about technology in a book, is the technology and costs will change faster than I can get this book published. Or as Susan Ayers Walker put it so perfectly, "Here today, gone tomorrow."

One of the things that won't change or go away is our need as caregivers to want to keep our loved ones safe. Falls are a major health risk for older loved ones. According to the Centers for Disease Control every 29 minutes an older American dies from a fall at home. And yet, caregivers cannot be hovering over their loved one 24/7.

"Maintaining dignity, mobility and quality of life is what is going to be important as we age," says Ayers Walker. "The most important thought for every caregiver is how do I keep my loved one safe?"

Home Safety and Security

Aging in place – living in our homes as long and independently as possible – goes hand in hand with the concept of universal design, which is the idea that products, services, homes, etc. should work for us whether we are age 18 or 80 (for more on universal design in your home see the chapter Cocoon). Many of the technology companies focused on addressing the needs of an aging population are beginning to embrace this concept of universal design. A great example of universal design, while not *techie*, is the OXO Good Grips® brand of home kitchen utensils. Originally developed by an engineer for his wife who suffered from arthritis, these gadgets, found in most U.S. kitchens, are actually beneficial to anyone at any age.

However, as Ayers Walker pointed out, "Safety first."

Personal Emergency Response Systems (PERS)

The days of the old TV commercial, "I've fallen and I can't get up" are as old as rabbit ears on your TV. There is an emerging category in the aging technology space called Personal Emergency Response Systems (PERS) and Mobile PERS (MPERS). Many of these products include a GPS-like tracking device and a service, typically through a cellular provider, to help family caregivers keep their loved one safe by alerting the caregiver immediately if a loved one has fallen. This is a huge leap for caregivers. Older electronic safety pendants worn around the neck required the loved one to push a button and talk to an operator for help. However, if your loved one hit their head or was unconscious, it made the device as powerless as Superman coming into contact with kryptonite.

These new PERS and MPERS devices come in different forms such as a watch, a belt clip, a lavalier or even a walking shoe. Companies in this category include Intel/GE Care Innovations™, Lifecomm™ (a joint venture among Qualcomm, Hughes Telematics and American Medical Alert), the Alzheimer's Association ComfortZone® location management service and device, and others. SecuraTrac® is one company that offers mobile technology to track an older loved one, a child or a lost pet – marketing itself as a safety device for the family member who is missing – a great example of universal design *and* messaging.

Many of these products are enabled for two-way communication so family caregivers and their loved one can agree to a set perimeter called a *geofence* or *virtual wall*. As opposed to older PERS devices, which do not work far from the home base they were connected to, GPS-enabled technology allows for the wearer to travel whatever set distance is desired – whether a few blocks to the local grocery store, or church or synagogue or even further – where everyone feels comfortable. If the perimeter is broken, a warning signal is sent to the caregiver's smartphone or computer via text, email or in some service packages, an actual phone call. Google Maps finds the GPS signal and gives the caregiver the exact location of their loved one. The stories on the TV news of worried families unsure of where their loved one has wandered off to are over – it is PERS and MPERS devices to the rescue.

Most of these products have three separate costs involved: the cost of the device, the cost of the service (typically a monthly service charge similar to a cable or cell phone service) and for some, an activation cost.

Robotics

In the blockbuster *Star Wars* movies, robotic droids such as C-3PO and R2-D2 assist their human counterparts, Luke Skywalker and Han-Solo, to save their planet from the Death Star. This futuristic vision dreamed up by genius filmmaker, George Lucas, is no longer the future; it is the present, especially when it comes to addressing the safety and health needs of an older population. We know 85 percent of senior Americans currently live at home, and more than 29 percent of them are living alone. Bring on the robots.

It should surprise no one that Japan, the country that leads the world in technology innovation and an ever-increasing aging population, would be ahead of the curve when it comes to robotic assistance in caregiving. By 2015, one in four Japanese citizens will be over age 65, which has shifted this country's focus into high gear to respond aggressively to the need for age-friendly technology.

"In the early days, I used to think, are you guys nuts? No way are older people going to be interacting with robots," was Dishman's reaction years ago to some of these prototype droids. "The reality has proved me wrong." Dishman says the goal is not to replace the human contact for aging or ill loved ones but he is also realistic with an ever-growing older population, some people may need robotic assistance.

There is a robotic bathtub to help people with disabilities wash without more than one assistant. Or you can trade in your live pet for Paro, a robot that resembles a baby seal and has sensors to react to touch, light, sounds and voice recognition. Paro is being tested on those with Alzheimer's and autism to act as a replacement for a real pet. In trial studies conducted among residents at Vinson Hall Retirement Community in McLean, Va., the Paro robot, which has been in therapeutic use since 2007, shows it reduces a patient's cortisone levels, an indicator of stress.

Pearl the Nursebot is being tested at Carnegie Mellon University as a replacement for a home health aide to lift a loved one out of bed or wheelchairs, feed a patient and help older loved ones exercise limbs to prevent atrophy. A special battlefield extraction and retrieval robot is being tested to lift wounded soldiers off dangerous battlefields. Panasonic has piloted tests with a hairstyling robot that has 16 fingers to shampoo, rinse, condition, blow dry and otherwise manage your older loved one's beauty salon needs.

And a robotic suit known as HAL (Hybrid Assisted Limb) is being tested in Japan on Parkinson's and spinal cord injury patients that will allow them to improve their strength by 10 times. The patient gets strapped into a robotic skeleton that uses sensors attached to the wearer's skin to react to nerve impulses and essentially move their arms and legs accordingly. A nursing home patient who has been wheelchair-bound for two years was able to walk with the suit.

"Even when robots become more affordable, I don't think they will replace a live caregiver, but they will supplement the activities caregivers perform," says Center for the Digital Future's Jeff Cole. "Assisting older people so they don't fall or transferring a loved one so a caregiver can avoid back pain in lifting a loved one is where robotics will make a difference."

While all these devices are still in trial, cost thousands of dollars and are not available to the masses, it is only a matter of time before C-3PO or R2-D2 will be helping us out at home. May the Force be with you.

Health and Wellness

When it comes to managing our health and wellness needs, Larry Minnix, CEO of LeadingAge, believes we are moving from an institution or product-centric model to a patient-centric model. "We want our health care delivered in the home." The era of doctor house calls may be returning it is just they will be *virtual* doctor house calls.

Remote Monitoring

Long-distance caregivers, those caring for loved ones in places where weather can be a deterrent for a loved one to keep a doctor appointment, and caregivers who want to skip the hours-long trip to the doctor with their loved one taking them away from work, after-school pick-ups and other activities will all love remote monitoring.

In a study conducted by the National Alliance for Caregiving and UnitedHealthcare, 7 out of 10 caregivers said they would like a product that can provide some type of remote monitoring to ensure their loved one is safe or so they can track their medication adherence and vital health statistics. On the care recipient side of this conversation, almost half of Americans age 65+ surveyed by AARP said they are interested in technology that keeps them safe – things such as preventing falls, turning off the stove if they forget, regulating the thermostat automatically, etc. Forty-six percent of these older Americans also reported they would be willing to give up a little privacy to have a monitoring device that alerted their family or others when they needed help.

While home safety monitoring is not a new concept (just think nanny cams for child surveillance), many seniors are rightfully resistant to being watched as if they have reverted back to being children who cannot be left alone. What I have told caregivers is when having the conversation with an older loved one about remote monitoring, you have to mind your *P*s (forget the Qs). You want to change the conversation from *privacy invasion* to *protection* and *prevention* for them and *peace of mind* for both of you.

Remote monitoring is a wide-ranging category with everything from sensor-infused carpets to check a loved one's gait and risk for falls, also known as magic carpets or smart carpets, to systems that can detect when a stove has not been turned off or a door left opened and will adjust the problem automatically.

Intel has been an innovator in this category and has merged its development efforts with another pioneer in this space, GE, to form Care Innovations™. One of its remote monitoring devices, the Care Innovations™ Guide, is the next generation in telehealth by connecting your loved one with her doctor or health care professional such as a nurse practitioner so daily monitoring of vital signs can be done remotely. Installed on any device that runs Microsoft® Windows® 7 with a secure digital (SD) card slot and a webcam, the Guide will take biometric measurements, provide instructional videos for more information on your loved one's condition and allow for virtual doctor visits through video chats in the comfort of your loved one's living room.

Care Innovations have also pioneered a motion sensor device, QuietCare®, which uses wireless monitoring technology to help caregivers stay informed of loved one's movements within the home environment. The system is unobtrusive allowing maximum freedom to your loved one while simultaneously providing you with data analyzing anomalies in her routine to allow you to identify accidents before they happen or respond faster to serious issues such as falls, which puts 2 million seniors into emergency rooms every year.

There are also everyday items that offer built-in safety features. Smart canes developed by the Oregon Health & Science University detect gait, pressure and other warning signs and sound an alarm if there is danger from a fall. Home for Life Solutions offers equipment that will turn off a stove, using a built-in motion detector, if the user forgets. Even slippers can have a safety feature. AT&T ran a clinical trial with Texas Instruments using SmartSlippers, produced by 24eight, designed for older Americans. The slippers cost about $100 and come with a cellular plan for $25 per month that allows the slippers to send messages to a caregiver. If the wearer's walk becomes wobbly, an accelerometer in the sole – the same technology that makes some smartphones' screen respond to moving it sideways – will send a text to a family member or the wearer's physician.

Companies such as Philips Lifeline, ADT®, MedicAlert®, LifeStation®, BeClose®, Grandcare Systems™ and others have created numerous offerings in the remote monitoring and safety segment of aging technology. Even Maxwell Smart and Agent 99 would be impressed.

Fitness Tech

When we think of Nintendo®, we think of Super Mario™ Bros. or Tetris® and only as they relate to boys under age 15; at least until the Wii Fit™ came along. Since the Wii Fit comes with a balance board and affords the type of low-impact exercise critical for older loved ones or caregivers who cannot get to a gym, it is a dream come true for more than kids.

The Wii Fit encourages the user to stretch and move joints that could otherwise become stiff. Because it has been designed as a game, participants receive stimulation that encourages them to continue and to return for more each day. There are also real social benefits. Assisted living facilities across the country hold Wii bowling parties for 80, 90 and 100-year-olds. The benefit is not just for kids or older adults – it's universal physical fitness for all ages.

However, Microsoft has upped the ante of its Nintendo competitor when it comes to Xbox® advantages. Announced in 2010 (with a Windows PC version announced in 2012), the Kinect® allows users to toss the game controller and use your voice or gestures to command activities in the software and on the screen – completely hands-free. Although marketed as a video game fan's dream come true, the Kinect is also being used to assist cardiac surgery rehabilitation patients through the Esoma Exercise System. Patients wear sensors while playing games to monitor heart rates and blood oxygenation that is then communicated to physicians for monitoring and health coaching.

In addition to remote monitoring and games for health, technology is making great strides in medication safety and compliance. Whether a pill bottle cap with a GPS chip that communicates to caregivers when medications are not taken, or a medicine cabinet that has facial recognition software to remind you to take your medications or that you already have taken it – technology will again make a difference for caregivers in avoiding the 125,000 deaths of older Americans that happen every year and the 1 million seniors who are hospitalized because they incorrectly took their prescription.

A company called Independa™ combines social connectivity such as Facebook, email and calendars of events like birthdays or church outings with safety reminders prompting loved ones when to take medications. Originally developed for computers and tablets, Independa is piloting a program with LG on new TV sets using the TV's remote control. You can read more about these specific medication safety technologies in the chapter Drugstore Cowboy.

Communications and Engagement

Did you know 48 percent of Americans over the age 75 have a cell phone, and that number grows every year? When it comes to communicating, technology is making it a lot easier for caregivers and older loved ones to stay in touch.

Call Me

The Jitterbug cell and new smartphone with Great Call® service is another example of a product known as great universal design. The phone meets the needs of an older customer but really offers features we all love – larger buttons, larger numbers on the screen, easy *on* and *off* buttons, powerful speakers for clear sound – even when using the phone with a hearing aid.

The phones are stylish in design and come in different colors – I love the red version created for the American Heart Association's *Go Red for Women* campaign. The Great Call service is something I wish all cell phones and smart phones would offer – no contracts, no cancellation fees and some safety features such as a 24/7 LiveNurse app, pre-scheduled medication reminders and the new 5Star Urgent Response for immediate 24/7 help in any unsafe situation – kind of like Onstar® in your car but this is *help in the palm of your hand.*

On an interesting note, when I talked to Martin Cooper, who consulted to his wife Arlene Harris the inventor of the Jitterbug, he says there is a myth that he was inspired to create the first cell phone for Motorola back in 1973 from watching Captain Kirk on TV's *Star Trek* use his communicator. In fact, the motivation for the invention of the handheld cell phone was a belief that people are fundamentally and naturally mobile; that belief preceded Star Trek by many years (a true case of art imitating life).

One tip about when the phone can be used as an early warning system for caregivers was included in a TEDMED presentation Eric Dishman gave in 2009. At this annual VIP gathering of the world's visionaries on health and medicine, he advised caregivers to be aware of *quiet voice* with a loved one. If you notice your older loved one is talking a lot lower or quieter than normal, this can actually be an indicator of early Alzheimer's or Parkinson's disease. The message here is to LISTEN to our loved ones – they may be telling us more than just what we think we hear.

Smile

Videochat and Skype™ are game changers for caregivers. One caregiver I talked to said she loves Skype because, "Now I can see my 84-year-old father-in-law and see if he is doing all right rather than just talking to him over the phone." He is using a Telikin computer with built-in easy interface and touchscreen technology that allows him to use a computer without having to manipulate a mouse with arthritic hands. This technology is also great for long-distance caregivers and for keeping families connected. One older woman I spoke to in an assisted living facility in New York told me she has weekly video chats with her college-age granddaughter who is studying in Italy.

Two other products that are communication devices disguised as a digital photo frame and an ink jet printer are Ceiva® and Presto, respectively.

Ceiva, started by two former Disney executives, is a simple way for family and friends to share digital photos with older loved ones. Anyone can send a photo and messages from Facebook, a smartphone or email to the Digital Photo Receiver and the service connects through the Internet or the phone line. Images and messages are automatically displayed in the frame. In addition to photos, Ceiva has different channels such as its Foodista.com channel from which recipes, such as those for diabetics, can be automatically delivered to the frame.

Presto is the perfect computer-less solution if you want to share emails or digital photos with your older loved one or ensure your loved one has email about important medication reminders or other health information. Even if your loved one is not computer-savvy, he can still receive or send digital photos without the hassle of a computer hook-up. Presto is a printing mailbox and mail service all-in one with everything automatically printed. Your loved one does not need to learn anything new. Each Presto printer/service comes equipped with its own email address and your loved one receives easy-to-read, beautifully formatted emails via the printer's telephone connection without interfering with your loved one's existing landline telephone line.

Contribution and Learning

While there are numerous products that fit into this category, including DriveSharp from Posit Science® for brain health and honing your driving ability as you age, the wonders of the digital age have opened up a whole new world for caregivers and their loved ones.

Tablets and eReaders including the iPad and Kindle are two devices Jeff Cole believes are making a huge difference for older Americans. "Being able to adjust font size on your eReader, having an audio function for audio books, using touchscreens instead of a mouse for dexterity issues – all these are keeping us connected and relevant to the world as we age."

One of the tough challenges caregivers face is isolation, both for themselves and their loved ones. Devices which keep older Americans connected and up-to-date on world events and news are essential to combating this issue.

It's not just older Americans who benefit from the latest technology. The HollyRod Foundation has a campaign to donate iPads with learning apps to children with autism. Fifty percent of children with autism spectrum disorder have extreme difficulty learning to speak and half of those actually never will. While these individuals have difficulty communicating, they have much to say. Traditional Alternative Communication Devices on average cost around $8,000 but the Apple iPad along with specially designed communication apps, allow those with autism the ability to speak for a total cost of under $1,000.

In addition to the technology, several organizations in different communities are connecting younger *tech tutors* with older Americans. The Motion Picture and Television Fund has computer tutors for its members; volunteers of all ages who help seniors create Facebook pages, create email addresses, search the Internet for information and troubleshoot tech issues in the home. Pace University has a nursing school program where college students are paired with seniors in assisted living facilities to help them navigate learning about the Internet and social networking online. When I produced and hosted my TV show, *Handle With Care,* for the RLTV cable channel we showcased this program. The star of our program was 84-year-old Tony who had never used a computer before meeting his college tutor, Daniel. Tony was a lifelong subscriber and reader of the *New York Times* but as soon as Daniel taught him about reading the paper online or going to CNN.com on his Telikin computer, Tony was hooked and cancelled his 60-year subscription.

When it comes to the many technology advances for how we will live better, longer and easier, our higher learning institutions are rallying behind the needs of a graying society including universities and innovation labs such as those found at Carnegie Mellon Quality of Life Technology Foundry, MIT AgeLab, Oregon Center for Aging and Technology and Georgia Tech University.

As Jim "Oz" Osborn, executive director of the Quality of Life Technology Center at Carnegie Mellon University, said at a boomer technology conference I co-produced, "Getting older is a challenge and the possible ways to mitigate that have to do with technology…we're big on robots, we're big on connectedness, we're big on mobile apps, we're big on virtual coaches."

There's an App for That

A survey from VibrantNation.com on Boomer age women (who make up the majority of caregivers) found they will pay top dollar for gadgets that make their lives easier – 28 percent planned to purchase an iPad and 83 percent are using smartphones for functions other than a telephone including apps and calendar features.

Several apps for smartphones are created specifically for caregivers such as Elder 411 and Elder 911 from Presto in collaboration with Dr. Marion Somers, offering caregiver tips and checklists; Caregiver Apps, is an aggregator of the best apps being offered for caregiving; Caregiver's Touch, an organizational tool for caregivers to store personal health records (PHRs) and medical professional contact information; Easy Connect coming from Early Bird Alert™, will offer an app that is a health care hotline including instant connection to health care providers, transportation services and other lifestyle activities personalized for your loved one.

Attention Caregiving Shoppers

My biggest frustration in this wonderful world of technology for caregivers is there is no Best Buy aisle for aging tech. When I spoke to the people I consider to be at the forefront of this aging technology revolution I asked each of them, "Where would you advise a caregiver to find these products or learn more about their options?" They all replied that nothing – amazingly – exists. Jeff Cole is sure that will change within the next five years. Eric Dishman is still amazed no one has at least aggregated the information in one location caregivers could find with a quick Google search. Laurie Orlov says, "There is no store – either brick-and-mortar or online; you just have to do a Google search." But how do you find something you don't even know about?

Peter Radsliff, CEO of Presto and co-founder of AgeTek Alliance, says the difficulty for today's caregiver is traditional retailers such as Best Buy or Walmart don't have a place for caregivers to browse today's products that will help them and help their aging or disabled loved one. However, he is hopeful. "Whether it's mainstream retailers like Target, pharmacies such as Walgreens, specialty stores like GNC for nutritional supplements, or online stores like firstStreetonline.com, HomeHealthTechStore.com or ActiveForever.com, you can find some – but not all – care-related products and their success will stem from people voting with their dollars."

In the same way Apple revolutionized the music and MP3 world as well as retailing with its Apple stores, Radsliff believes in the not-so-distant future there will be a one-stop place where caregivers can shop or at least more places pointing the way to the technology we know will make a difference for caregivers. My hope is by the time you read this book, some smart entrepreneur will have figured it out.

I end this chapter with a discussion I had with the father of the cell phone, Martin Cooper, when he was the keynote speaker for a Consumer Electronics Show (CES) conference I co-produced called SilversSummit. When I asked him about his philosophy regarding technology addressing the needs of older Americans and helping our family caregivers, he said his motto is, "The best way to get people to think out of the box is to avoid creating the box in the first place. And if there is a box that is to be especially avoided, it's the one we seniors are so often relegated to."

As the Trekkies say, "Live long and prosper."

Caregiver Checklist

- ✓ Use specific terms and words in your search engine when looking for devices or technology products to help you.
- ✓ Keep an eye on some of the web sites discussed and others in the Resource section – new technology breakthroughs are happening every day to help caregivers.

Twister

Disaster planning when caregiving

In the 1996 movie, *Twister*, stars Helen Hunt and Bill Paxton play *storm-chasers* trying to learn more about tornadoes in Oklahoma so they can create an advance warning system to save more people from impending doom. This chapter is hopefully going to do the same thing – provide you with important information you need to know to avoid disaster calamities for your loved one and to be better prepared to help in cases of emergency.

Very few of us are prepared for disasters even though just about every region of the country has some type of disaster-prone weather issue. In the Northeast it can be extremely cold temperatures, ice storms, blizzards and floods. For the Midwest it is tornadoes. For the Gulf states and southeast it is hurricanes and for the western states it can be earthquakes and wild fires. And of course it is not just Mother Nature we need to consider – there are those unforeseen man-made disasters such as 9/11.

In the aftermath of Hurricane Katrina, one of the most deadly hurricanes in recorded American history which struck the Gulf Coast in 2005, a *Houston Chronicle* investigation found at least 139 nursing home residents died because the facilities did not have the proper disaster plans or staff training in place. Forty percent of all the dead bodies found in the wake of Katrina were over age

70; 7 out of 10 fatalities were older Americans who could not evacuate on their own. More than 35 residents of St. Rita's Nursing Home just outside New Orleans died during Katrina, drowned in their beds. While prosecutors charged the owners of the facility with negligent homicide, saying they should have evacuated the home, a jury acquitted the owners of all charges. Regardless of verdicts, the result is the same – your loved one is gone and his death could have been prevented.

"Katrina became the poster child for everything bad that could happen," says Larry Minnix, CEO of LeadingAge, a nonprofit organization dedicated to supporting older Americans.

The Perfect Storm

Over the next several years, we have a perfect storm brewing: more natural disasters occuring each year; an aging population that either resides in a facility or is living at home but is more vulnerable at coping with a disaster crisis; and a lack of comprehensive planning both with family caregivers and health care facility administrators.

Scientists report a worldwide increase in the number of natural disasters over the past 25 years. In 1980, only about 100 such disasters were reported per year, but that number has more than tripled to 300 or more a year since 2000. The increase is expected to continue, and storm-related disasters are predicted to increase in intensity. According to FEMA (Federal Emergency Management Agency) records, the top 10 disaster-prone states, as ranked by historical statistics on major disaster declarations are Texas, California, Oklahoma, Florida, New York, Louisiana, Alabama, Kentucky, Missouri and Arkansas.

You may have an older loved one retiring to Florida or perhaps a disabled sister lives in Oklahoma or your father is in a memory care facility right near California's San Andreas earthquake fault line (Experts have been predicting the *big one* for California – the 8.0 on the Richter magnitude scale – for years. As a native Southern Californian I have my emergency stash in my car – water, good walking shoes, an epi pen for my asthma, sunscreen and peanut butter. I still have not figured out what I will do about my daily Starbucks coffee addiction…).

Nationally, more than 3 million people spent at least some time in a nursing home during 2009, according to the latest available data. Nearly 40 percent of them, 1.2 million, were in the top 10 disaster-prone states and 40 percent of those living in assisted living facilities have dementia and most likely will be confused in a disaster scenario unable to help themselves. A 2005 Harris Poll showed 13 million people age 50+ will need help evacuating during a disaster.

As caregivers, our expectations are if our loved one is residing in a facility – a retirement community, assisted living or skilled nursing facility – the administrators and staff of that facility will know what to do in a disaster and take care of our loved one. The reality is as caregivers, we have to ensure we ask the right questions of facility administrators and staff to determine whether they have the proper process in place and here is why.

An Office of the Inspector General report for the U.S. Department of Health and Human Services showed 92 percent of the 16,000 nursing homes in the U.S. meet federal emergency guidelines created by the Centers for Medicare and Medicaid Services (CMS). In addition, 72 percent met the training standards established after the Katrina disaster. That is the good news. Here is the bad news. An in-person evaluation where visits were made to 24 randomly selected facilities in top disaster-prone states showed a woefully different story – good on paper bad on execution. Of the 24 facilities visited:

- 23 of them could not describe how to handle a resident's illness or sudden death during an evacuation;
- 22 did not have a back-up plan for staff that called in sick or could not get to the facility during a disaster;
- 15 did not have information about how to handle specific medical needs of residents such as breathing tubes or oxygen tanks;
- 7 did not have a plan for identifying residents in an evacuation such as using wristbands or name tags;
- 0 facilities had adequate supplies of water, designated by federal guidelines to be at least a 7-day supply for all residents.

Iceberg Straight Ahead

In the same way everyone thought the Titanic was *unsinkable*, you cannot trust that a disaster may never happen where your loved one lives. How can you prepare to help your loved one in case of disaster? As Chris Bennett, founder of OneStorm.org, which provided comprehensive disaster planning advice to the Red Cross and FEMA after Katrina, says, "Preparedness can be a learned behavior, but it's not a switch that gets flipped overnight. Just ask yourself, do you want to be the fool who prepares for the storm that never comes, or the fool who never prepares at all?"

Apparently Americans are feeling less foolish these days. According to the Centers for Disease Control, the Ad Council in collaboration with the U.S. Department of Homeland Security conducted a study on disaster prep after Katrina and found the proportion of Americans who said they have taken any steps to prepare rose from 45 percent in 2005 to 55 percent in 2006. The Ad Council also found 54 percent of those surveyed in 2006 had put together an emergency kit, 39 percent had created a family emergency plan, and 40 percent had searched for information about preparedness.

The things for caregivers to plan ahead for are whether or not a loved one can:

- *Shelter in place*, meaning stay in their home to ride out a storm or disaster – do they have enough food, water, back-up power?
- If an evacuation is necessary – how will you get them to leave, what will they take with them and where will they go?
- If they are in an assisted living, nursing home or other facility, what are the emergency preparedness and evacuations plans?

The Day After Tomorrow (is too late)

First of all, you need to educate yourself on the weather-related issues of the region where your loved one lives. It is often difficult in disaster situations for caregivers to be able to communicate and help – whether you live across town or across the country.

If you live in the same area, you may be prohibited by law enforcement and authorities such as the National Guard from getting to your loved one. If you live cross country, phone line connections to emergency relief services and available information from organizations such as FEMA may be difficult to get. Either way, you need a plan. I am not advocating you hunker down like it is Armageddon but asking a lot of questions and putting a few plans in place will allow you to sleep at night.

According to Larry Minnix of LeadingAge, your first step is to understand the disaster plans for the facility where your loved one resides. He advises disasters can be nature-related, accidents such as residency fires or bomb threats. No matter the emergency, by federal law, a nursing home is required to have an evacuation plan should a disaster occur. The facility's disaster preparedness plan should be reviewed by staff, and staff should be trained on the procedures and drills. Minnix advises asking the following questions of facility administrators *and* staff caring for your loved one and making these observations during your visits to the facility:

1. Ask what the facility's disaster plan is and ask to see a copy of the plan.
2. Ask how often staff is drilled on the procedures (ask both administrators and staff and compare answers from both.)
3. Ensure there is no chain on any exit doors in the facility. Most locations that deal with dementia or mental health patients need ways to ensure their residents do not wander off. This means exit doors should have a punch code which most staff and administrators will know how to open in an emergency. Chains on doors are extremely dangerous during a panicked evacuation of a facility and should never be used.
4. What is the facility's supply of medications, food and water? Again, federal guidelines say at least seven days for water.
5. Ensure the facility has back-up generators in situations where there may be a power outage. This is critical for residents on life-saving machines that require electrical power.
6. Ask where your loved one would probably be taken in an evacuation situation or if there is a phone number where caregivers can call to get more information on that specific facility and its residents.

You can also find checklists of questions in addition to the previous list from these resources: the National Citizens' Coalition for Nursing Home Reform, the Centers for Disease Control (CDC), the American Red Cross, and the Department of Homeland Security.

One of the key points Minnix makes is family caregivers, especially those who live near their loved one's facility, can be a helpful part of the emergency team in a disaster situation. He advises, "Families should show up at the facility and ask what they can do to help. I've been involved in several disaster relief situations where family members became vital transportation providers or aided residents who were frightened during an evacuation." Minnix says when family and friends can lend a hand, then facility administrators and staff can do what they have to do more easily.

You may want to also prepare some information and communication plans within your family and circle of friends. This becomes even more critical if your loved one lives at home and has no other assistance. For instance:

- Have a list of contacts for your loved one. Let your network know if a disaster happens and your loved one cannot reach you, your loved one may call this person to check in. Ensure someone is on your list who lives more than 100 miles away –

sometimes it is easier to get a long-distance call through rather than a local call in an emergency situation.
- Have your loved one's prescription info and medical contacts written down, including their insurance information.
- Remind your loved one to always tell you about his travel plans and you will do the same. Always have a designated person in your network to help out if your travel plans call for you to be out of the country or far away.
- Create an *Emergency Information* list of instructions and put it in your loved one's purse or wallet. This becomes a lifeline if your loved one is unconscious and unable to communicate with emergency personnel. Have information such as:

1. Where to locate their oxygen tank, their refrigerated medications (such as insulin or gamma globulin), their cell phone or communication device and their wheelchair.
2. Conditions such as bad knees, deafness or partial blindness so rescuers know to write down what they are saying, or know to lead them by letting them take their arm.
3. Service animals? Have enough food and water for them as well as your loved one.
4. Where your loved one's emergency kit is located. Have a *go quick* kit with essentials such as a two-week supply of medications, flashlight, battery-operated radio, food and water for three days and special items (extra pair of contacts or eyeglasses, insulin tests, epi pens, copy of birth certificate, insurance card, Medicare/Medicaid card, and some cash $50-$100).

Transportation becomes one of the scarcest commodities in a disaster situation. If something like Katrina hits a community, there are only so many transportation choices available and everyone will be turning to them. If your loved one still drives, remind her to never park the car in the garage without having the fuel tank at least half full. If she no longer drives (or may be too injured to drive), have alternative transportation planned.

For many older Americans, pets are family members. If your loved one has a pet, you should investigate the emergency pet shelter options in the area. Most emergency shelters run by the Red Cross or local disaster relief organizations do not allow pets. In addition, you will want to prepare for the pet's survival needs:

- Determine whether pets can accompany your loved one to a shelter or other location for safety – such as a hotel or friend's home. If not, make alternative plans.
- Assemble a pet disaster kit to include leash and carrier, medications, health and vaccination records, water, and other necessities for the pet's well-being.

- Be sure the pet's ID tags are either on the animal or in the pet disaster kit. If your loved one has to evacuate, be absolutely certain the pet is wearing identification.
- Include a notation on your Emergency Listing Information that your loved one has a pet that you would like transported with them. Include the pet's name in the information.

Perhaps the most important thing you can do to prepare for a disaster situation is to have the conversation about the plan with your family and loved ones. Minnix calls this the "big family pow wow." Often older loved ones may refuse to leave their homes in an evacuation situation. They either may not feel the disaster is as serious as you are telling them or they may be fearful of leaving their home and all their possessions. This can be a big caregiver challenge where bringing in a professional – maybe a geriatric care manager, a local fire or police department personnel, anyone of authority – can help your loved one understand the seriousness of the potential issue. And of course, this conversation has to happen prior to a disaster so you avoid the calamites and panic of Katrina.

Also, consider a loved one may have to use a Medivac during an evacuation. You need to know what is covered and what is not by your loved one's insurance. It is always good to review this information before a disaster when insurance phones will be ringing off the hook. You may not have a moment to spare in a life and death situation. Again, this is why it is so critical to have copies of your loved one's medical and insurance information handy.

Perhaps the best example of disaster preparation is Noah – he heeded the warning and built the Ark before the flood. Time to get on board with your family's disaster plan.

Caregiver Checklist

- ✓ Know the emergency plans of the facility where your loved one lives.
- ✓ Have an emergency plan if your loved one lives alone or your parents are older and need help in a disaster.
- ✓ Ensure your loved one has a *go quick* kit and instructions to emergency medical personnel in their wallet.
- ✓ Have the conversation with loved ones about the family's emergency plans – *just in case.*

Planes, Trains and Automobiles

Traveling with a loved one, caregiving vacations, hotels & services

Taking a vacation is something most caregivers only get to do in their dreams. But just like Steve Martin found in the hilarious comedy he starred in with John Candy, *Planes, Trains and Automobiles*, whether traveling home for the holidays or taking a family summer vacation, where there is a will, there is a way.

Whether your loved one has dementia, autism, is in a wheelchair or uses a walker, has hearing or sight impairment, special health needs such as diabetes, or travels with an oxygen tank – taking a trip doesn't have to be a distant dream. Just read Sylvia Mackey's story to see traveling need not cease when your loved one is diagnosed with an illness or disorder – all you have to do in Sylvia's words is: Prepare, Prepare, Prepare.

There are some considerations that should be made when you are planning your trip. A great resource for those traveling with special disabilities or health care needs is the Society for Accessible Travel & Hospitality (SATH). Here are a few things this organization recommends you keep in mind which may affect the details of your itinerary:

Seasonal temperatures – When traveling during the winter when it is very cold or during the summer months when it can be very hot and humid, take into consideration your loved one's illness and how temperatures may affect her.

Crowds – Crowds can be a source of agitation and frustration for some travelers who have a disease or disorder such as autism, post traumatic stress disorder, dementia or Down syndrome. In addition, some travelers have mobility issues such as navigating in a wheelchair. Consider trips to amusement parks such as Disneyland, sporting events or carnivals or other crowd-heavy locations carefully and possibly plan your trip during *the off season* or *off times* when there will be fewer people to worry about.

Waiting in lines, walking far distances – Whether it is the airport, museums or other location, consider the impact to your loved one if you have to wait in long lines or walk far distances. Scope out resting places, ensure you have water to prevent dehydration from long walks and consider asking for a wheelchair or cart for a loved one to use.

Special dietary needs and medications – If your loved one is a diabetic, or has special dietary needs such as needing gluten or dairy-free meals, ensure you call ahead to plan where to eat, or order a special meal. You can also bring special foods with you.

Also, ensure you have your loved one's medications with you if you plan on being gone for a few hours or a few days, so prescribed medication schedules can be maintained. Always check on where the closest pharmacy is to your lodging or location in case you need to get an emergency prescription, and DON'T put your loved one's medications in checked luggage which can get lost. Always put it in your carry-on luggage. If the medications are liquid and exceed 3.4 ounces (the allowed limit according to TSA), then you may need to call ahead and ensure you have authorization to bring these on board with you. In addition, plan ahead and get to the airport early. Even with special arrangements and allowances, these medications may delay you going through security checks.

Insurance coverage and identification – When traveling, it is important to ensure you have your loved one's insurance information with you, especially if an emergency hospitalization or other crisis happens. Keep in mind Medicare benefits are NOT available outside of the U.S. Apart from leisure travel, you may be moving a loved one to be closer to you. In these situations remember to update her identification. As you will read in Jill Eikenberry and Michael Tucker's story, her mom had an expired passport and driver's license which they did not discover until they got to the airport to move her to New York.

In addition to being able to identify your loved one to airline and other authorities, if your loved one becomes lost – whether an autistic child or a parent with Alzheimer's – always ensure you have a recent photo to share with security or law enforcement who will search for him or her. You may want to also consider a location tracking management service such as ComfortZone from the Alzheimer's Association or SecuraTrac. Your loved ones wear the device which has an embedded GPS chip so if they wander off, your cell phone can find their location instantly.

When traveling I normally think of travel insurance as just another way for airlines and others to make money. But when traveling with a loved one where unexpected, last-minute issues can cause you to cancel, travel insurance may not be a bad idea. Knowing how unwilling travel services are to refund any money, this insurance allows you to not lose the entire cost of the trip.

Emergency services – It is always smart to become knowledgeable about the services that may or may not be covered in case of an emergency with your loved one.

An example of this is a story about a business associate of mine who is a major power player in Hollywood. Recently his mother, who is in her 80s yet hearty and hale, had flown to South America to visit a relative. While there, she had a heart attack which then almost gave my associate one as well. In a panic, he knew he wanted to get his mother back to the U.S. immediately to receive medical treatment in the states. Because this man is fortunate to have great financial resources, he wound up spending more than $100,000 to charter a private plane with a registered nurse on board to bring his mother home.

What he found out later was there are services which for approximately a $395 annual membership fee, would have flown his mom home in a similar private airplane outfitted with all the medical equipment needed (and a licensed registered nurse at a separate cost). Whether it is MedJet Assist, NetJets, which collaborates with the Mayo Clinic, or others, help is available you just need to know before a crisis hits what are your options for emergency medical transport. My associate had the means to get his mom home but the point is this – if he had planned ahead for her potential health emergency issues, he would have saved himself a considerable amount of money not to mention saved himself the anxiety and worry of having to act fast when emotions were running high.

This lesson should not be lost. By planning ahead – no matter how big your paycheck – you can save valuable pennies when it comes to planning travel for a loved one with special needs.

Come Fly With Me

As you learned by reading Sylvia Mackey's story, airports can become a dilemma if you do not think ahead. Most airlines and airports publish brochures or guidelines and helpful tips for travelers with special needs and disabilities. Check the web site or call the customer service line to see what you need to think about for your loved one.

Typically, when you make an airline reservation, you want to ensure you have provided information to the booking agent or online ticketing service that your loved one is traveling under a special code: "SSR" which stand for Special Service Request. It is also wise to call ahead and speak to the airport customer service representative about your loved one's special circumstance as Sylvia did. She advises to make this call at least one month in advance of travel to discuss any special needs to consider. Again, don't wait until the last minute when you are rushed and harried and may find you have to do some additional work to make everything happen smoothly.

Also, ensure you book your loved one into an aisle seat, especially if they have a wheelchair or need to get up to use the toilet frequently. And you should advise the airline if your loved one travels with an oxygen tank - you will have to have a doctor's prescription for it with you.

Now, Voyager

When booking a cruise, train trip or hotel lodging, make sure you ask about accessibility for your loved one who has mobility issues. You will also want to understand the emergency plans for your hotel, cruise ship or train. For instance, if power is lost but your loved one needs power for medical equipment, how will you ensure your loved one will be OK?

In addition, understanding the possible evacuation plans in case of an emergency is critical if you have a loved one who moves slower or uses an assistive device. For hotel lodging, it is always best to request a first floor room, especially if your loved one uses a wheelchair, walker or cane or has trouble with stairs. In emergencies, elevators will not be operating making it difficult for you to get your loved one to safety quickly if you are not on a ground floor. You may also want to ensure the hotel has a mini fridge in your loved one's room if refrigeration for medications or other personal items is required.

Easy Rider

While I doubt you will plan a motorcycle road trip with your loved one (such as Jack Nicholson, Peter Fonda and Dennis Hopper took in this 1969 movie), there are a few things to think about that can make your ride *easier*.

If traveling with a loved one with dementia or autism, music can be soothing but the playlist is critical. Create a playlist for your rental car from an earlier era for older loved ones – most dementia patients find music from their youth or younger days more enjoyable than even the soothing sounds of Enya. Do be careful though about tunes from the past that may evoke sad memories. Music has proven to also soothe those with autism, Parkinson's and other disorders. Put the tunes on an iPod that can plug into the dashboard, create a CD or ask if the car comes with Pandora playlist capability.

Also remember to hydrate. As opposed to plane travel where a flight attendant can help you out, if you are driving, you need to have water handy for both you and your loved one. Millions of children and elders die every year from lack of fluids. In older loved ones, signs such as irritability, confusion or poor skin elasticity are signs of dehydration. In children it may be temper tantrums, diarrhea or vomiting.

North by Northwest

A Genworth report *Beyond Dollars* found 40 percent of caregivers had reduced family vacation after taking on the care of an older loved one such as a parent or grandparent. While caregiving can overtake you, you should not let it take over you and your family from enjoying a little vacation. There are two ways to travel even if your loved one requires supervised care and you need to get a break. Both services are a form of respite care:

Respitality – An innovative concept where participating hotels provide you as the caregiver (and your family) with a room, dining and even entertainment while a local respite service provides the companionship care to your loved one in their home or another location such as an assisted living facility. This model was created by the United Cerebral Palsy of America.

Residential Facility Respite – More assisted living facilities are setting aside beds or facilities where caregivers can bring a loved one for a few hours, a weekend or even an extended stay. This gives caregivers an opportunity to take a business trip or even a family vacation and know their loved one will be looked after in a trusted, capable facility.

Plaza Suite

There is another type of travel – not the leisure kind but the necessary kind when your loved one becomes ill or is going through rehabilitation or special therapies and you do not live within reasonable driving distance: caregiving hotels. Similar to the Ronald McDonald Houses concept where parents of ill children have a place to stay near the pediatric hospital in which their child is getting treatment, several facilities now exist that are dedicated to caregiving family members of an adult.

For instance, The American Cancer Society Hope Lodges offer caregivers a free, temporary place to stay when their lived one is getting chemotherapy, other treatments or surgeries in another city.

If your loved one is a military veteran, there is The Fisher House™ Program, *comfort homes* built on the grounds of major military and VA medical centers. Annually, the Fisher House program serves more than 17,000 families, and have made available over 4 million days of lodging to family members since the program originated in 1990.

The concept behind these *caregiving hotels* is families are stronger when they come together, and this bond actually helps the healing process. It is a comfort to the loved one being treated and it gives peace of mind without tremendous out-of-pocket expense for family caregivers who want to be by their loved one's side during these emotionally trying times.

Up in the Air

Similar to the caregiving hotels, many disease organizations and nonprofit groups offer grants or help when a caregiver needs to find travel, especially airline flights, to be by a loved one's side. Angel Flight is a nonprofit organization that uses volunteer pilots and the donation of funds and planes to fly families and their loved ones for special medical treatment. Whether a child needs special cancer treatment, a veteran's family needs to get to a VA medical center, or other caregiver emergency, this national organization says it *gives hope wings*.

In addition organizations such as The Farrah Fawcett Foundation, which you will read about in Alana Stewart's story, provides travel assistance to families who are seeking special cancer treatment.

Parks and Recreation

Another form of respite for caregivers may be *caregiver camp*. Whether it is a weekend retreat with caregivers or a family camp where you and your loved one and other family members can get away, these camps help caregivers become like the Energizer Bunny – recharging your battery to keep the care going and going and going and going.

Camp Reveille – Operated by Joan Lunden (you'll read about this in her story) in the Maine woods every summer. Women age 22-72 refresh, renew and reconnect with nature and other women for fitness and wellness activities. Many female caregivers attend each year.

Challenge Aspen – Providing recreational, educational and cultural activities for those with disabilities, including wounded veterans and their families. One of the main activities is an annual skiing event.

Easter Seals – Offering a variety of camps for children and adults living with disabilities. The purpose of this program is to promote fun but also to meet emotional needs such as personal satisfaction, adjustment to new environments and education around healthy lifestyles. While your loved one is at camp, you can get a much needed respite break.

Hole in the Wall Gang – Started by the late actor Paul Newman (named after the gang of outlaws in his famous movie, *Butch Cassidy and the Sundance Kid*) for seriously ill children. This summer and weekend camp in Connecticut every year offers 20,000 children battling cancer, sickle cell anemia and other chronic conditions the opportunity to ride horses, canoe, sing around the campfire and otherwise forget their illness for a while all free of charge. This organization also runs the Painted Turtle Camps for terminally ill children and their families.

Project Sanctuary – Operates therapeutic retreats for military families, primarily from OEF and OIF, helping them avoid two of the biggest issues they face: divorce and suicide. This nonprofit organization is proud of the fact that since its founding in 2007, they have held 24 retreats helping 182 families, and 95 percent of couples are still married and there have been no suicides.

WomanSage – Empowering women age 50+, this nonprofit organization in Southern California has a philanthropic arm that partners with the local Alzheimer's Association chapter to offer a Caregiver Cruise. Scholarships are provided to caregivers (friends can join but must pay their own travel expenses) on a weekend Carnival cruise. Respite care is provided for the loved one while the caregiver is on the cruise.

Wounded Warrior Project – Offers weekend getaways to military service men and women who have service-related injuries since September 11, 2001. The retreats are provided for caregivers only or for the whole family. They have found the outdoor activities coupled with the support group discussions promote both health and healing.

Caregiver Checklist

- ✓ Ensure you call ahead to airlines, hotels and other locations to make advance plans for your loved one's travel.
- ✓ Understand if your loved one travels what the emergency services may be to help them if needed.
- ✓ Plan in advance for your loved one's needs during the trip – mobility, prescriptions, nutrition, etc.
- ✓ Know there are programs and services to provide respite care for your loved one so you can get a break and attend a caregiver retreat or camp or take a vacation without worrying about your loved one's care.

Dr. Doolittle and The Sound of Music

Alternative therapies: pets and music

When we think of alternative medicine and therapies we typically think of Eastern medicine such as massage therapy, acupuncture, holistic medicine and herbal remedies. Two of my favorite alternative therapies now have numerous studies to back up their effectiveness in addressing a variety of illnesses and disorders including autism, Alzheimer's, cancer, MS and Parkinson's.

Snoopy to the Rescue

My favorite cartoonist the late Charles Schulz of *Peanuts* fame wrote, "Happiness is a warm puppy." I wonder if he knew happiness is just the start when it comes to enhancing the lives of older loved ones in nursing homes or assisted living, terminal patients such as those suffering from AIDS, children with special needs and even caregivers looking to improve their own health. Known as Animal-Assisted Therapy (AAT), there is a growing movement to increase animal/patient interactions for health and wellness benefits.

The notion of pet therapy all began in the 1860s although most of the studies were conducted in the 1980s. Famous nurse Florence Nightingale recognized more than 150 years ago that animals provided a level of social support in the institutional care of the mentally ill. In an effort to prove the therapeutic benefits of pet therapy, the National Institutes of Health has funded grants to study scientific evidence-based research in therapeutic effects on children.

You may have read about the dogs that can smell cancer in their owner long before a formal diagnosis is made, help calm children who have an epileptic seizure or even bring people out of comas. Pet Partners (formerly known as the Delta Society) tells a story about its visit to a terminally ill patient. When the handler arrived with her cat, the patient had slipped into a coma. As the handler put the cat into the bed, the patient suddenly awoke, removed his arms from under the sheets and started to pet the cat. I truly believe animals have special healing powers and a sixth sense. To back up my notion, I read an article with Dr. Edward Creagan of the Mayo Clinic Medical School who observed, "If pet ownership was a medication, it would be patented tomorrow."

While dogs, cats and rabbits are most commonly used with older patients, dolphins and horses have also proved effective with children affected by mental health issues, epilepsy, physical disabilities or autism. The biggest benefits of cozying up to a "warm puppy" are:

Socialization – older loved ones often feel isolated whether living alone at home or in a facility such as a nursing home or assisted living. In fact, Human-Animal Interactions published a study of elderly dog owners revealing 75 percent of men and 67 percent of women considered their dog their only friend.

Some studies have found just a few minutes a day petting or visiting with an animal lowers the stress hormone of cortisol and increases the feel-good hormone of serotonin. The results can range from lowered heart rates and blood pressure to decreased depression. For older loved ones still living at home, who can manage the daily needs of a pet (feeding, walking), some surveys have found the interaction and companionship of a pet can improve your loved one's health through increased physical activity and even lower pain levels in some arthritis patients.

Emotional - for older patients depression can be common, especially if they recently lost a spouse, received a terminal diagnosis or had to move from the comforts of home. Pet therapy or even a new pet can provide the unconditional love and comfort that helps reduce anxiety, particularly noted in nursing home patients.

Some assisted living facilities now have a Pet Care Coordinator to help seniors care for their own pets. If an owner forgets to feed the pet or it becomes too difficult to walk them or care for their other needs, the Pet Care Coordinator can help keep pets up-to-date on veterinary visits, grooming and vaccinations. Silverado Senior Living which includes memory care assisted living communities for Alzheimer's and dementia care residents, encourages pets in the community including privately owned pets, resident pets and visits from pet therapy organizations. Pet therapy for those with Alzheimer's or dementia has also proven to be a powerful tool for what is known as *sundowners*, a symptom where paranoia and irrational behavior occur at dusk or sundown.

"When we first opened our doors, our goal was to make this community as much a home as possible," says Steve Winner, co-founder and chief of culture for Silverado Senior Living. "Since we are all animal lovers and we realized how important pets were to our residents, this became a home for not just people but the animals they love."

This was at a time when animals in a community were thought to be dangerous and unclean. Silverado became a pioneer in seeing the benefits outweighed the risks. Winner says he knows some Silverado residents would not be doing as well as they are if they had to leave their pets behind when they moved into their new assisted living home.

Animals have even proven to be valuable members of the hospice team for a terminally ill loved one. There is a famous cat in Providence, Rhode Island known as Oscar who is one of the critical members of the hospice team in the local nursing home. Patients and family members have reported when Oscar enters a room, there is a sense of calm—even though Oscar is known by residents as visiting a room when someone is dying. As opposed to a bad omen, Oscar brings comfort and peace to both the patient and the family members. Oscar stays with the patient, sitting quietly in her lap or on her bed where he remains until the loved one has passed.

Children with autism can improve their communication skills, which can often be stressful, by owning or visiting with pets. Because animals are non-judgmental, special needs kids relax and are able to absorb other benefits during their pet therapy sessions. Animals' nonverbal communication and profound acceptance can be soothing for those who struggle with language.

Hippotherapy, which is therapeutic horseback riding, is practiced in 24 countries and benefits those with physical, psychological, cognitive, social, and behavioral problems. In fact, the American Speech and Hearing Association now recognize hippotherapy as a treatment method for individuals with speech disorders. While some benefit from the connection and the relationship built with the horse, other riders benefit physically from the movements that help build core strength, body awareness and muscle memory. When I spoke to Alan Osmond, he shared a story with me about his friend, Ann Romney, wife of Mitt, who manages her multiple sclerosis through frequent horseback riding activity.

Pets can also benefit the caregivers. Caregiving can make you feel like you are all alone. While adding a pet to the list of loved ones you have to care for may seem like overload, having that happy face and wagging tail or a purring kitten to give you some unconditional love when you return home can benefit caregivers as well. Studies have found caregivers are twice as likely as the general public to develop chronic illness due to the prolonged stress of caring for a loved one. If having a pet can increase your exercise, lower your blood pressure and bring a smile to your face – maybe finding a Lassie, swimming with Flipper, holding Thumper or riding Mr. Ed is just what the doctor has ordered.

Following are organizations where you can find pet therapy handlers/animals or participate in caregiving pet events:

Pet Partners Therapy Animal Program trains and screens volunteers with their pets so they can visit patients/clients in hospitals, nursing homes, hospice and physical therapy centers, schools, libraries and many other facilities. Over 10,000 handler/animal teams have been trained and accredited through Pet Partners. The Pet Partners Service Animal Program provides information and resources for people with disabilities, as well as their friends and family, who are considering getting a service animal or who are currently partnered with a service animal.

Pets for the Elderly Foundation match seniors with cats and dogs by underwriting the pets' adoptions.

Therapy Dogs Inc. is a national registrar with a listing of more than 12,000 handler/dog teams in U.S. and Canada. The organization provides registration, support and insurance for volunteers who want to provide pet therapy services.

American Cancer Society Bark for Life is a fundraising event to honor the caregiving qualities of our canine best friends. Canine caregivers are canine companions, guide dogs, service dogs, rescue dogs, therapy dogs, police dogs, cancer survivor dogs and diagnostic dogs who, with their owners, are joining the American Cancer Society as relay teams and participants.

Numerous organizations in local communities, including Pet Therapy, a nonprofit organization in Southwest Florida bring pets into nursing homes for weekly visits with puppies and dogs brought by adult and even child volunteers.

A Little Night Music

Is music one of the keys to a longer, happier life – despite your health issues?

Although music has been with us since the dawn of time, in the last few decades studies have proven music as a therapeutic tool can increase cognitive function in Alzheimer's patients, help premature infants gain weight, encourage autistic children to communicate, lead stroke patients to regain speech and mobility, control pain for dental, surgical and orthopedic patients and manage anxiety and depression for psychiatric patients.

Dr. Oliver Sacks, a renowned neurologist and psychologist at Columbia University Medical Center best known for his 1973 book *Awakenings* – which became an Academy Award-nominated film starring Robin Williams and Robert De Niro, and who also wrote *Musicophilia: Tales of Music and the Brain* – testified at the hearing before the Senate Special Committee on Aging titled, "Forever Young: Music and Aging," and issued this statement:

> "The power of music is very remarkable… One sees Parkinsonian patients unable to walk, but able to dance perfectly well or patients almost unable to talk, who are able to sing perfectly well… I think that music therapy and music therapists are crucial and indispensable in institutions for elderly people and among neurologically disabled patients."

Since music is associated with one of the five senses – hearing – which is controlled by the brain it makes sense we should exercise our brains with music listening to spur cognitive function in the same way we use physical therapy to exercise our limbs, muscles and joints to regain mobility and physical function.

When it comes to Alzheimer's patients, studies have shown music reduces agitation or improves behavioral issues such as violent outbursts. In one pilot program, 45 patients with mid- to late-stage dementia had one hour of personalized music therapy, three times a week, for 10 months, and improved their scores on a cognitive-function test by 50 percent on average. One patient in the study recognized his wife for the first time in months. Another music therapy study showed stroke victims can learn to walk and use their hands again.

And music therapy is not just used with older patients. When it comes to those children diagnosed on the autism spectrum, music therapy allows these children to develop identification and appropriate expression of their emotions – music becomes the universal language. Many people with diagnoses on the autism spectrum have innate musical talents so music therapy can give these individuals a sense of accomplishment and success.

As you will read in Holly Robinson Peete's story, she told me how her son R.J., who was diagnosed at age three with autism, loves music and he has even recorded a song. In fact, Holly finds music a great way for her entire family to connect with R.J. and to enter his world. She told me, "I think music makes him more comfortable – it is a way for R.J. to communicate without being judged."

Music as therapy is not just for your loved one. We know caregivers encounter increased stress over caring for a loved one. Since studies show listening to music can lead to increased secretion levels of melatonin, a hormone associated with mood regulation, lower aggression, reduced depression and enhanced sleep – using music to cope with these common caregiver complaints can be a welcome relief to caregiver burn-out.

Although the 2008 documentary *Young@Heart*, showcased a chorus of 80-year-olds singing Beatles, Rolling Stones and Sonic Youth cover songs, most experts agree with an older loved one it is best to choose music that reminds them of an earlier, happier time in their lives. Following are some ways to bring more music into your life and the life of your loved one:

1. **Discover the happy times tunes:** Talking to your loved one about happy times in their life and understanding the music associations with that time are essential. Whether it is big band, gospel, rock 'n' roll, country, opera or blues, find out what made your loved one happiest. Most older loved ones, especially Alzheimer's patients who retain long-term memory rather than short-term memory, find tunes from their youth the most joyful. But be careful. Music can also evoke sad memories. One Holocaust survivor in a pilot program reportedly became very upset upon hearing a Wagner opera which reminded him of that traumatic era of his life.
2. **Engage younger generations**: You can help create emotional intimacy when spouses and families share creative music experiences. Whether it is downloading songs from iTunes, creating a Pandora play list or using the latest technical creation for digital music files, engage your kids in interacting with their grandparent or sibling with special needs to choose their favorite music.

3. **Pick the right setting**: It may not be as simple as turning on a radio. The radio can be distracting with constant advertising that breaks the peace of music. Instead, try internet radio like Pandora channels, or use an iPod or CD player instead. And be careful with headphones – some may take comfort in the privacy of headphones while others will become irritated or uncomfortable. Also, consider live music situations carefully. For author Gail Sheehy, being able to take her husband, who was suffering from cancer, to a last jazz night out on the town, was a gift she will always treasure. But for special needs children and some older adults – the unsettling activity of a live concert or band can be frightening.

4. **Let your music play**: As a caregiver music is your therapy as well. Whether it is creating your own playlist to lift your mood when you have a *down day* or just taking pleasure in watching your loved one become engaged, music can make your heart soar. Celia Pomerantz, author of *Alzheimer's - A Mother-Daughter Journey*, found her mother, who grew up in Puerto Rico, loved a certain era of salsa music from such celebrated artists as Tito Puente. She created song lists of her mom's favorite tunes while her mother was in the nursing home. Celia became enchanted as her mother blossomed into the woman residents called "the dancing queen." The joy of music and watching her mother dance lifted Celia's spirits about her mother's Alzheimer's diagnosis.

The Music Man and Mary Poppins

The American Music Therapy Association (AMTA), a nonprofit organization that represents over 5,000 music therapists, corporate members, and related associations worldwide offers information about music therapy studies and a listing of credentialed music therapists who offer services in institutional, residential and private home settings.

Music can both evoke and create memories that last forever. I close with this heartwarming story from the AMTA web site:

> When a couple danced together for the first time after five years of the husband's deterioration from probable Alzheimer's disease, the wife said: "Thank you for helping us dance. It's the first time in three years that my husband held me in his arms." Tearfully, she said that she had missed him just holding her and that music therapy had made that possible.

Caregiver Checklist

- ✓ Understand the therapeutic benefits of pets and the pet therapy services available.
- ✓ Learn how to use music to soothe or help your loved one and lift your spirits as well.

Curtain Call – How Will You Prepare for the End?

I intend to live forever, or die trying.

– *Groucho Marx*

When it comes to the days and weeks right before and after *the end*, caregivers go through a variety of emotions. There may be relief and there is certainly grief. There may be guilt and a sense of unfinished business with your loved one who is gone forever. There can be continued conflict with siblings or other family members which may make peace hard to find. This is typically a period of time where caregivers may go through a *coulda, shoulda, woulda* period.

Whatever your emotions, Doug Bates, a palliative care social worker with the Motion Picture and Television Fund (MPTF), says, "Give yourself permission to have your feelings – whatever they are."

Beyond the Bucket List

End-of-life wishes

Did you see the movie *The Bucket List* with the exceptional actors Jack Nicholson and Morgan Freeman? While both men faced terminal illness they found comfort and companionship in connecting with one another to check off their wish list of things to do before they died. They ended life the way they lived it – their way.

One of the hardest things you will do as a caregiver is let go of your loved one. But it is also a great gift to honor your loved one's end-of-life wishes and help him do it his way or what I would call *beyond the Bucket List*.

When Jiminy Cricket sang "When you wish upon a star" 72 years ago in the Disney animated classic film *Pinocchio*, it was about bringing a wooden puppet to life. However, it is the end-of-life where we need to ensure our wishes will come true. The only way to make this happen is to ensure two things:

1. Our desires are legally binding.
2. We have communicated our end-of-life wishes to close loved ones.

One of the most important things we can do – at any age – is to have our legal paperwork in order outlining how we want our last days and wishes to be carried out. Many people spend a lot of money in legal fees to develop a Living Will, Advance Directive, Durable Power of Attorney for Medical and Financial, DNR order (Do Not Resuscitate) and other legal documentation. An affordable yet legally binding alternative is to create a Living Will at one of the many online legal documentation sites. While creating the paperwork is the easy part (and you will read more about legal documentation in the chapter Raiders of the Lost Ark found in Casting Calls), having the conversation with loved ones so everyone understands our wishes is the hard part.

There is a tool available that is not only affordable, valuable and legal but helpful in starting the conversation. It is called *The Five Wishes*. In 1997, Jim Towey, who had served as Mother Teresa of Calcutta's friend, volunteer AIDS worker and legal counselor, created a nonprofit organization, Aging with Dignity. At the core of the organization was a document Towey created that was in his words a "living will with a heart and a soul." Essentially, the document asks five questions that cover medical, personal, emotional and spiritual needs that help you communicate how you want to be treated if you are too ill to speak for yourself:

3. Which person you want to make health care decisions for you when you can't make them.
4. The kind of medical treatment you want or don't want.
5. How comfortable you want to be.
6. How you want people to treat you.
7. What you want your loved ones to know.

To date, the $5 document (either downloadable to your computer or mailed to you) has been filled out by millions of people worldwide and has been translated into 26 languages and Braille. It is used in all 50 states and meets the legal requirements for an Advance Directive in 42 states (in the remaining eight states you can attach *The Five Wishes* to the forms that state requires).

Because *The Five Wishes* has interesting origins with the principles of Mother Teresa infusing its purpose, this can be the conversation starter with your family. While the emphasis is on aging boomers and older generations to ensure these wishes are in place, having a Living Will is smart for everyone.

It is the legacy of the Terri Schiavo case that shows us the agony and antagonism that can happen to tear families apart when someone's decisions about end-of-life care are unknown. Schiavo was only 27 when she was put on a ventilator and feeding tube after cardiac arrest left her brain dead. She lay in a vegetative state for 14 more years while her husband battled her parents over whether or not to keep her alive on machines. If she had a Living Will, there never would have been a battle. While you or your loved one may believe casual conversations about end-of-life wishes are sufficient, this proves having those wishes written down in a legally binding document are essential to avoid any conflicts.

Another great resource for ensuring your last wishes are legally binding is Caring Connections, a program of the National Hospice and Palliative Care Organization (NHPCO). This program is a national consumer and community engagement initiative to improve care at the end-of-life. Since 2004 Caring Connections has provided more than 1.3 million Advance Directives to individuals free of charge. It also provides free resources and information to help people make decisions about end-of-life care and services before a crisis and brings together community, state and national partners working to improve end-of-life care through a national campaign called *It's About How You LIVE*.

Since this book has a movie/TV theme, yet another avenue is to turn to the movies. There is an educational DVD called *Consider the Conversation™: A Documentary Film About a Taboo Subject*. Created by two men, one a hospice worker, the other a teacher and filmmaker, the film explores the fact that dying is a topic Americans do not want to discuss but must. As our society has evolved to showcase reality TV shows and cable news constantly tackling previously *off limits* conversations about religion, politics and sex, dying is a topic we need to address. This thought-provoking film, which can be purchased as a DVD or seen occasionally on local PBS affiliates nationwide, can also spark thoughtful conversations with loved ones about end-of-life wishes and is just another way to have the vital conversation that most of us avoid. Rather than provide the answers, the film probes the questions we should all be contemplating and discussing when it comes to *the end* of our lives.

Forty years ago people did not live as long as we do now, because we did not have the technology or medical interventions to keep people alive. But dying today can be a long slow process and this requires a lot more dialogue.

The reality is if you do not have the conversation, family members can be confused and conflicted which can lead to emotional exchanges you do not want. Dying is not a choice but how the end will be is. We owe it to our families to share those wishes. So often caregivers feel guilt over having to make tough decisions because a loved one has not had the conversation or created the documentation. If a caregiver has to decide to *turn off the machines* or literally *pull the plug*, the guilt can remain with you for years. It is a gift we give to our loved ones to ensure our end-of-life legal wishes are written down. Once done, it is time to start talking.

The other side of end-of-life wishes is for aging parents of a child with special needs. The reality today is many special needs children – those with autism, Down syndrome or cerebral palsy – have longer lifespans than they did 20 years ago. A special needs child may live into her 50s, 60s or even 70s with varying degrees of care needed depending on the condition. Because longevity is now a factor for all of us, parents of special needs children need to meet with an estate attorney to establish the proper custodial care for their adult child to prepare for the day they are no longer here to care for their child.

The Real Bucket List

While having the conversation and getting legal paperwork in order for end-of-life is critical, there are also other wishes loved ones may have. Actors Jack Nicholson and Morgan Freeman called it *The Bucket List*, Thomas Rollerson calls it the Dream Foundation.

In 1993, Rollerson was seeking an organization to fulfill an end-of-life wish for an adult but all he found were groups, such as the Make-A-Wish Foundation and the Starlight Foundation, which provided these dreams for children. One year later he started the Dream Foundation, dedicated to fulfilling those wishes of dying adults. Thousands of wishes are granted every year ranging from a terminal cancer patient meeting an Olympic athlete, to a family devastated by astronomical medical expenses having their heating bill paid for a few months. *When you wish upon a star* doesn't have to just be for children.

Twilight

Hospice and palliative care

In the hit film and book, *Twilight*, which launched a thousand vampire imitators, Edward Cullen and his *undead people* avoid daylight and embrace the night. While this makes for intriguing mystery and romanticism, it is the mystery of death and dying that continues to confuse and conflict us. The end stage of life for our loved ones, their *twilight*, is one that is often hard for caregivers to accept. There are many taboos associated with dying, just like it is a taboo for Bella to love Edward. But this chapter will shed light on the mystery, taboos and despair that can be those dark hours for caregivers and bring end-of-life into the light.

"The rules of the universe won't be changing for you," says Rabbi Arthur Rosenberg, the chaplain for the Motion Picture and Television Fund (MPTF) palliative care team. "As we get older and closer to dying, we have a longing for spirituality because we start to realize life is finite…Spirituality is not about God it is about your individual spirit."

As we near end-of-life, Rabbi Rosenberg says regardless of religious beliefs or lack of beliefs, we all have the same three questions, "Where did I come from?" "Where am I going?" "What am I supposed to do while I am here?" It is in this phase of caring for a loved one we encounter hospice and palliative care.

Hospice and palliative care are the compassionate care services a loved one receives when facing a terminal diagnosis. Also known as *comfort care,* this team-oriented approach provides the emotional and spiritual guidance so important to patients and their family caregivers. The purpose is to eliminate pain and fear during our last days and to help the families through the process.

The difference between the two services is hospice is about *caring* not *curing.* It typically is administered the last several weeks or even months of a person's life whereas palliative care can be provided at any time and duration after a loved one has received a diagnosis. Hospice and palliative care can be provided in the privacy and sanctity of your loved one's home, in your home or in hospice centers, hospitals, nursing homes and other long-term care facilities.

While caregivers must continuously seek to be seen as part of the primary care team along with a loved one's physician, surgeons and other experts when caring begins, it is in the hospice and palliative care phase that the health care professionals recognize the needs of the caregiver and family as much as the person who is dying.

Rabbi Rosenberg advises that a hospice chaplain, such as himself, is an essential part of the care team taking the family's *spiritual temperature* and reconnecting the patient and caregiver on the patient's last journey. He says the concept of chaplains began with the U.S. Armed Forces when wounded and dying soldiers needed comfort on the battlefields, far from home and separated from their own pastor, rabbi or minister.

"We go on the journey with the person and their caregiver – we don't abandon you and regardless of what you believe in terms of your individual faith, a hospice chaplain is trained to guide the family through this transition to your loved one's ultimate *home* and bring peace to the family about the loss."

Rabbi Rosenberg also states it is through the palliative and hospice care experience that many caregivers and loved ones find forgiveness and acceptance.

"Many families are in turmoil, they are complicated and to some degree fractured and this creates a lot of alienation," says Rabbi Rosenberg. He advises in the hospice environment is where inclusion can be created to bridge those issues for families.

"We can create a circle around the bed where everyone joins hands, to pray in our own words, to say what we want to say and to seek forgiveness. It can be very healing because it is much harder to let a loved one go when there is unfinished business."

To enter hospice care your loved one's primary care physician will make a referral to a hospice care provider and team. A physician has to sign on for six months or less of hospice care for the course of life for the patient to qualify for benefits under Medicare. Palliative care does not have time restrictions on the length of care and can include treatment such as clinical trials or chemotherapy.

According to the National Hospice and Palliative Care Organization (NHPCO), hospice and palliative care have been provided to more than 1.2 million patients and their families each year over the last 30 years. In addition, more than 460,000 volunteers participate on hospice teams every year. Volunteerism is an essential part of the hospice service and 20 percent of these volunteers are new to hospice care.

One such volunteer is hospice stand-up comic, Jim O'Doherty who has won Emmy and Golden Globe awards for shows such as *Seinfeld*, *That 70's Show* and *Two and a Half Men*. While humor and hospice seem strange bedfellows, O'Doherty has found that levity, even in the face of a chronic illness, can bring relief to the person who is dying. It can also help the family and even the health care professionals. He learned this lesson through his personal experience of having a 16-year-old brother with terminal brain cancer. Putting his stand-up comic career on hold, he joined his family at Memorial Sloan-Kettering Cancer Center in New York. He watched as his brother used humor as a tool to fight for his life, and that is when O'Doherty discovered that humor was much more than just telling jokes. He created a unique humor workshop for The Cancer Support Community. This international cancer patient support organization was formerly known as The Wellness Community and in 2011 merged with Gilda's Clubs Worldwide, which was formed to honor the passing of the gifted comedienne and actress Gilda Radner of *Saturday Night Live* fame who lost her battle with ovarian cancer in 1989. The humor workshop became one of the best attended programs offered and has been presented in hospitals across the country to show people facing life-threatening diseases that understanding humor is a vital element in their fight to be well.

Perhaps this is the lesson of hospice care. When you understand that the body knows when it is time to go, even if you are not ready, you have to let go of the physical aspect of caregiving and focus on the connection with your loved one from an emotional and spiritual perspective.

"So many caregivers get so lost in the physical aspect [of caregiving] they end up putting their emotions on the backburner and it's so easy to do that," says Doug Bates, a palliative care social worker with the Motion Picture and Television Fund (MPTF). "Sometimes my role is coaching them through that emotional process, helping them see they are powerless over a loved one's illness and help them to be more present with their loved one."

In addition to reconnecting with our loved one in a special way, it is through caregiving that we reconnect with the faith in ourselves according to Vic Mazmanian, director of faith outreach for the Mind, Heart & Soul Ministry of Saddleback Church and Silverado Senior Living. He advises caregivers should acknowledge it sometimes takes pain or problems to make changes in our lives. After going through a caregiving experience with a loved one, we start to reconsider our own choices and future path and Mazmanian believes this is the special gift of caregiving.

Sequels

Life after caregiving – coping with loss and paying it forward

So much is written and discussed about caregiving but so little is written about *after the caregiving* has ended. While writing my blog, I had several readers who asked me to write about what you do once your caregiving role is finished. This chapter is for you.

During caregiving, your life is focused with activity, consumed with responsibility. In some ways, caregiving becomes your *constant*, your anchor in life. It grounds you though it can also grind you into dust. It is something to which you belong – you have a purpose. After the loss of a loved one, your life is quiet. All of a sudden there is this void where once there had been no time for anything other than caregiving. While caring for a loved one, you had no time to eat – now you have nothing but time to eat. Your caregiving life may have been a constant merry-go-round some days flashing by so fast and furiously you felt dizzy. Now, all of a sudden, everything has stopped. This can be very unsettling for some caregivers.

Many adult children who lose a parent, especially a second parent, report feeling like an *adult orphan*. A widowed spouse who had his identity wrapped up in being a couple now suddenly feels desperately alone, a ship without a rudder. And yet, some caregivers report feeling relief after their loss. After months or even years of watching a loved one decline – stricken with cancer and suffering through painful chemotherapy or enduring the *slow motion death* of a loved one with Alzheimer's who not only may have forgotten who you were but may have been frightened by you or angry at you for months – your grieving process did not start at death it started at diagnosis.

"We are *human beings* not *human doings*," says Rabbi Arthur Rosenberg, chaplain for the Motion Picture and Television Fund (MPTF). "Healing from grief takes time but eventually you will learn to let it go."

In their groundbreaking book, *On Grief and Grieving*, Elisabeth Kübler-Ross and David Kessler, state, "As a society we are all unprepared for loss…things feel unfinished." Their book identified five distinct phases for grieving a loss:

1) Denial
2) Anger
3) Bargaining
4) Depression
5) Acceptance

They explain the process of grieving is very personalized. It is well-meaning friends and family who want to *cheer you up* or rush you to get over your grief similar to Cher's Oscar-winning performance in the movie *Moonstruck* when she slaps Nicolas Cage and tells him to *snap out of it*. The reality is no one can tell you or get you to just snap out of it. Everyone will move through the five stages of grief but how fast or slow is dependent on a variety of factors. A grieving person is like a snowflake – each one is unique.

As you move through Stage 4 Depression (which I explore more in the Misery chapter) and enter Stage 5 Acceptance, the authors recommend, "Lean towards solace and soothing for yourself." In other words, if there was ever a time to focus solely on yourself – this is it. If you want to eat ice cream in bed, do it. If you want to watch endless hours of bad TV (or constant re-runs of *Law and Order* which can be seen just about anywhere in the world 24/7), do it. This is the time to truly indulge yourself in whatever way you please.

On the flip side of indulgence, Kübler-Ross and Kessler also advise to postpone, if possible, any life-altering decisions. Things such as selling your home and moving, quitting your job, joining the circus. It is not to say you cannot do all those things, just give it some time.

If you absolutely feel you cannot wait, get advice from friends, spiritual advisors, professional therapists or others you trust and who can help give you some perspective and clarity at a time when your emotions may still be fragile. Heal yourself and then decide what is next. There is no set time period for this but a professional therapist I worked with always advised to give things *the four seasons* – in other words, give it at least a year. There is something about moving through each season that gives you perspective on the future – you can see and feel forward motion.

Beyond grief, another side effect from caregiving is the chronic stress and possible neglect of your own health and wellness needs that can make you ill. In fact, illness after caregiving is very common. Stress has suppressed your immune system and now your body is under attack with no reinforcements in sight. This is a time to take all the focus you put on caring for your loved one and put that focus back on you. You need to restore your health – physically and mentally. Often we don't realize the toll caregiving has taken on us. When you read Alana Stewart's story about caregiving for Farrah Fawcett, she talks about not realizing the impact to her own health – and being astounded that it was in her chest near her heart where most of her subsequent health issues were emerging. Her heart was grieving and it was where her health issues with bronchitis decide to reside.

Very often, especially if you are over age 60, the loss of a spouse can result in the caregiving spouse developing shingles. If you have a sudden painful, blistering skin rash, this is shingles. You are particularly susceptible if you had chicken pox as a child – shingles and chicken pox share the same virus. While the virus was dormant in your system all these years, the chronic stress of caregiving and a weakened immune system can trigger shingles. The good news (because there always is some) is typically you will only have one attack which will last 2-3 weeks when the scabs from the blisters will flake off like a bad sunburn. Anti-viral medications or anti-inflammatories can help alleviate the pain and duration.

As you move into Stage 5 Acceptance Kübler-Ross and Kessler explain that does not mean you are "OK" with the loss of your loved one and what you both went through. The truth is we may never feel OK about it. However, we do need to get to a place where we create a new normal – where we can accept a world without our loved one. Full acceptance and healing will come in how you answer this question to yourself, "You are alive but are you *living*?" If you can find joy again in certain life activities, even if it resides side-by-side with your loss, then you are healed and whole again. Not the same whole person you were; the new whole person you are now.

Paying It Forward

One of the interesting responses to life after caregiving is many former caregivers actually volunteer to help current caregivers. Because I am a baby boomer, whenever I think of the essence of volunteering I think of the Peace Corps. The Peace Corps was the brainchild of then Senator John F. Kennedy as a challenge to American college students but was really brought to life by the late Sargent Shriver. Celebrating its 50th anniversary in 2011, the Peace Corps was about cultivating education, awareness and understanding of different cultures and helping to train others.

In caregiving today, there is a type of Peace Corps emerging which I will call the *Care Corps*. Whether mentoring new caregivers, volunteering online to help a friend who is caregiving, conducting in-person or webinar-based support groups, joining a chat room, becoming a hospice volunteer or volunteering through your church or synagogue to provide senior transportation, caregiving is ushering in a new wave of volunteerism for the baby boom and other generations. It is about cultivating understanding and training for our nation of caregivers.

As America faces an increasing percentage of people who are older and needing care, there will be more and more caregivers created who also need help to avoid the burn-out and stress that comes with caregiving or to refresh themselves once caregiving is completed.

According to Steve French, managing partner of the Natural Marketing Institute, a global consulting firm for health, wellness and sustainability, "Boomers are volunteering at a higher rate than the previous generation did at the same age." In fact, French says 39 percent of boomers report volunteer work is an important part of their life. According to the Corporation for National and Community Service, the federal agency that engages more than 5 million Americans in SeniorCorps, AmeriCorps and other projects, volunteers age 65 and over will increase 50 percent over the next few years, with just under 9 million volunteers in 2007 growing to 13 million by 2020.

You would think once a caregiver has been through the journey of caring for a loved one, she would be ready to relax and take a long break. Not all caregivers, according to a study published in the *Journal of Gerontology*. Researchers from the University of Massachusetts found older adult caregivers were more likely to be volunteers than non-caregivers.

The study found caregivers become *embedded in networks* once they become a caregiver, making them more likely to continue to seek these social interactions with like minds. They also have a routine of performing tasks for others – something they do not abandon even after caregiving ends. The study concluded caregivers are more likely to become involved in social networking and organizational memberships. And they may become very passionate about a cause that affected their loved one. Celebrity examples of this are David Hyde Pierce who is a tireless advocate for finding a cure for the Alzheimer's disease that devastated his family and took both his father and his grandfather, and Holly Robinson Peete who created the HollyRod Foundation to support families facing Parkinson's disease and autism, which affected her father and son respectively.

Also, older adults find volunteering an integral part of their desire to give back to society – a strong trait that ties us baby boomers together. Thus, caregivers uniquely combine their *obligatory* activity (caregiving) with later *discretionary activities* (volunteering).

The good news about volunteering is it can actually improve your health. A survey conducted by UnitedHealthcare and VolunteerMatch found volunteering can have the following health benefits:

- 34% of volunteers have *average* or *normal* BMI versus only 27% for non-volunteers
- 68% said volunteering made them physically healthier
- 73% said volunteering lowered their stress levels

Similarly, HomeInstead – an international organization that provides senior home care – conducted a poll that found 74 percent of older Americans who volunteered overcame feelings of isolation and 70 percent drove away depression through volunteering. Eight out of 10 volunteered to *occupy their free time.*

Since 1989 when President George Herbert Walker Bush launched his *thousand points of light* initiative for volunteerism, Americans have stepped up; there has been a 60 percent increase in volunteers since that time. Baby boomers and older generations have increased volunteerism by 40 percent since the '80s, according to a 2009 report from Hands On Network, part of the Points of Light Institute. One of the largest online volunteerism sites, Care2, has more than 20 million people of all ages who volunteer for a variety of causes, some of which include caregiving. They call themselves the *online dating service for good causes,* as they bring together volunteers and match them up with the cause closest to their heart.

Following is a quick snapshot of different ways to volunteer to help caregivers and their loved ones:

Create an online community of care: There are a few online sites where you can create private communities around the caregiver. One of my favorites is Lotsa Helping Hands. This free service allows you to send emails out to the caregiver's inner circle asking them to sign up to be volunteers. There is a sophisticated calendar tool, Help Calendar, where you list tasks to help the caregiver. Tasks may include picking up the caregiver's kids at school because she is at the doctor's office with her mom, or dropping off a meal for her family because she is at the nursing home that night visiting her loved one or sitting with her dad so she can get her hair done or go to the gym. What I like is the focus is on helping the caregiver. By giving the caregiver a *break*, also known as respite, this type of volunteering is a personal gift every caregiver needs.

Another online site is CaringBridge. Originally conceived to provide well-wishes and updates to the network of friends and family involved in a loved one's illness, the site has recently added a calendar tool to coordinate and perform tasks. You will find more on both of these sites and others in the LOST and Found chapter.

Faith-based organizations: Many local churches, synagogues and mosques offer support groups and other ways to help caregivers. An inter-faith nonprofit organization that has a plethora of volunteering opportunities is the National Volunteer Caregiving Network (formerly known as Faith in Action Network). Typical services include transportation, grocery shopping, minor home repairs, friendly visiting, bill paying, light housekeeping and respite for the caregiver.

While the National Volunteer Caregiving Network has affiliates across the country, there are many local faith-based organizations that perform similar tasks to help caregivers such as the Center for Volunteer Caregiving, a nonprofit faith-based organization formed in 1992 in Wake County, North Carolina.

Home meal deliveries: Approximately 7-8 million caregivers live long-distance from their loved one and cannot be there every day to ensure she eats properly or at all. Meals On Wheels has more than 2.5 million volunteers who pack and deliver 1 million meals *every day* to those who are homebound – many of them over the age of 60.

Hospice: According to the National Hospice and Palliative Care Organization (NHPCO), more than 22 million hours of hospice care are performed by volunteers every year; average time per volunteer was 46 hours.

In-Person Community Volunteers: Numerous local organizations provide community volunteers for caregivers. Many can be found through the Area Agencies on Aging (AAAs) and the Elder Care Locator. Here are a few stand-outs, some are member organizations while others are open to all:

Parker Jewish Institute for Health Care and Rehabilitation created the Willing Hearts, Helpful Hands program to connect caregivers with community volunteers helping thousands of caregivers and their loved ones in Nassau and Queens counties in New York.

WomanSage – Headquartered in Orange County, California with a handful of chapters around the country, this group for women age 50+ provides caregivers with a much-needed respite vacation by taking several caregivers on a local cruise and providing respite for their loved one while they get some *me time.*

The Transition Network was started by Charlotte Frank, a former senior vice president at McGraw Hill primarily to help women age 50+ through life-changing situations such as caregiving. Volunteers in New York City help each other through the Caring Collaborative.

Motion Picture and Television Fund (MPTF) has a program called Phone Buddies – volunteers who call seniors every week who may be lonely to cheer them up and socialize. Other MPTF volunteers shop for groceries; partner up for fitness or pool exercise at the Saban Center for Health & Wellness at the Woodland Hills, California campus; and tutor older MPTF members in their homes about computers and technology.

Mentoring: One way for former caregivers to get involved in their communities by helping other caregivers is through the National Family Caregivers Association Caregiver Community Action Network (CCANers). Located in 68 communities across the U.S., this caregiving *mentor/ volunteer* network helps to spread the word about caregiving through interaction with private and public agencies especially during November's National Family Caregiving Month.

In Melbourne, Florida, Dr. Rosemary Laird runs a mentoring program called the *Give Back Club* for the Health First Aging Institute. The program connects former caregivers with current caregivers to provide respite care, giving caregivers a break and providing companionship to the caregiver's loved one. There are also several support groups for caregivers who have recently experienced a loss to continue to meet and share their grieving journeys with each other.

Transportation and Senior Driving Safety: Getting around is a key concern for older Americans who no longer drive and family caregivers who struggle to provide the transportation their loved one needs. The following is a short list of organizations that provide volunteer drivers:

ITNAmerica is a nonprofit organization that matches caregivers and their seniors with volunteer drivers in 27 communities across the country. Providing what they call *door-to-door* and *arm-through-arm* service, this is not just doctor visit drop-offs, the Ride & Shop program will help your loved one carry packages from shop to car to home. You can volunteer to drive, donate an old car or participate in walk-a-thons across the country to raise funds for older Americans to get a ride.

National Center for Senior Transportation offers a web site powered by Easter Seals and the National Area Agencies on Aging that is a clearinghouse for senior transportation needs across the country. Their site provides information on where to find both paid and volunteer drives for your loved one.

CarFit is sponsored by the Automobile Club of America, AARP and the American Occupational Therapy Association to help older drivers remain safely in their cars and on the road longer. CarFit Technicians and Event Coordinators are volunteer-based, and hold CarFit activities at senior centers and other locations around the country to adjust an older adult's car to fit their aging needs.

Veterans' Caregivers - While the Department of Veteran's Affairs offers a variety of services to help caregivers of veterans, there are numerous veterans service organizations (VSOs) that have volunteer services to do the same.

Wounded Warrior Project (WWP) solicits volunteers to help with annual caregiver respite camps where caregivers gather to support each other and get a break. The WWP also has an online site, My Care Crew, where anyone can volunteer to help caregivers with a variety of tasks.

Joining Forces is an initiative to encourage institutions, businesses and individuals to do more to help military families that is championed by First Lady Michelle Obama and Jill Biden, wife of the Vice President. So far some of the programs and ways you can help include:

- The YMCA, National Military Family Association and Sierra Club Foundation offered free summer camp to 7,000 military kids at camps in 35 states.
- Wal-Mart and Sam's Club will guarantee a job at a nearby store for military family members who have been transferred to another part of the country.

- The U.S. Chamber of Commerce will hold 100 hiring fairs around the country to help 50,000 veterans and military spouses find jobs outside government.

ReMIND is the nonprofit organization that is part of the Bob Woodruff Foundation to provide resources and support to injured service members, veterans and their families. Its Stand Up for Heroes annual event is held in November or you can donate to the cause through the ReMIND Web site.

Help Our Wounded is a nonprofit organization started by Rosie Babin, a Texas-based mother of an Operation Iraqi Freedom (OIF) veteran who suffered traumatic brain injury (TBI) and who cares for her wounded son at home. She started the organization to provide support and direct assistance for veteran's families in need. The volunteer help are mentors who know how to navigate the VA and military benefits system – those caregivers who have been through the experience of caring for a veteran.

Caregiving and volunteerism are inherently tied together. As our nation faces more and more caregiving needs, the spirit of volunteerism will thrive for as Ralph Waldo Emerson expressed, "It is one of the most beautiful compensations of life that no man can sincerely try to help another without helping himself."

Refreshments – How Will You Overcome Stress, Burn-out, Guilt and Depression?

"I have to look after myself first. I think that is being self-full."

– Maya Angelou

When it comes to caregiving, there are two people in the relationship – your loved one and **you**. Each person is equally important but one tends to get short shrift – you. It is easy to do; you have multiple demands on you – work, spouse or partner, kids, other family members, friends and of course, the loved one who needs your care. Once you are through taking care of everyone else, there is no time left in the day for **you**. This entire section is just for **you**.

> **I am a caregiver and I am not alone.**

While this section will focus on your self-care, what may help is to know you are not alone. What you will find through these chapters will become you daily mantra:

I am a caregiver and I am not alone.

There are people, organizations and services that can help you. Think about it for a minute – there has never been a movie or TV show with just one person – you need a star, a director, a cameraman, a sound operator, etc. At most sporting events, there is not just one person – even if it is not a team sport like football or baseball, let's say it is boxing, tennis or horseracing – you still need two opponents (or a jockey *and* a horse). Caregiving is no different – you may feel like you are in it all by yourself but there is no need to make it a solo act.

When it comes to caregiving, there is no Triple Crown or a Super Bowl match-up, but there are major challenges most of the caregivers I have spoken to face when it comes to their own self-care. I call these caregiving challenges – the Final Four because if you don't outrun them, they will overrun you:

- Stress
- Burn-out
- Guilt
- Depression

As I have talked about throughout this book, stress is a caregiver's biggest challenge. A study by the Commonwealth Fund found caregivers are at twice the risk as the general population to develop multiple chronic illnesses due to the prolonged stress of caring for a loved one. And we know from the caregiver health risk study conducted by the National Alliance for Caregiving, stress is the caregiver's No. 1 complaint. If you read the Casting Calls chapters of this book, each chapter ended with a spotlight on the impact of stress on you: the caregiver. We need you to care for yourself as much as you care for anyone else.

I start this section on balancing self-care with caregiving by giving you tips on how to eliminate stress. I call the following pages Refreshments because *refresh* is what caregivers need and because it happens to be a ritual of mine whenever I go to the movies or a football game. I have to have my snacks or refreshments (popcorn and Milk Duds please!). These are your refreshments for taking back the control over caregiving.

In addition to managing stress, I will give you tips and techniques on how to avoid burn-out, how to get rid of guilt and how to defeat depression. If you can learn how to overcome these four caregiving obstacles, you will have developed the self-care tools so essential to your caregiving success.

Self-care is about self-help and the journey always begins with knowledge. Learning is a lifelong endeavor. When you take on caregiving, you take on college crash courses in a variety of areas, mostly your loved one's health. But this is also the time to learn more about you – your physical and emotional health. Explore your emotions over the relationship you have with your loved one, understand how to care for yourself while you care for others. These are the lessons of caregiving. You will learn how to find balance so you don't feel dizzy, dazed and confused like Jimmy Stewart in *Vertigo*.

In an interview with *Aging Today*, Maya Angelou discussed self-care,

> "I learned a long time ago the wisest thing I can do is be on my own side, be an advocate for myself...If I do that well enough, then I will be able to look after someone else – the children or the husband or the elderly. But I have to look at myself first. I know that some people think that's being selfish, I think this is being self-full."

Love, Actually

What you will also learn is caregiving is about love – the love we give away and the love we give to ourselves. Caregivers tell me they are performing a "labor of love." They are. They also will learn self-love and the power of this universal emotion.

There is a great opening to one of my favorite movies which is now part of my holiday DVD viewing ritual (along with *The Sound of Music*, *The Holiday* and of course, *It's a Wonderful Life*). The movie, *Love, Actually*, opens with a voiceover from actor Hugh Grant who says:

> "Whenever I get gloomy with the state of the world, I think about the arrivals gate at Heathrow Airport. General opinion studies make out that we live in a world of hatred and greed, but I don't see that. It seems to me that love is everywhere. Often it is not particularly dignified or newsworthy but it is always there – fathers and sons, mothers and daughters, husbands and wives, girlfriends, old friends. When the planes hit the Twin Towers, as far as I know none of the phone calls from the people on board were messages of hate or revenge, they were all messages of love. If you look for it, I've got a sneaky feeling that you'll find that love actually is all around."

As a caregiver you will see, you are not alone – love is all around you.

From Ghostbusters to Stressbusters

Learn to relax, reconnect

Remember the scene in the movie *Ghostbusters* where Bill Murray and Dan Aykroyd have to destroy the huge Stay-Puft Marshmallow Man? Well, that marshmallow man in a caregiver's life is called Stress and this chapter will help you become a Stressbuster.

If you are a caregiver stress is something you can't live with, but you can't seem to live without it either. As you read at the end of each Casting Calls chapter, stress comes in all shapes and sizes. It attacks each of us differently, but the impact almost always takes a toll on you emotionally and physically. Dr. Alice Domar and Dr. Susan Love in their book, *Live A Little!* state it is not caregiving that makes you stressed, it is how you perceive its burdens.

In a *Forbes* article, Debbie Mandel, a stress-management author said, "Women tend to say to the world, 'Look what I can do,' since they've been raised to please others and define their self worth according to the way others perceive them." She calls this gender phenomenon *stress addiction*. "Women who are addicted to stress are suppressing feelings of unattractiveness, unworthiness and inadequacy," says Mandel in the article. "[They're] always moving forward, living in the future or worrying what will happen later. It's a survival mechanism."

In addition, another *Forbes* article on working women discussed the impact of stress with no relief, especially for women juggling careers, children and caregiving. "Cortisol build-up can create memory loss and a lower attention span," says Sandra Chapman, the director of the Center for Brain Health at the University of Texas at Dallas. "It's particularly toxic to the memory area of the brain."

Conversely, while men feel stress they also may have better coping mechanisms than women when it comes to caregiving. A study conducted by Bowling Green University researchers looked into gender differences during caregiving and found men were able to balance their lives better than women.

"They see caregiving as just one of the tasks they have to complete instead of the main or only task approach of the female caregivers," says I-Fen Lin, the associate professor who headed up the study.

In addition, when it came to men caring for an ill spouse, the researchers found men received more praise from their spouse and from others for their caregiving role, and this positive feedback also contributed to them feeling less stressed. The caregivers who were sons caring for an older parent also asked for more help than their female counterparts.

"They approach caregiving from a problem-solving perspective and don't internalize their performance which the female caregivers tended to do which increased their worry and thus, increased their stress levels," continues Lin.

Robert Sapolsky, PhD, professor of neurobiology at Stanford University explained in a recent WebMD article that cortisol, long believed to be the culprit when it comes to stress hormones, is not the enemy for men. Rather it is the hormone oxytocin.

"In women, when cortisol and epinephrine rush through the bloodstream in a stressful situation, oxytocin comes into play," he says in the article. "It is released from the brain, countering the production of cortisol and epinephrine, and promoting nurturing and relaxing emotions. While men also secrete the hormone oxytocin when they're stressed, it's in much smaller amounts, leaving them on the short end of the stick when it comes to stress and hormones."

All this stress can spell serious health concerns for both women and men who are caregivers. A University of Michigan study found men who were more physiologically reactive to stress (as measured by high blood pressure) were 72 percent more likely to suffer a stroke.

In their book, *So Stressed*, Dr. Stephanie McClellan and Dr. Beth Hamilton recommend testing yourself on these questions to determine how stressed you may be:

- Can you drop your shoulders?
- Is your brow furrowed?
- Is your tongue pressed against the top of your mouth?
- Is your breathing rapid and uneven?
- Is it hard to focus on things like reading this page – do you find yourself distracted thinking about aches or pains in your body?

If you answered "yes" to most of these questions, your muscles are tensed and poised for an attack. However, having muscle tension in your body for a prolonged period of time will put pressure on your joints and reduce your blood flow which decreases your energy and eventually makes you feel fatigued and strained.

According to the American Medical Association, roughly 80 percent of all doctor visits are stress-related with prolonged stress contributing to everything from ulcers to heart disease. Robert Sapolsky stated in his book, *Why Zebras Don't Get Ulcers*, long-term stress can suppress the immune system and send it plummeting 40 to 70 percent below normal.

Stress is your body trying to talk to you. You need to listen. Do not blow yourself off because you just don't have time. Your body is one of your best friends. If a best friend were crying out to you that she needed help and could you just listen for a few minutes, wouldn't you do it? After hearing what your body has to say, your response should be to advise it how to relax and reconnect.

In the latest edition of his best-selling book, *The Relaxation Response*, author and meditation research pioneer Dr. Herbert Benson, founder of the Mind/Body Institute at Massachusetts General Hospital in Boston states, "By taking advantage of the cost-free, healing resources within all of us, the United States, by conservative estimates, stands to save more than $50 billion in wasted health care expenditures each year."

Test Your Stress

Stress tests are very popular these days. Banks and financial institutions go through them. So do software programs, hardware servers and nuclear power plants. The point of a stress test is to determine the stability of a system when it is pushed to the breaking point.

For caregivers, if you feel you might be at your breaking point, taking a stress test and discussing it with your doctor becomes essential. As stated in other chapters in this book, if stress takes you out of the picture, who will continue to care for your loved one? If you feel ongoing stress, known as *chronic stress*, there are a couple good Caregiver Stress Tests you can take.

The American Medical Association has a Caregiver Self-Assessment Questionnaire in both English and Spanish that probes stress-related issues. The Alzheimer's Association has also developed a specific Caregiver Stress Test for those caring for someone with dementia. Both of these tests can be found on web sites listed in the Resources section of this book. If you research stress tests online, be sure to choose one that specifically states *caregiver stress test* – otherwise you will find stress tests from the Mayo Clinic and others that test for heart health but may not include questions specific to your caregiving situation. Some of the questions on the two Caregiver Stress Tests I mentioned are:

Q: Have you withdrawn from family and friends since you began caregiving?
Q: Do you feel grief or sadness your relationship with your loved one is not the same as it once was?
Q: Do you suddenly have more trouble making decisions?
Q: Do you have lower back pain?
Q: Do you feel anxious about money and health care decisions for your loved one's care?

Other warning signs include: Are you constipated or have frequent diaherra? Do you feel dizzy or have you fainted recently? Do you have an upset stomach or bloating? Have you lost your interest in sex?

After you have taken one of the tests, if you score off the charts it is important to discuss it with your doctor. Stress can increase your blood pressure, raise your cortisol level which is the hormone responsible for belly fat, create tension headaches, exacerbate lower back pain and lead to other serious health issues.

Stress also has been linked to asthma, acne and alopecia (sudden baldness where your hair falls out – something Princess Caroline of Monaco suffered from in recent years). Another side effect of stress is the possible impact to your physical appearance: dull, lifeless hair, a destruction of the collagen fibers in your skin and breakdown of the elastin leading to sagging and wrinkles which can make you look years older than you are.

Stress is a bi-partisan offender – take a look at any President of the United States before he entered the White House and look at the photos of him after he leaves office. The stress of being the supreme leader of the free world has a price, and it ain't pretty.

Caregiving: Foe or Friend?

We know the No. 1 complaint for caregivers is stress – and if not managed can cause serious health issues – but the risks might be even greater than we knew. In a study published in the *Journal of the American Medical Association* by Richard Schulz and Scott Beach, both PhDs and researchers at the University of Pittsburgh, their findings suggest the mental and emotional strain experienced by a caregiver is an independent risk factor for mortality among elderly spousal caregivers. After adjusting for other factors, caregivers who report strain had a 63 percent higher incidence of death than non-caregivers.

While caregivers definitely fight stress that can increase certain health risks, the flip side to this is two more recent studies found caregiving may actually be *beneficial* to your health and longevity. The Boston University School of Public Health studied stress effects on caregivers and found a surprising benefit: better physical functioning among those *high intensity* caregivers who helped with bathing, dressing and other activities of daily living (ADLs). These caregivers had better walking speed and grip strength and may actually get more exercise or physical benefit from caregiving than non-caregivers.

A different study by AbT Associates in Cambridge, Massachusetts, found caregivers scored better on tests for memory and processing speed than non-caregivers. While there is no definitive link to the study findings, researchers believe caregiving is about multi-tasking and solving problems which improve these cognitive functions. As well, in a recent study published in the journal, *Stroke*, it was reported a full 90 percent of those caring for someone who had suffered a stroke said their caregiving enabled them to appreciate life more. Many also reported it helped them develop a more positive attitude.

In addition, Dr. Domar and Dr. Love say, "Stress also has side benefits. For example, your body will be stronger if you have both times of calm and periods of heart-pounding excitement." They go on to say the only people who are completely carefree are people under the age of twelve (and I'm not even sure about that given the amount of stressful homework my 12-year-old nephew goes through and the stress school-age children experience who may be bullied).

Australian social psychologist Dr. Charmaine Saunders says in her book, *Women & Stress*, stress can be harnessed in a beneficial way. She explains that sports psychologists help athletes build winning mentalities by using the stress response of an adrenaline rush that increases your heart rate and respiration and then turning that into increased energy. "Let stress give you the winning edge," says Dr. Saunders. "Instead of thinking 'I've got so much to do, I can't get it all done,' let the pressure stimulate you to be more efficient. Turn the stress into a challenge to be conquered not tolerated or controlling you. It will make your life more enjoyable rather than a struggle."

So much depends on the duration of the stress and how we deal with it. Caregivers spend on average 4.6 years in their caregiving role, and if stress, with no outlet, is experienced on an almost daily basis for this long period, then it is more likely your health will be impacted. Stress is inevitable so you can only control how you manage it. One of the ways to bring balance back into your life is to acknowledge you will encounter some stress and it may not always be bad. While chronic stress is to be avoided, putting pressure on yourself to create a stress management plan may just add more stress. Some of the following stress management techniques will help you become more of a *go with the flow* person.

How do you spell Stress R-E-L-I-E-F?

Just as there is no *one size fits all* for caregiving, different people have different ways to deal with stress. Sometimes we cannot control the disorders or diseases that attack our bodies. But learning to manage your stress will go a long way in keeping both your body and mind strong, so you can avoid the health risks we know are associated with stress.

There are many ways to address stress: better diet and exercise, adequate sleep, ensuring you have balance in your life. All of that sounds easy, right? When I have spoken to groups of caregivers, they all ask me, "I know I'm supposed to take better care of myself – BUT HOW?" A little discipline and faith is all it takes (and anywhere from 5 to 60 minutes a day – depending on how much time you have – but it is critical to give it at least five minutes a day).

While stress and burn-out can seem very similar, I address the nutrition, exercise and sleep and other ways to avoid burn-out in the chapter called Backdraft. For this section, I have found stress relief can be poured into two buckets: Relaxation and Reconnection.

Relax

According to the American Psychological Association (APA), 36 percent of Americans experience chronic work stress. If you couple work with caregiving, the statistics increase as the National Alliance for Caregiving (NAC) found. In the 2009 NAC study, more than half of working caregivers reported feeling *more stressed* about their caregiving situation and 50 percent were less comfortable discussing their caregiving responsibilities with their supervisor.

The Molotov cocktail for many caregivers is the combination of pressures of work and the exhaustion or time commitment of caregiving – compounded by the anxiety of how you will cover all the responsibilities and costs associated with *life as we know it.*

The APA is working with companies to find ways to de-stress employees without the use of prescription drugs. It has created a Family Caregiver Briefcase to help psychologists and other health care professionals better help family caregivers. The *tool kit* includes statistics, research and advocacy efforts, tools for helping caregivers cope with stress and the data reinforcing the critical help psychologists can play in helping family caregivers so professionals gain better understanding of their role in the world of caregiving.

For example, one company working with the APA, is holding a meditation class. Some companies are bringing in massage therapists and I worked for a company that brought in free yoga instructors for end of work day classes in an effort to help employees feel the *Zen* instead of the *burn*.

In today's fast-paced, stress-filled, slow economic growth, multi-tasking world – the art of relaxation is like speaking Latin – an almost forgotten, dead language. Dr. Benson's meditation technique, called the Relaxation Response, is one way to revive this forgotten language of relaxation. His technique is comprised of these steps and he prescribes doing this twice daily:

1. Choose a word, sound, short phrase or prayer you will repeat continuously for 10-20 minutes.
2. Sit still and comfortably.
3. Close your eyes and relax your muscles.
4. Focus your attention on your breathing, simply observing the in-and-out breaths.

5. Begin repeating your word.
6. As other thoughts may enter your stress-filled mind, don't force them away or become annoyed, simply, gently ignore them and continue your repetitive word or phrase.

What he found is this simple exercise when done daily can help with a host of health issues including fatigue, hypertension, asthma, constipation, infertility, insomnia, rheumatoid arthritis, chest pain, allergies, allergic skin reactions and more. You should notice improvement in your health and stress levels in less than one month.

Most de-stress tips deal with meditation offering a variation of Dr. Benson's technique. Here are some of the best I have found:

Breathe deeply – America's favorite MD – Dr. Oz – says relaxation can be as simple as breathing and only takes five minutes a day. Here is how: lie on your back, put one hand on your stomach and one hand on your chest. As you inhale, push your stomach way out to the count of 5. After five seconds, a comfortable breath should be held and then exhale slowly – letting your stomach come down and really pushing that stomach down until your belly hits your spine. Repeat this 10 times in the morning and 10 times at night. You will feel amazingly relaxed and it helps with drainage of your lymphatic system which removes the toxins from your body.

Visualize – The art of visualization is something that fascinates me and professionals say can really work. When you were a kid did you ever lie on your back and just stare at the clouds imagining their shape as animals or other objects? "I see a car, I see a lion, I see a four-leaf clover." That state of Zen is what you are going for here.

What makes visualization difficult is all the noise pollution we have in our lives. Constant interruptions by texts, emails, cell phones, crowded trains and traffic congestion all challenge you when you are trying to focus. If you are in the office or at home, take a little walk to a spot where you can sit and escape for a few minutes. Turn off your cell phone – it will only be a few minutes, and the world will not end in just those few minutes. Maybe do some window shopping – imagine yourself in that adorable dress or shoes, hitting that perfect putt on the golf course, or look into a bakery window and imagine the warm, hot chocolate being baked into the soft croissant. You can also sit on a bench and people-watch, and make up your own movie about the strangers walking-by.

Or, you can just sit and close your eyes and imagine a place you would like to be – a hammock in the Bahamas, a gondola in Venice, a mountain top in the Himalayas. My favorite? I'm in a red convertible cruising down Pacific Coast Highway along the beach in California between Santa Barbara and Carmel with Mark Harmon (I feel better already!).

Focus on one true thing – We are all juggling multiple activities: you have to pick the kids up from school, return that call at work, schedule the carpet cleaners, send that birthday card to your sister, get to the grocery store before they close – and on and on. Take 5 minutes all to yourself and just zone out.

Read a magazine, go for a walk and listen to the rustle of the tree leaves or the tweeting of the birds, plug into your iPod or radio station and sit or drive around for a few minutes with no destination in mind and really think about the song lyrics and how they move you. Remember the scene in the movie *City of Angels* where Nicolas Cage asks Meg Ryan how a pear feels and she describes the sweet, sugary sand that dissolves in your mouth? By focusing on one sensory activity – seeing, hearing, tasting, touching – your brain relaxes and sends impulses to your other muscles to relax as well.

Try yoga or tai chi – These relaxation activities are not just for the *new age* lovers – there are real health benefits to performing at least one of these activities just a few minutes a day. I know what you may be thinking – I thought it too when I took my first yoga class, "Why am I here? I'm too busy and this is just the latest Hollywood fad – the touchy, feely stuff I don't have time for!"

In my first yoga class, I could not relax AT ALL – I kept thinking about my deadline for an article I was writing, my nephew's birthday gift I had not bought yet, the credit card bill I forgot to mail, etc. All I wanted was a Starbucks coffee. But after one class, I was convinced. I left feeling warm and relaxed and…blissful.

Yoga is not a trend, it started in India more than 5,000 years ago, and more than 11 million Americans practice some type of yoga. Because yoga incorporates breathing techniques, it not only helps relax your body but it also has the meditative benefits of relaxing your mind. You will read in the stories of Marg Helgenberger, Jill Eikenberry and Alana Stewart yoga is something that gets them through the day.

Don't try yoga on your own for the first time – it is always helpful to take a class at your gym or local community center to learn the proper techniques and have an instructor advise you on poses and breathing. The health benefits beyond stress relief include:

1. Better flexibility – many first-time yoga participants noticed a 35 percent improvement in flexibility after just eight weeks of twice weekly yoga classes.
2. Release of the lactic acid in your muscles which contributes to tension, stiffness, pain and fatigue.
3. Lubrication of your joints giving you better range of motion.
4. Lowering of your heart rate as well as your blood pressure, which many doctors believe can be one solution to helping you prevent heart disease.

Some researchers have also found yoga can eliminate certain symptoms of arthritis, asthma, insomnia and help those with multiple sclerosis minimize pain.

The Mayo Clinic describes the ancient practice of tai chi (pronounced tie-CHEE) as *meditation in motion*. This ancient Chinese ritual of self-defense, when performed as exercise, is actually a serene, peaceful way to connect gentle motions with clearing your mind. Tai chi is not only good for caregivers but it can be good for our older loved ones as well, because the motions are slow and easy and it is considered a low impact exercise with little physical exertion, since emphasis is placed on graceful movement not strength or power.

You may have seen people gathered in a park or outside to practice tai chi – many believe it is best done outside because it can help you connect your spiritual self with nature for metaphysical benefits. In fact, many of the more than 100 poses are named for animals or nature.

The best part is no equipment or special dress code is needed to practice tai chi – this is a *come as you are*-type of activity. You may have to pay for a class, but many senior centers and parks and recreation locations offer low-cost or free tai chi classes. I saw a businessman in a suit in New York City join a tai chi class just by taking off his Brogue shoes and jacket. This is a *no excuses* type of exercise and relaxation. The health benefits are similar to yoga – it can lower your blood pressure, improve your posture and circulation, relax your muscles, provide headache relief and boost your immune system.

Yoga and tai chi can also help you and your loved one improve your balance, which can reduce the risk of falls – a serious health risk that puts 2 million seniors in Emergency Rooms (ERs) every year. Both yoga and tai chi create *homeostasis* – a steady state of harmony, balance and equilibrium in the body – which dates back to the ancient Greeks and Chinese. As Master Po said to David Carradine's character in the 1970s TV show *Kung Fu*, "I can only point the way, Grasshopper, you must walk the path yourself."

Massage - There is also the ancient art of massage. In BC 460, Hippocrates wrote, "The physician must be experienced in many things, but assuredly in rubbing" and massage therapy become widely used in Europe during the Renaissance. In the latest data available, which is 2007, the National Health Interview Survey found 18 million U.S. adults had received massage therapy. Sometimes we think of massage as an indulgence rather than the therapeutic health benefits. It is time to shift our thinking.

While massage therapists may be expensive on a regular basis, a 5-10 minute self-massage solution comes from Darrin Zeer, author of *Lover's Massage and Office Yoga*. The following self-massage technique from his book will help take you on the Zen Express Train:

1. Place both hands on your shoulders and neck.
2. Squeeze with your fingers and palms.
3. Rub vigorously, keeping shoulders relaxed.
4. Wrap one hand around the other forearm.
5. Squeeze the muscles with thumb and fingers.
6. Move up and down from your elbow to fingertips and back again.
7. Repeat with other arm.

According to the Mayo Clinic, massage can lower blood pressure, boost immunity, and provide therapeutic effect for those suffering from MS and cancer. It can also aid in alleviating lower-back pain, increase join flexibility, decrease anxiety or depression, relieve migraines and improve immunity.

Reconnect

In his best-selling book, *The Blue Zone*, author Dan Buettner advises social networks are one of the principles to living a long and happy life. When it comes to caregiving, your social network is your lifeline. This network may be friends or family members who make you laugh, give you a break from caregiving or just listen to you. It may also include a support group where you can vent and let it all out with other caregivers who know exactly what you are going through. I talk more about support groups, the power of friendships and even professional help in the chapter called LOST and Found.

Dr. Gary Small, author of *The Alzheimer's Prevention Program*, advises that becoming and staying socially active can reduce your risk for dementia by as much as 60 percent. His colleague at the UCLA Longevity Center, Dr. Steven Cole discovered, "Chronically lonely people overexpress genes linked to inflammation, which can cause brain cell damage and neural degeneration." Even if you like being alone, these researchers found one of the benefits of being social is in protecting your brain health.

The message here is to avoid disconnecting from your social network – no man (or woman) can survive as an island, even the reality TV show, *Survivor*, has taught us that. The tribe has spoken.

Backdraft and the Magnificent Seven – 7 Ways to Put Out the Flames of Burn-out

Sleep, sunshine, sustenance, sweating, soothing, sex, setting limits

In the world of firefighting, a backdraft is when a fire is starved of oxygen and tiny puffs of smoke are being pulled back into an enclosed space through small holes like those in a doorframe. When a door or window is opened, suddenly oxygen is released into the room and creates a spontaneous combustion and – kaboom! In the 1991 film, *Backdraft*, Kurt Russell and William Baldwin play two of the most experienced Chicago firefighters, who miscalculate an escalating threat of a backdraft.

When it comes to caregiving, your backdraft is the blow back of your own health neglect called *burn-out*, also known as *compassion fatigue*. When you are focused on caring for a loved one 24/7 for a prolonged period of time with no break, no oxygen, no breathing room – you may miscalculate the impact and suddenly it's – kaboom!

Caregiving typically means you are in a marathon not a sprint. A world-class runner who can finish the 100-yard dash in 9.1 seconds cannot keep up that pace for 26 miles – it is simply impossible. Caregivers need to learn how to train for a marathon. Even though your caregiving race may begin with a crisis event (a sprint), very often it lasts far longer than you may anticipate – not days but weeks, months or years (a marathon). When it comes to staying in the race, you first need to know the signs of burn-out. The symptoms can vary but here are some typical red flags:

- Fatigue
- Not getting enough restorative, uninterrupted sleep – frequent insomnia
- Cranky, irritated, frustrated – often not just one isolated incident
- Depressed or often sad, feeling hopeless or alienated
- Cannot focus or concentrate, easily distracted
- Missing appointments or cancelling them all together
- Frequent emotional outbursts – crying, yelling
- Excessive use of alcohol, medications, sleeping pills or rekindling old bad habits such as smoking
- Appetite change – eating a lot more or a lot less

Often, burn-out and stress are linked together. I would define the difference between the two this way: stress is the cause and burn-out is the effect.

When I spoke to former First Lady Rosalynn Carter, it was part of her pioneering efforts in support of caregivers that identified burn-out as a serious caregiver issue.

"One of the first things we focused on back in the 1980s was based on a survey we did that showed the significance of caregiver burn-out," remembers Mrs. Carter. "We did our first conference on burn-out and people were crying in the audience saying this was the first time someone understood what they were going through."

Mrs. Carter says what they learned is if caregivers do not take care of themselves, then the quality of care they can give to their loved one is diminished. Mrs. Carter also advises, "They [caregivers] also have to recognize the need for help and be willing to receive help."

She realizes this is easier said than done. Rosalynn speaks from personal experience. She was a young caregiver of only 13 when she looked after a father with leukemia and after his passing, cared for her younger siblings while her mother worked. She also cared for her mother who lived to age 94 as well as a brother and other in-laws. I asked her if she had identified herself as a caregiver through the years and she laughed, "No, I didn't realize I was a caregiver until I got involved in this work."

The Magnificent Seven

Once you realize you are a caregiver and burn-out is the enemy, one of the ways to fight burn-out is with what I call *The Magnificent Seven*. In this 1960 Western film starring some of the most macho men on the planet including Steve McQueen, Yul Brynner, Charles Bronson and James Coburn, seven gunmen are hired to protect a small village. Seven is the number that has meant something magical and powerful through the ages: the seven figures in Greek mythology (the Pleiades which are heavenly stars at night), the first seven movie studios in Hollywood; and the *Seven Sisters* – seven of the leading women's magazines in the 1970s-80s. In the fairy tale, Snow White has the Seven Dwarfs to help her find her prince and protect her from the evil Queen. In your caregiving story, your Magnificent Seven that will help you put out the flames of burn-out are:

1. Sleep
2. Sunshine and Supplements (vitamins, nutritional supplements)
3. Sustenance (good nutrition, hydration)
4. Sweating (exercise)
5. Soothing (soothing baths, aromatherapy)
6. Sex
7. Setting Limits

Sleeping Beauty

Sleep is not just for beauty it is actually one of the easiest and best ways to improve your health. Getting restorative sleep – uninterrupted for 7-9 hours is recommended by most experts. If you suffer from insomnia and sleep deprivation, you are at risk for numerous health issues. Lack of sleep can cause you to be forgetful, increase your appetite and cause you to be drowsy or distracted – which are how high risk events such as traffic accidents can occur. In fact, one study conducted by Australian researchers found losing two hours of sleep impairs your performance equal to having 0.05 blood alcohol level and the National Highway Traffic Safety Administration estimates there are 100,000 crashes each year based on driver fatigue.

More than 50 percent of people over age 65 suffer sleep disorders that ultimately shorten their lives and 70 million people in the U.S. have sleep problems. As if we don't have enough debt in our lives, this deprivation of sleep is called *sleep debt*. In an interview she did with WebMD, Susan

Zafarlotfi, PhD, clinical director of the Institute for Sleep and Wake Disorders at Hackensack University Medical Center in New Jersey, says, "Sleep debt is like credit card debt. If you keep accumulating credit card debt, you will pay high interest rates or your account will be shut down until you pay it all off. If you accumulate too much sleep debt, your body will crash."

A study done at the University of Washington at St Louis Medical School found people who had a lot of awakenings during the night – more than five per hour – were more likely to have pre-clinical Alzheimer's disease (which means they have normal mental skills but their brain changes are associated with the degenerative disorder). Another study published in *Stroke – The Journal of the American Heart Association* found the risk of heart attack in people with insomnia ranged from 27 percent to 45 percent greater than for people who rarely experienced sleep awakenings during the night. Other studies have shown healthy adults allowed to sleep just 5.5 hours a day quickly developed abnormal insulin levels and slowed metabolism. The researchers estimated the metabolic changes could translate into 12 extra pounds a year.

Eve Van Cauter, who directs the research laboratory on sleep at the University of Chicago, has been doing sleep research for 25 years and has found there are two hormones, gherlin and leptin, which influence our eating and weight in different ways. She calls these hormones the "yin and yang of hunger…One is the accelerator for eating (ghrelin), and the other is the brake (leptin)." Lack of good restorative sleep causes these hormones to be out of balance and thus, your body gains weight.

Insomnia typically is a function of not being able to relax our minds and our bodies. You will read more about relaxation techniques in the Ghostbusters/Stressbusters chapter. However, if frequent insomnia or trouble with a good solid 7-9 hours of sleep is eluding you, there are three things to think about:

1. Try the sleep hygiene tips listed in the next few paragraphs – in the same way we need to keep our personal hygiene maintained, our sleep hygiene is just as important.
2. Try the quick relaxation technique you will read about in the previous Stressbusters chapter.
3. If all else fails, seek a doctor who is a sleep specialist and can give you a sleep evaluation says Dr. Lawrence J. Epstein, head of the division of sleep medicine at Harvard University.

Here are four sleep hygiene tips that can help you become Rip Van Winkle:

1. Create a sleep-inducing environment: a dark, quiet, comfortable and cool room.
2. Do not use your bedroom for anything other than sleep or sex. (that's right, I wrote *sex*, more on that below). Ban TV watching, using your laptop or iPad and no reading in bed.

3. Make sure you do not eat at least two to three hours before bedtime, and avoid caffeine or alcohol close to bedtime. Smoking can also cause you to have trouble sleeping. If you find you are tossing and turning at night and you cannot get those eyes closed, try drinking green or chamomile tea before bed or put a lavender pillow near your head which aids relaxation. A glass of milk also works (unless you are lactose intolerant; if so, go back to tea).
4. Create consistent sleep cycles. Establish consistent sleep and wake schedules, even on weekends. Our bodies have internal clocks called circadian rhythms that synchronize our active and rest states with biochemical reactions in our bodies. Circadian rhythms are based on light/dark cycles – with light having the most impact on our ability to get to and stay in restorative sleep.

"Even if you get enough sleep, it may not be healthy sleep," says Dr. Don Harden, medical director at the Sleep Wellness Institute. "About 40-50 million people in the U.S. suffer from chronic sleep disorder and another 20-30 million have intermittent sleep-related problems related to stress, anxiety and depression."

Little Miss Sunshine

In a report from the Natural Marketing Institute, a global consulting firm for health, wellness and sustainability, 21 percent of baby boomers said they are "always looking for the next fountain of youth remedy," and 3 out of 5 are turning to nutritional supplements to ensure they get the proper nutrients they don't get in their normal diet.

According to Gale Bensussan, president of Leiner Health Products, one of the world's largest manufacturers of vitamins, nutritional supplements and over-the-counter drugs, vitamins and supplements help relieve physical stress, but scientific studies have yet to prove their impact on mental stress.

"Thirty-five years ago most physicians ignored the positive effects of supplements, but the more we have learned over the years about nutrition, you see doctors embracing a combination of prescription drugs, supplements and vitamins for greater health," says Bensussan. He observes nutritional supplements are enjoying a similar evolution that baby boomers created with natural foods. In the 1960s, *natural foods* was a term coined to mean *good for you* – at the time it was seen as a fringe movement associated with hippies; now it is mainstream.

He advises everyone should take a daily multivitamin, and there are studies showing women can multi-task better and have improved mental acuity after an increase of B-complex. Bensussan also supports the theory behind increased dosages of Vitamin D, also known as the *sunshine* vitamin, in helping with reducing the risk of falls and improving bone strength.

For those caregivers who have been mostly housebound with a loved one or living in areas where there are fewer days of sunshine (Anchorage? Seattle? Portland?) you can become SAD. Not the sad like in a sad clown, the sad as in seasonal affective disorder (SAD). According to the National Institutes of Health, SAD is a type of depression that occurs at a certain time of the year, typically in winter and affects more women than men. Vitamin D can help. As you will also read in Alan Osmond's story, he believes higher doses of daily Vitamin D have helped him manage his multiple sclerosis.

Super Foods for a Super You

As stated in our Rehearsals chapter called Breakfast at Tiffanys, we know 4 out of 10 caregivers report weight management due to chronic stress as a big challenge. There are many diets – some fads, some not – that come along to help us lose weight. For caregivers, it is not always a matter of losing weight (or gaining weight if you are anemic or prone to being underweight) – it is about having the stamina and the strength to be a good caregiver to your loved one.

If your body was a car, you never want to overfill the tank or let it hit *empty,* you want to try to keep at least ½ of good premium fuel in your engine to keep it running like a Ferrari.

Most importantly, you want to eat properly so not only do you have endurance and power but you maintain a healthy body mass index (BMI). We know BMI can be a risk factor in developing type II diabetes, heart disease and even a predictive factor for Alzheimer's disease. While you can get a calipers test or underwater test (also called a hydrostatic test) or other BMI measurement from a health care professional or your doctor, you can do a simple math equation – which factors together your height and weight – to calculate your current BMI measurement. The number should be between 18.5 and 24.9 for both women and men regardless of age (see the box).

> ## How to calculate your Body Mass Index (BMI)
>
> 1. Take your weight
> 2. Divide it by your height in inches
> 3. Divide this new number by your height in inches again (yes, a second time)
> 4. Multiply the new number x 703
>
> The result is your BMI. Remember, for both men and women the number should be between 18.5 – 24.9 to maintain good health.

Research shows most Americans gain 1-2 pounds every year after age 20 and while that does not seem like a lot, by the time we hit age 50 – two-thirds of all Americans are overweight. Now factor in issues such as not dropping the baby weight after childbirth or stress eating over caregiving, and you have a real health issue when it comes to your weight.

For women, weight gain over time is a serious health risk. A National Cancer Institute study found women who were at a normal weight and BMI at age 20 and increased their BMI by five points (essentially a 30-pound weight gain for a 5-foot 4-inch woman) had nearly double the risk of developing breast cancer after menopause than women who had maintained a healthy BMI range through the years.

One study found different impulses and emotions can cause us to crave different foods. For instance, if you need comfort, you will turn to a food that made you happy as a child. It may be the soothing cool of ice cream or it may be the warm blanket of a good soup. If you are feeling stressed, we have a tendency to grab something salty – french fries, potato chips, dill pickles, saltine crackers. If all this focus on food and weight is making you hungry or even more stressed, do not panic and run to the fridge for an ice cream sandwich!

In his book, *The Alzheimer's Prevention Program*, Dr. Gary Small, director of the UCLA Longevity Center, tells of a study UCLA conducted with the think tank, the RAND Corporation, which showed adopting one healthy lifestyle behavior (one of these seven activities) can lower your risk for Alzheimer's. In fact, their study concluded if everyone in the U.S. chose to eat omega-3 fatty acids found in fish such as salmon twice a week, or took a brisk walk every other day, we could expect 1 million fewer cases of Alzheimer's than otherwise anticipated.

While many *diets* profess *do this but not this*, according to experts at WebMD, a diet of *super foods* should be part of your daily intake. Here is their rundown of seven super foods (note the powerful number 7 again):

1. Blueberries are great anti-oxidants and an anti-inflammatory that can lower your risk of heart disease and cancer as well as other chronic illnesses.
2. Omega-3 rich fish such as salmon, herring, sardines and mackerel help your heart, joints and memory. Some medical professionals believe it can also reduce depression, another common caregiver complaint. If you are not a fish fan, you can also find Omega-3 in walnuts and flax seeds.
3. Soy such as tofu, soy milk or edamame, as well as almonds, oats and barley lower cholesterol. In addition, oatmeal can help regulate blood sugar levels which are important for those who have diabetes or are pre-diabetic. However, if you have a family history of breast cancer, it is not recommended you add soy to your diet.
4. Fiber keeps cholesterol in check and can aid weight loss since you will feel fuller. Look for beans, whole grains, fruit and vegetables. I try to *eat the rainbow* daily – one food a day that is red, orange, yellow, green and blue – which makes it fun and easier to remember to add these super foods to your daily diet.
5. Tea has been shown in several studies to lower cholesterol. While the antioxidant power is the same in black tea as green tea; the green version has an added element which studies have found helps inhibit the growth of cancer cells.
6. Calcium found in dairy foods, salmon (again), leafy green veggies, almonds (again) or sesame seeds, asparagus and figs build strong bones, help reduce the risk of osteoporosis and avoid brittle teeth. Women over age 51 should have 1,200 mg of calcium daily. Keep in mind Vitamin D aids in the absorption of calcium.
7. Dark Chocolate – hallelujah! Chocolate with at least 60 percent cocoa content has eight times the antioxidants as strawberries, and can help lower bad cholesterol (LDL) by up to 10 percent. But do not overindulge; 2-3 oz. a day will do it. How happy are you I can say "you must eat chocolate?"

Like Water for Chocolate

Since we ended the last section on the happy note of chocolate, let's segue into what makes your body happy: water. How important is water in avoiding burn-out and maintaining good health? Think of your body like the globe. The earth's surface is 70 percent water. So is most of your body. Here is the percentage of water composition throughout your body according to Watercure.com: lungs (90%), blood (82%), brain (76%), muscles (75%) and bones (25%). You can see why staying hydrated is so essential for your body to continue working properly.

According to EverydayHealth.com drinking enough water every day throughout the day will help you prevent heartburn, it will help ease the pain in joints caused by issues such as rheumatoid arthritis, it will decrease heart pain (angina is lack of water in the heart/lung axis), it can help reduce or eliminate migraines (which can sometimes mean there is lack of water in the eyes and brain), it reduces bouts of colitis related to constipation in the large intestine and can help manage asthma (when combined with salt), which affects 1 in 12 Americans, including 14 million children. Water also helps the kidneys flush the toxins from your body.

Although the latest Institute of Medicine report shows eight glasses of any liquid is beneficial, try to stay away from diet sodas, which are typically high in sodium and can cause bloating. These sodas also contain phosphoric acid a major contributor to the development of osteoporosis. In addition, diet soda has high levels of acidity which are thought to be one of the major causes of chronic inflammation, and creates a plethora of health issues that are the major contributor to a host of chronic illnesses such as arthritis, diabetes, heart disease and even Alzheimer's disease.

You should also consider swapping coffee for hot tea (I know I love my iced mocha, too). Coffee can raise your levels of cortisol – the notorious stress hormone according to Nicholas Perricone, M.D., author of *7 Secrets to Beauty, Health, and Longevity.* Instead, a University of London study found participants who drank regular black tea displayed lower levels of cortisol, and reported feeling calmer during six weeks of stressful situations. However, I can offer some good news for coffee drinkers: a 2012 study of 42,000 people published in the *American Journal of Clinical Nutrition* found regular coffee drinkers had a lower risk of Type 2 diabetes and had no higher risk of heart disease or cancer than non-coffee drinkers.

Water can help you lose weight because it fills you up. A study done in Germany showed subjects who drank 17 ounces more water increased their metabolic rates (rate at which you burn calories) by 30 percent. However, you can drink too much water, so don't become Esther Williams yet. People with certain heart conditions, high blood pressure and edema (swelling in lower legs) need to be careful about adding too much water before consulting a physician first.

While different experts vary on the amount of water you should drink every day, the consensus has been 64 ounces a day (8 glasses at 8 ounces each). However, more recent reports are advising another measurement: take half your body weight and drink that much water in ounces. If you drink 64 ounces, you should only weigh 128 pounds – while that is what it may say on your driver's license, the reality is if you are a 140-pound woman, you need to drink at least 70 ounces of water a day and if you are a 180-pound man you want to increase your water intake to 90 ounces.

Let's Get Physical

You just cannot feel at your best if you live a sedentary lifestyle. And although caregiving may leave you exhausted and without any time to get to the gym or exercise on your own, you have to find ways to fit some type of physical exercise into your daily and weekly routine. Staying physically fit actually gives you more energy, and finding these minutes for your body health improves your mental health as well. It is a 1-2 punch that will help you banish burn-out. Here are some non-gym rat ways to get physical that only take a few minutes a day:

Walk the dog. This gets you outdoors and walking – it not only gives you a cardio workout but it also allows your mind to relax. Being outdoors and away from your caregiving duties for a few minutes can help with stress relief as well as physical endurance. And Lassie will thank you too. One weight management program calls it *Use the Hound, Lose a Pound.* If you don't own a dog, go it alone – solitude can clear the mind.

Stretch. While stretching may not make you sweat, it has tons of physical benefits such as improving your flexibility, circulation, alleviating lower back pain and lowering your blood pressure. Stretching also helps your balance and coordination. Make sure you go slow and don't overdo it – there is no gain in pain.

Strength training. You don't have to become Arnold Schwarzenegger to help build strong bones and muscles. According to the National Center for Health Statistics, every year we lose 1 percent of our bone and muscle mass. Lifting light weights will not only help prevent osteoporosis as you age but also boosts your energy levels and improves your mood. If you don't own weights or have a gym membership, you can lift soup cans or do isometric exercises like lunges and squats in your own living room.

Just dance. In ancient times dance was ceremonial and a spiritual and celebratory form of self-expression. Why argue with history? Whether you sign up for ballroom or salsa or take a cue from Tom Cruise in *Risky Business* and rock out in your underwear in the living room, the benefits of dance are tremendous. Dance improves your core strength and your endurance – especially important when it comes to a long caregiving journey.

Get in the swim. Hydro-exercise – which provides natural resistance without weights – can be an extremely effective way of exercising and tones your whole body. It is essential to those who lack good balance, have joint trouble or may be managing a chronic illness such as MS. Michael Brazeal, former head of the fitness program at the California Health and Longevity Institute and now owner of his own personal training service, Brazeal Fitness, advises hydro-exercise can help manage heat sensitivity of other types of exercise that so many MS patients suffer from. In addition, the buoyancy of the water helps with balance – another MS challenge.

Scents & Sensibility

Besides working up a sweat, you also should do something that soothes you physically. A warm bath is great for combating burn-out. A study done in Japan showed the stress relief from baths helps you fight colds through vascular and lymph system stimulation, which encourages bacteria-destroying properties in the immune system. If you do not have the time for a bath, just running your hands under warm water for a few minutes can truly relax you. AAAHHHH.

Another solution for soothing body and soul is to literally *stop and smell the roses* or at least the flowers. For those naysayers who chalk aromatherapy up to *new age* trendiness get ready for a whiff of reality. According to the M.D. Anderson Cancer Center at the University of Texas in Houston, a bubble bath can improve memory, a scented handkerchief can calm a patient during an MRI, a kitchen cleaner can ward off nausea and even energizes another person.

Aromatherapy is just what it says – *therapy* – and using essential oils can have amazing healing affects. Lavender was used by the ancient Egyptians 2,500 years ago and is still used to treat insomnia, migraines and stress relief. Rosemary relieves muscle pain. Spearmint aids digestion and can even help with nausea. Men tend to like more masculine scents which can have the same impact. Bay laurel and ylang-ylang treat rheumatism, skin rashes and stomach ailments. You will read in the story about Alan Osmond he believes in the healing power of frankincense for his multiple sclerosis. Don't worry – this is one time it is all right to inhale.

Sherri Snelling

Sex and the City

One of our basic human functions is sex. Yet when you are caregiving you may feel like the *40-Year-Old Virgin*. This is a problem on multiple levels. Since the dawn of time sex has been a fundamental human need but unfortunately there is no *Kama Sutra* for caregivers. In our still somewhat Puritan society, we typically think of sex as titillating – more like something out of *9 ½ Weeks* or *Fifty Shades of Grey*. The reality is sex is not just about intercourse, using food as foreplay, or getting tied up. It is about intimacy, it is about sharing, it is about tenderness, comfort and connection. It is about life force and it is about physical touch. And all of these things are important to nurture caregivers – whether you are a Carrie, a Miranda, a Charlotte or a Samantha (or the men who loved them).

In their book, *So Stressed*, authors Dr. Stephanie McClellan and Dr. Beth Hamilton found one-third of women ages 18-59 suffer from a loss of interest in sex due to stress. Since many caregivers fall into this age range and they suffer from increased stress, we already know stress can kill off good health. Now it looks like it's killing our sex drive as well. Much of how we respond to sex is based on a variety of factors. For more in-depth exploration on sex between partners, read up on Dr. Ruth, Dr. Laura or Dr. Pepper Schwartz. For our purposes, I am going to examine sex in the context of physical touch, compassion and connection – all things caregivers need.

When we are caregiving, we are often witnessing the decline or dying of a loved one. That process may be slow and take years, but intellectually we know the outcome. To be a witness to this process day in, day out is emotionally exhausting. It is also frightening and fear is an emotion that can mess us up in many ways. When you are caregiving, you may be grieving – grieving the loss of a once vital and superhuman parent who is now frail and vulnerable; grieving the inevitable abandonment over the impending loss of an ill spouse; grieving over the great expectations that must change when you have a special needs child. This grief makes us crave physical and emotional contact and intimacy. But sex – or any activity where we derive enjoyment and pleasure – while grieving is taboo or so we were raised.

Men have been raised to avoid thoughts such as, "I feel alone and I need to be held." They may have been taught these emotions are weak and childish. In fact, it is the scared inner child watching a parent decline that brings out the fear in many male caregivers.

Women might be facing empty nest syndrome (*losing my kids*), menopause (*losing my femaleness*) and caregiving (*losing my loved one*) all at the same time. These intense changes in our bodies and lives can leave us feeling isolated and fearful. The thought of intimacy is frightening, so we avoid physical closeness because if we don't have it we can't lose that as well.

Physical touch at these tough caregiving times is something vital to our existence. You may need to make love or just lie in bed with your spouse or partner because you yearn for the intensity and warmth of life as you watch the coldness of approaching death.

You may need to be hugged by a friend. You are watching a loved one battle painful cancer chemotherapy leaving them so weak they can no longer wrap their arms around you. But the void of having no physical contact has to be filled. As a caregiver, don't be afraid to initiate the hug and as a friend or family member, don't be afraid to give a hug to a caregiver. Scientific studies have shown babies in neonatal units who were held and cradled for a few minutes a day thrived and survived versus babies who did not feel human touch. It is more than physical – it is soulful to get and give hugs. It can even be hugging your dog or cat or hugging your kids as they jump out of the car to get to school.

Just Say No

One of the best things caregivers can do to avoid burn-out doesn't have anything to do with nutrition, fitness or staying connected. It has to do with disciplining your mind and resolve to *set limits*. Caregivers have to resist the urge to take on more than they can handle. Learning how to set boundaries on your time is not easy. If you are a list keeper, it makes it easy to check your schedule and simply see you do not have time to add one more thing to your list of caregiving responsibilities. But just saying "no" does not mean you simply leave your loved one or friend or co-worker at a loss, and it also does not have to make you feel guilty.

Instead, have your list of family or friends who can step up for that activity or have your list of paid resources – whether it is respite care or help from a hospice volunteer – who may be able to handle this new or added request or look after your loved one while you take on this additional activity.

Two for the Seesaw

Caregiving is all about balance. Think of yourself standing in the middle of a see saw. One end is all about your loved one's needs, the other end is all about your needs. Neither side of the see saw is more important than the other. If you step too far to either end, the see saw tips and everything is out of balance and you fall off and possibly hurt yourself. Your goal is to maintain balance in the middle of see saw.

Two for the Road – Get Off the Guilt Trip

Seek forgiveness, let go gracefully, find kindness

In the classic 1967 movie, *Two for the Road*, a couple played by Audrey Hepburn and Albert Finney struggle with their marriage. We watch their marriage unfold in flashbacks over a 10-year period during annual road trips along the southern coast of France. They both have guilt over things they have done to hurt each other, but in the end the love they have overcomes their fears and guilt.

Guilt can come in many forms. It can be brought on by feeling you are not doing enough for your loved one, you may have made promises you can no longer keep. You may be so focused on caregiving you are neglecting your other responsibilities. It can also emerge from anger – you lose your temper over little things because caregiving has you anxious, confused and exhausted and then you feel guilty over the blow-up.

"Our family lives are fraught with guilt at every stage of the lifespan," says Sara Honn Qualls, professor of psychology at the University of Colorado at Colorado Springs. "Guilt is a consequence of not being able to let go of idealized roles – having unrealistic ideals, and caregiver guilt is not a lot different from other categories of guilt – it is just different in context." She adds a personal recollection, "I will never forget the first day I took my son to day care, the guilt I felt was really not much different from the first day I put my mother in a facility for dementia care."

The reality of guilt is it typically is a response to fear and lack of control. When loved ones become ill or have disorders that impact their lives, you are fearful for their future and also how it will ultimately impact you. You also want to be able to solve it and in many ways you cannot. We don't have control over how our loved ones have lived their lives or managed their health and even if we could, many diseases and certain disorders, especially those we are born with, are not within our control. Our health is our own responsibility – we have control over that but we still may not be able to prevent certain health issues. Life just happens and so do illness and accidents.

When I spoke to former First Lady Rosalynn Carter, she said feeling guilty is a universal emotion for caregivers. Having been one of the pioneers of identifying caregivers as a population that needs more support and help, Mrs. Carter says caregivers have to learn how to let go of guilt.

"I don't want caregivers to feel guilty for taking some time for themselves," says Mrs. Carter.

She told me the story about a woman she interviewed for her caregiving book who had given up gardening when she cared for her mother. Mrs. Carter encouraged her to find time for herself even though all her focus was on caring for her mother. The woman took Mrs. Carter's advice and began to take a few minutes each day to go back to her gardening. Then she began to take photographs of the flowers in the garden to show her mother. Friends and family told this caregiver how beautiful her photographs were and bought some of them. The woman was soon selling her garden photography from her home. She was able to create an income stream, bring a smile to her mom's face and give herself a much-needed break all in a few daily minutes of finding her *me time*. You will read more about how to find your *me time* in the chapter, Reality Show – Me Time Monday.

Blame is Guilt's Middle Name – and It's Bad

The difference is whether you blame yourself or others or even your loved one for their condition. Blame is a bad, bad emotion – it's like all those bad boys (or girls) your mom warned you about in school. Nothing good will come of it. Blame will keep peace at arm's length. Blame can also inhibit something all caregivers need to adopt: knowledge and learning. Blame is the opposite of discovery. If you let blame soak up all the sun in your life, there is no *enlightenment*. The light that can be shone on discovering new therapies, new diets, new ways to care for your loved one will get ignored, because you are spending all your energy chasing blame. Blame is the bad boy – let him go.

We may also be feeling guilty because of past hurts. Often when caring for a parent, our childhood experiences are brought into sharp focus. When spending more time with a parent, dormant memories can resurface, and they may not all be good memories. Perhaps you felt mom loved your brother more than you, yet here you are providing the hands-on daily care for her while he calls her once every two weeks despite living only 30 minutes away. This makes you resentful and angry and you may lash out at her or get irritated over things that normally would not set you off. It isn't what she just did, it's the past bubbling up to the surface.

Perhaps an ill spouse slighted you or hurt you somehow in the past and even though you forgave him, now he is vulnerable and you realize you did not really get past the hurt – you paid it lip service and buried it. Well, like a cake that rises in the oven, the hurt is back and it's gone from a mole hill to a mountain. Your anger over this old incident is compounded by the fear you may lose your loved one. This hurt and fear makes you angry; you say or do something and the ultimate result is you feel guilty.

To move past your guilt, you have to come to terms with past hurts and wounds. You have to forgive your loved one. If you are struggling with this forgiveness, you have to seek help from a support group, a spiritual advisor or a professional therapist, because in the end it is you who is suffering with guilt, and that is cargo you don't need to carry around while you are caregiving.

Regrets and Realistic Expectations Only Please

Often we confuse guilt with regret. Guilt is typically linked to a purposeful act – you did something with intent to hurt someone. Regret is the emotion when we feel we did not do enough – it is brought on by sadness or disappointment over something we cannot change. Either way, guilt is the trip you are probably on as a caregiver, and I'm going to help give you some detours to go from guilt to gratitude.

"Having regrets after the fact is very typical of caregivers," says David Solie, author of *How to Say it to Seniors*. "We feel guilt because we thought we were right about something and yet we could not change our loved one's mind or the situation."

Besides control and fear another factor that can help guilt grow is unrealistic expectations. As a caregiver, you want to provide the best care to your loved one. Of the hundreds of caregivers I have spoken to, many of them tell me no one can take care of their loved one as well as they do. I agree and disagree. I agree that the love and personalized care you give your loved one is special and something no one else can replace.

However, I disagree because there are others – family, friends and professionals – who can perform some of the caring tasks just as well as you do. For instance, you may be buying groceries and cooking meals for your loved one. Someone else can lend a helping hand and certainly with input from you, the task can be accomplished just as well as if you had done it. That extra 30 minutes to the grocery store and 30 minutes to cook a meal just gave you one hour back. You can either spend the hour having more quality time with your loved one or you can find another friend to sit with your loved one for one hour while you get a break. This is just one *exit* off the guilt highway you can take.

Guilt can also be like a hit-and-run driver after the loss of a loved one. In the book, *On Grief and Grieving*, there is a section about *hating* a spouse for dying and leaving you all alone which creates enormous guilt in widows and widowers. In addition, the authors, Elisabeth Kübler-Ross and David Kessler, go on to say any unresolved anger or resentment toward a parent will make guilt your constant companion even after the parent is gone. They write, "Death has a cruel way of giving regrets more attention than they deserve."

The best way to avoid all these obstacles on the guilt highway is to have the conversation with your loved one. If your spouse is ill, you need to ensure you understand the details of his end-of-life wishes. You also should discuss his opinions on your remarriage. I have spoken to many spousal caregivers who did not have this conversation before their loved one died – as hard as this discussion is – and then they lived with guilt when they fell in love again. They felt they were betraying their deceased loved one. If they had the conversation with their spouses at least they would not be wondering, "Would it have been OK with my first husband?" If they knew the answer, they may have been released from their current guilt.

"Guilt is HUGE – I wish I had a good answer for how to let it go," says Vic Mazmanian, director of faith outreach for the Mind, Heart & Soul Ministry at Saddleback Church and Silverado Senior Living. "No one can tell you how to stop feeling something, but what I have found works for me, and others I have counseled, is to give it to God."

Mazmanian says if we can remind ourselves, as a caregiver, the time and care we are providing is making a difference in our loved one's life, then the guilt should lessen. "It is not about us, it is about the person we love and just being there to sit near them or touch them is important to them."

If you can embrace this concept as a caregiver – small gestures and just being there can be enough – it will go a long way to getting you off the guilt trip.

As stated earlier, you also must resolve past hurts or issues with parents or siblings or friends before they pass. This is for your sake. Your inability to resolve anything after they have gone may cause you to be stuck in a traffic jam of guilt for the rest of your life. Have the hard conversation, engage a professional to help facilitate the dialogue if you need to but don't avoid the conversation – it will only mean your life will be stuck on the guilt highway forever.

Good Guilt, Bad Guilt

Believe it or not, there is good guilt and bad guilt. Good guilt is when something has happened you regret but you take the time to reflect on it. One key tip is to always look forward and not backward. It is like driving – you have to keep your eyes on the road ahead or you will crash and burn. You cannot change the past but you can steer towards a better future. When you have a regret in caregiving, examine how you can address it differently next time. It may have made you feel powerless – how can you take that power back?

For instance, your loved one may have been given a medication that had terrible side effects and created even more problems for him and for you as his caregiver. You find at the next doctor appointment there is an alternative to the medication prescribed which does not have the same dramatic side effects. Rather than beating yourself up for not asking more questions the first time, simply make a mental note any time a medication or treatment is prescribed (for anyone, not just your loved one), ask a lot of questions, ask about alternative measures or treatments, discuss it with your loved one after doing a little Internet research and then make your decision. This gives you your power back and guess what? Guilt is gone – like Elvis it has left the building.

Another aspect of good or *normal* guilt is something professionals call *survivor guilt*. It is a common emotion for those who experienced something traumatic and survived when others did not live through it. The horror of surviving a concentration camp in World War II or walking out of the rubble after the 9/11 attacks creates survivor guilt. This is also normal when caregiving. You may feel guilty your loved one is sick or disabled and you are not. You want to change it but you cannot. You must go from guilt to gratitude. I know it seems impossible, but gratitude for health and life allows you to do things in the honor and memory for those who cannot. Your health allows you to be a caregiver. Surviving the death camps like those at Auschwitz allows those survivors to tell the world their story to hopefully ensure another holocaust will never happen. Survivors of September 11th can take some comfort their efforts to rebuild and honor the memory of those lost helps all of us be hopeful again. The road from guilt to gratitude, particularly when facing these levels of tragedies, is not easy. Often it requires years of professional help and a strong spiritual faith to see any good from such pain and suffering. But in the end, what we come to realize – and this is important for caregivers to understand – we can neither control the outcome nor prevent the problem. We can only respond to it.

Bad guilt is when you are adrift in an endless sea of guilt. It is ongoing – wave after wave. You are drowning in guilt with no rescue boat in sight. Bad guilt is when we have unrealistic expectations as discussed previously. Caregivers often feel they have to do it all alone. This is unrealistic. A typical characteristic of the baby boom generation who are facing caregiving today is we want *more, more, more*. As applied to caregiving, this means we want more time with our loved ones. We want more solutions for their illness or disorder. Not being able to get more makes us feel powerless and it is somehow our fault. And again, powerlessness leads to guilt. Loss of control, feeling powerless, having unrealistic expectations, being fearful of the future – just like all roads lead to Rome – all these emotions will lead to guilt – bad guilt.

Detours for Your Guilt Trip

Now that you know guilt is a two-lane highway with good and bad, here are some suggestions about how to exit your bad guilt trip during caregiving:

Seek forgiveness. Understand everyone is only human. Your loved one who is suffering or coping with an illness or disability is only human – he can only do so much. We expect the doctors to be gods and have all the answers. That is not possible; they are only human and giving you their best educated guess. It does not mean they are always right, which is why it is so important to arm yourself with as much knowledge as you can to be your loved one's advocate and champion.

You are only human – you cannot do it all with a smile every day. You may have moments of anger or frustration, you may lose your temper, say something you regret, forget something important. When you do, ask yourself, "Was my intent to help or harm?" If it was to help then ask your loved one for forgiveness and then forgive yourself. If it was to harm, then seek immediate professional help to overcome these feelings because something darker is at play.

Let go gracefully. A great quote from a play called *The Torch-Bearers* written by George Kelly, the uncle of actress and Princess Grace Kelly, states: "The art of living is the art of letting go gracefully." One example of literally letting go gracefully of your guilt is from a book called *Happy* which has secrets on how happiness is sought in different cultures.

I like this idea from Thailand which is about letting your sadness or guilt go – it is called The Lantern Festival. The Thai people gather on one day in November (you can do this alone or with friends any day although November is National Family Caregiver Month and a good time to try this). They write down in notes to people whose forgiveness they seek – telling them they did not mean to hurt them or they are sad they cannot change things. They put the notes in candle-fueled paper lanterns. As the notes burn inside, the lanterns are released into the sky and float away. It is a very spiritual symbol for the Thai to see all these lights lifting away the bad and creating a warm glow in the sky.

Since I'm sure the local fire department hates this idea – I am recommending you use the concept not the pyrotechnics. Write down your regret or something you are feeling guilty about. Read it out loud. Give it a moment for the words to evaporate into the air and then scrunch the note into a ball and throw it into the fireplace or tie it to a helium balloon and let it go outside. Feel the sensation of the guilt floating away.

Be kind to yourself and give yourself a break, literally. You know you cannot do it all alone. Seek help from friends, family, neighbors and professionals. Remember – be realistic and set reasonable expectations for what you can and cannot do. Ask yourself this, "If I were hiring a professional to care for my loved one, would it be OK with me that this professional caretaker always seemed frazzled, exhausted or irritable?" The answer is, "Of course not."

If you are feeling any of these signs of burn-out, get help so you can be at your best as a caregiver. You can read more about putting out the flames of burn-out in the Backdraft chapter. Balance is essential to avoiding health issues *and* the guilt of not being at the top of your game.

Another way to be kind to yourself is to take the time to write yourself a thank you letter for everything you do – the patience, the time, the love you are providing your loved one. Take this letter out and read it on days when you feel down or like you cannot go on. Congratulate yourself for the wonderful gift of care, the gift of giving you are doing every day.

Misery – Dealing with Depression

Finding nature and words

In her Oscar-winning performance in the film, *Misery*, Kathy Bates plays Annie Wilkes, a psychopathic fan who cannot deal with the fact there will be no new additions to her favorite series of novels when the author, Paul Sheldon, played by James Caan, decides to end the book series by killing off the main character. I'm sure many Harry Potter fans felt the same way when our Hogwarts heroes ended their run but none of them tried to kill J.K. Rowling for *closing the book* on her popular characters like Annie Wilkes attempts to do to Paul Sheldon in the movie.

This is the difference between mild, situational depression (the Harry Potter fans saddened Harry, Hermione and Ron will create no more magical spells) and clinical depression or mental illness (Annie torturing and trying to murder Paul.)

Many caregivers worry when they encounter the fourth stage of grief – Depression – as identified by authors Elisabeth Kübler-Ross and David Kessler in their book, *On Grief and Grieving*, they may be suffering from mental illness. The depression envelops them like the fog along San Francisco bay, and they cannot lift their spirits or feel the sunshine in their lives. While approximately 9 percent of the population suffers from some type of depression according to the Centers for Disease Control (CDC), a survey conducted by Caring.com found more than double the national average – 1 in 4 caregivers of older loved ones – experiences depression.

According to the American Psychological Association (APA), depression is more than just sadness or grief – it is the most common mental disorder but it is also treatable. People with depression experience a lack of interest or pleasure in daily activities, significant weight gain or loss, insomnia or excessive sleeping, lack of energy, inability to concentrate, feelings of worthlessness or excessive guilt and recurring thoughts of death or suicide. The APA also warns social isolation increases the risk of depression. Since caregivers often feel isolated, the slippery slope of grief becoming long-term depression may be a real risk.

In his wonderful book, *Spontaneous Happiness*, Dr. Andrew Weil, relates a personally painful memory of depression,

> "In 1972, I spent a month in a cottage on the shore of Lake Atitlán in the highlands of Guatemala…In any direction I looked I saw beauty: the deep blue mirrorlike surface of the lake, snowcapped volcanic cones, colorfully dressed Mayan Indians…And I was miserable, unable to shake my dark mood. The contrast between my mood and my surroundings made me feel somehow contaminated and unworthy of the place. Not only did that add to my despair, but it made me even more averse to venturing out and seeking social contact. I told myself that I shouldn't subject others to my negative emotions or risk 'infecting' anyone with them."

Throughout our caregiving journey, we may experience varying degrees of depression. It is hard to watch a loved one suffer or face death, even harder after we lose him to illness. It is difficult to be a parent to a special needs child or be caring for a loved one with an illness or disorder that has social stigma attached such as AIDS, post traumatic stress disorder (PTSD), bi-polar disorder or schizophrenia. The National Alliance for Caregiving study, *Caregivers in Decline*, found among those caregivers who felt their health was impacted by caregiving, 91 percent reported suffering from depression. The World Health Organization predicts by 2030 more people worldwide will be suffering from depression than any other health disorder. And 1 out of 10 Americans, including many children, are currently taking anti-depressant medications.

Yet depression during the decline and after the loss of a loved one is a *normal* response during the grieving process – it is called *situational depression*. It only becomes a serious mental health issue when it continues beyond the normal limits of mourning.

What is normal? The APA identified a spectrum of depression disorders with the most severe type being major depressive disorder. Clinical depression is defined as the inability to defeat depression and get to the last stage of grief – Acceptance – or when depression comes on suddenly for no apparent reason and will not depart.

Sara Honn Qualls, professor of psychology at the University of Colorado at Colorado Springs, says, "A clinical state of depression is different from grief and there is no strong evidence that the stages of grief occur sequentially – they tend to cycle or occur simultaneously." She goes on to say caregivers who are not getting any pleasure from their lives are at risk for depression. She advises any caregiver who is struggling to care for herself or cannot let go of her loved one even after death needs professional intervention.

Charles Darwin, the renowned English naturalist and author of *On the Origin of Species* (1859), was a depressive with a different take on the periods of sadness and gloom that would hold him in its grip. He suffered greatly from the death of his 10-year-old daughter Annie and yet he seemed to find some positive light in the middle of his darkness. He wrote it is sadness that "leads an animal to pursue the course of action which is most beneficial." His depression became part of his belief in his famous *survival of the fittest* theory.

Some researchers believe some bouts of depression may spur creative thinking. They point to Socrates, Plato, Mozart, Michelangelo, Shakespeare, Isaac Newton, Edgar Degas, Hans Christian Andersen, Ernest Hemingway, Virginia Wolff, William Styron, Sylvia Plath and Woody Allen just to name a few famous names who have suffered from depression at some point in their lives.

Whether you believe depression has positive elements (the scientists and researchers are still debating this one), most caregivers want to move on from grief and depression. One of the first steps in doing this is to identify that you need to take care of yourself as much as you cared for your loved one.

In 2011, the Oscar-winning actress, Catherine Zeta Jones, announced she had bi-polar II disorder, also commonly known as manic-depression. According to the National Institutes of Health, "Bi-polar disorder is a condition in which people go back and forth between periods of a very good or irritable mood and depression. The *mood swings* between mania and depression can be very quick."

In Zeta-Jones's case, she checked into a mental health facility for a few days rest when they made her diagnosis. The respite came on the heels of a year-long stressful and traumatic episode where Zeta-Jones was caregiver to her husband, Oscar-winner, Michael Douglas, as he battled throat cancer. As he announced his remission from the disease, his wife announced her repercussions as his caregiver. My take away from this story is two-fold:

1. I applaud Catherine for her courage in coming forward to announce her struggle with depression and a mental health issue that still has much stigma attached to it.

2. I also give her my *caregiving award* for recognizing the need to take care of herself for both her role in helping her husband with his ongoing battle to stay healthy and for her two small children – all of whom need her. Her self-care statement of spending a few days to get treatment is a lesson all caregivers should learn.

"There was a poll done recently that showed the stigma is lifting around depression but we have a long way to go," says former First Lady Rosalynn Carter, a lifelong caregiver and mental health advocate. When I spoke to her about caregiving, she talked about her concerns for those with mental health issues and their caregivers despite the strides made in public awareness.

"The polls are showing that the more people learn about certain issues – schizophrenia, bi-polar disorder, depression – they become more uneasy about it."

She is also concerned certain events, such as the shooting spree in summer 2012 in a Colorado theater that killed 12 people followed almost a month later with another shooting at the Sikh temple in Milwaukee, only increases people's fears about people with mental health issues. This in turn makes it difficult for caregivers of those with mental illness or who may be suffering from their own depression to reach out for help.

The Rosalynn Carter Institute for Caregiving at Georgia Southwestern State University is dedicated to taking evidence-based research to understand caregiver needs and then translating that research into programs. Since 1987, RCI has been a leading advocacy, education, research and service unit for caregivers and has recently created a Wounded Warrior Family Caregiver Program and conducted research, REACH (Resources for Enhancing Alzheimer's Caregiver Health), all to support caregivers.

Message in a Bottle

A pitfall of depression is a dependence on substance abuse to assuage the pain. In the National Alliance for Caregiving study on caregiver health risks, it was reported 10 percent of caregivers are turning to prescription drugs and alcohol to cope. We also know caregivers often rekindle bad habits such as smoking to deal with the stress or depression of caregiving. While these measures may seem to help a caregiver's mental anguish, they are a crutch for coping with caregiving and they are simply creating other negative health issues down the road.

Another way to cope, rather than abusing prescription drugs or alcohol, is to write your thoughts down. Journaling has been known to have strong therapeutic effects for many people struggling with emotions they cannot express verbally. In an interview with the *New York Times*, Andy Thomson, a psychiatrist at the University of Virginia believes one solution outside of prescribing anti-depressants is to write down your thoughts and feelings.

Thomson said in the interview, "…a recent study that found *expressive writing* — asking depressed subjects to write essays about their feelings — led to significantly shorter depressive episodes." The reason, Thomson suggests, is writing is a form of thinking, which enhances our natural problem-solving abilities. "This doesn't mean there's some miracle cure," he said. "In most cases, the recovery period is going to be long and difficult."

Death Takes a Holiday

The 1934 movie, *Death Takes a Holiday,* was remade in 1998 as *Meet Joe Black* with Brad Pitt as *Joe Black* (aka Death) who visits earth to understand why he is so unwelcome in people's lives. No one welcomes Death but he visits anyway and with him he brings depression. Authors Kübler-Ross and Kessler advise, "See Depression as a visitor – invite him in – embrace him – and he'll be on his way."

Even after a loved one is gone, the spectre of death becomes a pall on once celebratory events and can easily trigger depression. The way caregivers respond to facing the holidays after a loved one is gone – or in cases of Alzheimer's, a loved one who is gone in mind but not body – depends on the individual caregiver's personality.

Some caregivers celebrate the life of a departed loved one by singing mom's favorite Christmas carols or lighting a candle for a sister whom breast cancer took too soon; others decide not to feel the absence of a lost loved one by taking a trip or volunteering to help others.

A friend of mine who lost her father to cancer cannot think of Thanksgiving without her dad carving the best turkey in town. Now, instead of spending Thanksgiving stuffing herself like the rest of us, she volunteers to feed the homeless at a local shelter. "Dad fed me all those years, now I'm paying it forward by feeding someone else," she told me.

In Holly Robinson Peete's story you will read how her family celebrates her father every January 1 – his birthday – with stories and by watching his old TV shows so her younger children, who never knew their grandfather, can feel connected to him.

What is essential is to acknowledge that special occasions – whether birthdays, anniversaries or holidays – are changed forever. You must find ways to redesign your holiday to accommodate the way you wish to remember your loved one. The first season of holidays and special events without a loved one may evoke an episode of depression, but learning how to recreate these events is part of the path to Acceptance.

"Learn to let your life be informed by the lessons you received from your loved one," says Rabbi Arthur Rosenberg, chaplain for the Motion Picture and Television Fund (MPTF). "You can still have a conversation with your loved one after they are gone; it just becomes a one-way conversation."

On Walden Pond

In his famous 1854 book, *Walden*, transcendentalist Henry David Thoreau immersed himself in nature by living in solitude in a cabin in the woods outside Concord, Massachusetts for two years in order to gain a better perspective on society. Perhaps he was on to something. Experts in the field of psychology today point to a new phenomenon called *nature deficit disorder*. Originally coined by Richard Louv in his book, *Last Child in the Woods*, nature deficit disorder was meant to highlight the behavioral problems with modern children but also points to a lack of connection to nature as the root cause of ailments, both physical and emotional, in people of all ages. In fact, there is a higher incidence of depression per capita among people who are city dwellers than those who live in rural areas.

Dr. Andrew Weil expands on the hypothesis of nature deficit disorder by identifying some key sources that contribute to depression: lack of physical exercise, reduced human contact, overconsumption of processed food and an endless desire for distractions. He further explains our disconnect from nature and our evolution of modern conveniences as enablers of depression:

1. We are a more sedentary society – Stuck behind a desk all day, whether at work or at school, and still sitting on our bums in the evenings watching TV, checking out Facebook or playing video games. Lack of physical exercise is a known contributor to depression.
2. We stay inside too much - Staying indoors and not getting outside deprives us of sunshine and the natural Vitamin D he says is critical for brain health. He also points to modern conveniences such as air conditioning as keeping us cooped up and isolated from society. In days gone by when summer weather was sweltering, people would gather outside on the front porch and socialize with neighbors.
3. Let there be light (but not all the time) – Our circadian rhythms, based on periods of light and dark, are our bodies' natural way of regulating healthful sleep patterns. The *artificial* light we have on at nighttime – whether that is a bedroom table lamp, glow from the TV or computer screen – all conspire to throw off our natural rhythms, and don't allow our bodies the natural *healing* of restorative sleep, which can also affect our emotional health.
4. Vision is tied to brain health – Instead of staring off into beautiful vistas and landscapes like our forefathers of yesteryear, our eyes are concentrated on reading books, emails and texts. Modern vision problems can be connected to brain health issues such as depression.

The answer is not to *Go Thoreau* and become a recluse in a wood cabin like the Unabomber. But there are ways to incorporate more nature into our lives.

- Taking walks has twin benefits – you are getting physical exercise and you are outdoors listening to the rustle of the trees, smelling the flowers and hearing birds chirping. Try to leave the iPod at home.
- Making time for family and friends helps us avoid the isolation that contributes to depression.
- Go jump in the lake – literally. The late, great actress Katherine Hepburn who lived to be 96 years old, attributed her longevity and her positive outlook on life to many things but one of them was taking a frigid dip in a lake or pool every morning. If you cannot jump in a lake, try taking a warm bath – no music, no interruptions, just you and the sudsy water.

On a Clear Day You Can See Forever

One caution most health care professionals make is depression, and any side effects such as substance abuse, must be treated with a trifecta of solutions and not just one bandage in isolation. Here are your three prescriptions for treating ongoing depression:

1. Professional therapy typically provided by a licensed psychologist —After diagnosis, the psychologist may prescribe an anti-depressant. Professor of psychology Sara Honn Qualls recommends caregivers first get a physical exam from their primary care physician to ensure there are no other health issues impacting emotional health. Your doctor can make a recommendation on seeing a specialist if needed. A psychiatrist is a health care professional with a medical degree who has studied disorders of the brain. Typically psychiatrists will treat patients with medications. In contrast, a psychologist is someone who has studied the pyscho-social behavioral aspects of emotional health. They will be more focused on problem-solving techniques through therapy and counseling. Whichever type of health care professional you choose, ensure he understands caregiving, as this is the core of why you need help.
2. Prescription drugs to treat depression – The most common antidepressant pharmaceutical category being SSRI (selective serotonin reuptake inhibitor).
3. Support group help – It is important to find and join support groups specific to your caregiving situation. For instance, if your loved one has dementia, join an Alzheimer's Association support group. If you are misusing alcohol to cope, then perhaps try a group specific to your substance abuse issue such as Alcoholics Anonymous. See more about support groups in the chapter LOST and Found.

Qualls states national studies on the effectiveness of support groups are not always impressive in helping caregivers through depression. She says the data shows caregivers value support groups and feel they definitely get something from the experience, but when it comes to dealing with the issues of depression, the outcome data is not as impressive and support groups are not enough to treat the distress of the caregiver's depression. Qualls says there is some evidence in research literature that self-help books, sometimes called *biblio-therapy*, and guiding your way through the depressive episodes has benefits in treatment of depression. Qualls recommends caregivers do best when they can work from a menu of options and use an assessment approach to create what the caregiver needs from that menu.

The most succinct summation of how to deal with depression I believe comes from the brilliant, lightning sharp mind of Winston Churchill who was the deliverer of democracy during the dark days of World War II. He called his depressive periods, his "black dog of depression." But when called to lead, there was no other statesman who could have galvanized Great Britain to help defeat the Nazis. Churchill, in one of his more famous quotes, said, "If you're going through hell, keep going."

Cue Cards – How Will You Find Happiness and Support?

My mother wanted us to understand that the tragedies of your life one day have the potential to be comic stories the next.

– Nora Ephron

When you become a caregiver finding happiness and support are not easy tasks. But without both you will find it harder to carry on caring for your loved one.

Whether your musical tastes run to the '70s TV show with the Partridge family singing their theme song, *C'mon Get Happy* or the 1950s song that inspired it, *Get Happy* made famous by Judy Garland, the message is happiness is in our hands – not something we are handed.

Happiness is not about making more money, buying more shoes or having the biggest house or coolest car. It is about what is inside you and clearing the hurdles of things you fear. Whether it is humor, hope or having fun, happiness is right around the corner.

Getting to happy is sometimes easier when you have friends and circles of support. As I have written, caregivers often feel all alone. They may have family, friends and others around them but somehow they can't overcome this feeling of isolation. Reaching out and learning how to ask for help and receive help is not easy but think of it like a hug – it's like a boomerang – you get it back right away.

The Pursuit of Happyness

Humor, Hope, Having Fun

What is happiness and how can caregivers be happy? Typically, we accept our caregiving role as something we should do, we may even want to do it or in some situations we have to do it. But no matter how you enter your caregiving role, happiness it not something you naturally associate with caring for a loved one who is ill, has a disability or disorder or is getting older and more frail. However, it does not mean you can't find happy moments, times of joy or satisfaction in your caregiving role.

Lately there have been a lot of books and articles written about how we achieve happiness but the reality is the definition of happiness is inside each of us – it can't be handed out like candy at Halloween. This means, if you have a day, a month or a year when happiness is elusive, have no fear – happiness is still inside of you, it is just trapped and you must learn how to let it out.

Researcher Sonja Lyubomirsky, a psychology professor at the University of California at Riverside and author of *The How of Happiness*, calls happiness the "Holy Grail of science." With a grant from the National Institute of Mental Health, she has spent years researching what makes us happy. One of her projects found by thinking about happy events for just 8 minutes every day for three simultaneous days, study participants felt their *life satisfaction* levels increase for the following four weeks – levels they did not feel prior to the study.

Another philosophy comes from Gary Zukav, author of *Spiritual Partnerships*, who writes, "Happiness is temporary … Joy is permanent … Joy versus happiness is a choice." He argues happiness depends on what happens outside of you, it requires you to try to change other people and situations around you (such as a loved one's illness) and that is not possible. He believes joy is about changing yourself – facing your fears, removing those obstacles that are holding you back from being *your authentic self* and allowing joy to fill you up rather than pursuing something elusive and short-term such as happiness.

I see it slightly differently. I do believe happiness is a good thing. Little steps give you a temporary lift – especially as fuel to keep you going on your caregiving journey. While joy might be the deeper, more fulfilling emotion, it requires a lot of soul searching and is a lifelong effort. So both happiness and joy need to find a place in your life, especially as a caregiver.

Happiness is just like health. Health is 50 percent genetics and 50 percent how we live our lives (good eating, physical fitness, positive outlook on life, etc.). Lyubomirsky found in her research happiness is 50 percent driven by our biology (we're predisposed or have *set limits* for happiness), 10 percent is connected to life circumstance, such as a unique talent for playing piano which gives you satisfaction, and 40 percent is left up to us. Think of maintaining your happiness in a similar way you maintain your weight. You know you have to eat a nutritious diet and stay active to maintain physical health. Happiness is the same. You have to constantly pursue your happiness. You can't take a happy pill and be blissful the rest of your life. If joy is the goal line, happiness steps are the first downs on your way to a winning life.

Gretchen Rubin, author of the best-selling book, *The Happiness Project*, spent a year test-driving a variety of happiness theories and one she feels is important comes from doing simple tasks such as making your bed every day. When applied to caregiving, you may find happiness in performing simple tasks for your loved one: bathing them, taking them to the doctor, watching a TV show together you both love.

AARP conducted a survey among older adults, *Beyond Happiness: Thriving,* that found having good relationships with friends, family and even pets was a key driver to finding happiness. Nancy Davis, who has lived more than 20 years with multiple sclerosis and started the Nancy Davis Foundation for Multiple Sclerosis to find a cure faster, told me she wears orange because it is her *happy color*. In fact, scientific studies have been done around colors, and wearing yellow tops the list of bringing a smile to our faces (just think of the Smiley Face icon from the '70s).

The Girl Scouts have even gotten in on the happiness bandwagon. They teamed with Martin Seligman, PhD, former president of the American Psychological Association and head of the Positive Psychology Center at the University of Pennsylvania, to develop the Science of Happiness badge. The teen girls spend one month coming up with strategies for how to improve their happiness quotient. The new badge was part of a revamp of the program in 2012 – the first in 25 years – to mark the 100th anniversary of the Girl Scouts of America.

When it comes to happy countries, Denmark tops the list for global happiness surveys attributed to the fact the Danes know how to *go off grid*. They eliminate the noise pollution in their lives, turning off smartphones, unplugging from TVs, computers, iPods and video games and practicing the ancient Danish art of *hygge* (pronounced HOOgah) which loosely translated means *cosiness*. They curl up with a good book in front of the fire or make life simpler by spending a day fishing or cooking with friends and family.

For caregivers, happiness may not be the first emotion you would associate with caring for your loved one. You may be overwhelmed, frustrated, sad and exhausted. But caregiving is an outside force. You need to tap into your inside force to find your happiness. If you find your happiness is hibernating, it's time to wake the bear. Just like Winnie the Pooh, it's time to grab the *hunny* jar that makes you happy. In the following section, I suggest several ways to think about your happiness *hunny* jar.

Laugh Track

I remember my mom telling me as a kid, "Laughter is the best medicine." Mom was right (I know she is happy I just wrote that). Scientific studies show laughter is a powerful elixir for stress and pain. As a caregiver, laughter can lighten your load, connect you to your loved one or others when you most need an emotional break and it keeps you grounded. There is a lesson to be learned in the statistic that young children laugh on average 350 times a day and adults only 15 times a day. Children tend to be carefree and full of joy – a lesson is to be learned from finding your inner child (read on for more about this).

Actress, producer and laughter advocate Goldie Hawn has focused on the healing powers of laughter for years. Known on the 1960s hit TV show, *Rowan and Martin's Laugh-In* as the *giggle girl*, today she has created The Hawn Foundation and a program called MindUp to cultivate happiness and the power of positive thinking in young school age children.

One of the lessons Goldie learned about happiness, she wrote about in her book, *Ten Mindful Minutes,* which she said she wrote for parents and caregivers. The giggle girl follows what the Guru of Giggling, Dr. Madan Kataria, taught her, which is how to practice laughing through a series of physical exercises created to elicit fits of hilarity. It is estimated more than 250,000 people in 36 countries follow Dr. Kataria's laugh lessons. He is also a star for corporate human resource departments where he leads employees through laughter sessions to improve productivity on the job. In fact, a growing trend among yoga devotees is Hasya yoga – known as the medicinal magic of laughter yoga.

You can smirk at all this but consider the health benefits of laughing:

Laughter relaxes the whole body. A good, hearty laugh relieves physical tension and stress, leaving your muscles relaxed for up to 45 minutes after your laugh-fest.

Laughter boosts the immune system. Laughter decreases stress hormones and increases immune cells and infection-fighting antibodies, thus improving your resistance to disease.

Laughter triggers the release of endorphins. These natural feel-good chemicals in our bodies promote an overall sense of well-being and can even temporarily relieve pain.

Laughter protects the heart. Laughter improves the function of blood vessels and increases blood flow, which can help protect you against a heart attack and other cardiovascular problems.

One humorous tale of caregiving actually involves my mom who cared for my grandma after she had a stroke. One day, they both slipped as mom was transferring grandma from wheelchair to bed. Rather than be sad or upset, they both sat on the floor laughing at the absurdity of the situation. Caregiving can be what you make it and that day two women I admire and love decided to make it funny.

You will also read how humor became part of the stories of Alan Osmond and David Osmond, Michael Tucker and Alana Stewart as they faced chronic illness – whether their own or that of their loved one.

Charlie Chaplin said it best, "A day without laughter is a day wasted." If you need some inspiration to tickle your funny bone, watch some re-runs of *I Love Lucy* or *The Three Stooges.* I dare you not to laugh.

Funny Face

Of all the things Michael J. Fox is known for (brilliant comedic actor, Parkinson's advocate, dad, husband, author, guitar and hockey player), being an eternal optimist is at the top of the list. In fact, he filmed a documentary about optimism in Bhutan called, *Michael J. Fox: Adventures of an Incurable Optimist.* Traveling to this remote kingdom in the Himalayas, he found this country is ahead of the curve when it comes to happiness – they actually measure the gross national happiness of their citizens. In an interview with Oprah talking about the Parkinson's disease he has lived with for more than 20 years and his trip to Bhutan he says, "I don't know whether it was the altitude or the thinning of the blood or whatever, but I had much less symptoms [of Parkinson's]. It was just an amazing place."

Bhutan may not be the only country focused on its public happiness levels. Great Britain's Prime Minister, David Cameron, suggested polling residents of the United Kingdom about their subjective well-being on an annual basis. At a time when global leaders are struggling with financial woes and anemic economies, Cameron said, "It's time we admitted there's much more to life than money, and it's time we focused not just on GDP but on GWB – general well-being."

The Mayo Clinic actually did a study tracking participants over a 30-year period and found the optimists had a 19 percent higher chance of still being alive and they suffered less from depression. Other studies have shown optimistic people have less chronic stress because they view setbacks as minor incidents that can be overcome. We know ongoing stress is the No. 1 factor causing caregivers to develop chronic illness at twice the rate as the general public according to a study by the Commonwealth Fund.

What is optimism and how do you get it? Are you born with it or can you cultivate it? Experts say one of the characteristics of an optimist is the power of a smile – remember how good you feel when someone smiles at you? You inevitably smile back and for a few seconds all seems right with the world. Even though you may be blue or having *one of those days* – try smiling. It is hard to be mad or sad when you have a smile on your face. Lyubomirsky's research found people tend to mirror each other and she found smiling is truly infectious – it catches on faster than the flu.

When I think of someone who is happy, I think the best example is actually from the beloved *Winnie the Pooh* books. Bouncy orange tiger, Tigger, is the ultimate optimist. He is super-cheerful, always trying to make others laugh. Unfortunately, he doesn't have much luck with friend, Eeyore. This sad, gray, gloomy donkey is extremely intelligent but unable to pull himself out of the doldrums. You decide – are you a Tigger or an Eeyore?

Sherri Snelling

Find Your Inner Child

Why is it that once we hit age 21 (or 51) whenever we do something silly, someone inevitably tells us to "Grow up!" Well, the secret to happiness may just be to ignore these killjoys and tap into what author and self-help guru Louise L. Hay calls "loving the child within."

I recently took the Real Age Test, an online evaluation developed by those famed doctors, Mehmet Oz and Michael Roizen of the best-selling *You – The Owner's Manual* book. What struck me as I took the test is so much of what is truly good for our bodies, our minds and our souls are things most of us did when we were kids. As you will read in Joan Lunden's story, she says she tries to find her inner child when I asked her how she finds her *Me Time*.

While all childhoods are not alike, here are my eight tips for caregivers on how to tap into the kid you once were and embrace that youthful, carefree time once again. Trust me it will improve your health and wellness and increase your happiness score:

Naptime: Remember taking naps as a kid? While health experts say we should get 7-9 hours per night, if you are a caregiver, the luxury of uninterrupted sleep can sometimes be elusive. How about an afternoon nap? If you think this is just for kindergarteners, Winston Churchill, Albert Einstein, Thomas Edison, John F. Kennedy and Ronald Reagan were all avid afternoon nappers.

Some people feel naps can disturb your circadian rhythms – the sleep/wake cycles in our bodies that typically have us on a regimen of 16 hours awake time and 8 hours of sleep time. However, many people don't realize our bodies also have two distinct dips in alertness – typically at 2 a.m. and 2 p.m. A study in the journal *Sleep* found a 10-minute afternoon nap can reduce sleepiness and improve cognitive performance. If you nap longer than 30 minutes you may encounter *sleep inertia* which is the groggy feeling that sometimes follows sleep. Try to plan 10-20 minutes of naptime a day as if you were four-years-old again.

Bath time: Remember how we used to hate taking baths as a kid? As a stressed out adult caregiver, baths are a luxurious dream for which you typically don't have time. Baths – especially those taken with Epsom salts and fragrant oil like lavender – help reduce stress, improve circulation and aid relaxation. A study done in Japan showed the stress relief from baths helps you fight colds through vascular and lymph system stimulation which encourages bacteria-destroying properties in the immune system. Take 10 minutes for a bath at least three times a week and don't forget the bubbles and the rubber ducky.

Playtime: It sounds silly but playtime can actually help caregivers avoid the burn-out they so often face. While escaping to summer camp may not be feasible, ride your bike, go ice skating, find a local summer fair to ride the carousel or roller coaster, or jump into your backyard or local community pool (doing your best cannonball!) or a pile of leaves at the beginning of fall. Playing can give you the mental health break you need. Find a few minutes every day or at least once a week to *play*.

Outdoor Fun and Sun: Ten minutes of sunshine a day is enough to boost your natural levels of Vitamin D – which promotes calcium absorption needed for strong bones and has been proven to aid prevention of health risks such as diabetes, multiple sclerosis, cancer, allergies and osteoporosis. In addition, sunshine boosts your mental health – brain functionality and optimism all improve with increased levels of Vitamin D. One study in the *Journal of Finance* found stocks traded on sunny days were more profitable than those on cloudy days.

Seashells by the seashore: One of my favorite childhood memories is collecting seashells along the beach with my mom and brother. We would walk for what seemed like miles to find special colors and shapes. Since heart disease is the No. 1 killer of women and men, walking 30 minutes every day gives you the cardiovascular exercise you need to keep your heart healthy, according to the American Heart Association. If you don't live near the beach, find a hiking trail or just take a brisk stroll through the neighborhood.

Daydream: Remember lying on your back and looking up into the clouds deciding which shapes you could find? A lion, a car, or even hearts? If you can find a patch of ground – whether it is your backyard or your neighborhood park, take a few minutes each week to just lie on your back and watch the clouds float by. If you can't find a patch of grass, just lie on your back in your living room – no TV, no music, no external disturbances allowed. I found a great app on iTunes called iClouds – lie back and watch the clouds roll by on your smartphone or iPad. As a variation of meditation, cloud gazing ensures you have the mental stamina to keep going as a caregiver.

Take a time-out: If you find you have a short fuse and caregiving has you frustrated or stressed, time to give yourself a *time-out*. Take 5 minutes to walk outside, blow off steam, even yell (but not so loud all the neighbors come running). Our extraordinary third president of the United States, Thomas Jefferson, once declared, "If angry or upset, count to 10 before responding, if really angry, count to 100." Whatever gets you past the moment of pent-up anger, give yourself a moment to address the emotion and then calmly move on.

Hold hands: Remember the first time you held hands with someone you liked? Your heart beat faster, your oxytocin levels (*cuddling hormone*) surged and a warm feeling of happiness came over your whole body. The National Alliance for Caregiving found most caregivers feel all alone. Hand-holding can be the prescription caregivers need. A University of Virginia study showed wives who held the hands of their spouse or a friend reduced their stress levels.

Real Age Calculator

As we grow older and start to care for aging parents or other loved ones, what is our risk as caregivers for being *older* than our real age because we often neglect our own health and wellness needs?

Take the scary leap with me (make sure you put your knee brace on first) – there is an online calculator developed by the well-known authors of *You – The Owner's Manual* books, Dr. Mehmet Oz and Dr. Michael Roizen. It is called the Real Age Test and it takes about 15 minutes to complete the online questionnaire. Be prepared – it will ask you about your cholesterol levels, blood pressure reading, eating habits, fitness routine, sleep patterns, etc.

What you get is an *estimated age* based on your health and wellness answers as well as tips on how to improve your age score (meaning scoring younger than you really are) in the various areas.

See RealAge.com to take your test.

Play It Again, Sam

One way you can get happy and healthy is to adopt *fun* behaviors. Volkswagen actually offered grants to people around the world who came up with ideas to make health more fun, called *The Fun Theory*. My favorite idea is called *Piano Stairs* (you can watch it on YouTube). It was led by a research group in Sweden that filmed the entrance/exit to a busy subway system. This group realized almost everyone coming and going to the metro took the escalator instead of the stairs which were right next to each other.

Late one evening they painted the stairs to look like piano keys and wired each step with piano keys sound. The next morning and all day long something amazing happened. People gravitated to the piano stairs and noticed by stepping on them they would make piano sounds. People of all ages began walking, jumping, laughing and climbing up and down the stairs to *play*. Almost without exception, everyone took the stairs that day. In fact, researchers found 66 percent more people took the stairs than the escalator. Fun, health, happiness – what a concept.

Higher Powers and Hope

In his book, *Happy – Simple Steps to Get the Most Out of Life*, Dr. Ian K. Smith identified the principles for finding more happiness in our lives. One of the key principles is to develop a spiritual life and practice forgiveness. When we search for deeper meanings in life, believe in a higher power or just want to understand our and other's limitations, we are on the path to more happiness in our lives.

Numerous studies have shown our spirituality increases as we age. Forgiving your loved ones for their behaviors – whether crankiness, obstinance or constant neediness - is hard for caregivers. Take these trying times and forgive your loved one, because in the end he is probably afraid and that often changes our personalities. For your sake, find an expert who can suggest techniques on how to cope, so you can maintain your happiness level.

Vic Mazmanian, director of faith outreach for the Mind, Heart & Soul Ministry of Saddleback Church and Silverado Senior Living in Southern California, told me, "Caregivers need to appreciate the small daily miracles with their loved one – a smile or the fact a loved one with Alzheimer's is calmer in their presence – these are the things that can help caregivers feel happier and alleviate their stress."

In many instances, caregivers have found comfort in talking to a spiritual advisor, whether your pastor, minister, reverend or rabbi. You will also find many faith-based organizations have support groups for caregivers, some with volunteers who can help you in some of your caregiving responsibilities. Reaching out to your faith-based community can give you an overall feeling of belonging that helps remove that happiness killer: feeling all alone. It will ultimately bring you hope…and happiness.

Nostalgia and Riding the Roller Coaster

Many of the caregivers I have talked to characterize their caregiving as an *emotional roller coaster*. One way to cope with the ups and downs of caregiving is to focus on *being present*. Rather than be concerned about the physical aspects of caregiving, think about the emotional side of caregiving. You are helping your loved one through a frightening journey. You have said by your presence, "I will be here for you."

Another principle from Dr. Smith's book is to strengthen and deepen relationships. Practice this with your spouse or partner, your kids, your friends or even with the person for whom you are caring.

We know from numerous studies isolation is bad for our older loved ones – it impacts both their health (such as not eating properly or enough) and their wellness (sometimes leading to depression). By spending quality time with your loved ones – time talking and sharing – not time helping them get to the doctor or dress themselves – you are helping them achieve better happiness which will ultimately increase your happiness as well.

Many older loved ones like to talk about days gone by. Nostalgia is important to them, it is a happier time than perhaps the present where they are unable physically to do things they once loved and they feel powerless to change it.

When I would spend time with my 80-year-old grandpa – he loved to talk about his early childhood growing up in Cleveland. I was fascinated by our family's genealogy, so I encouraged him to remember as much about his childhood as he could, and I scribbled these stories into notebooks (this was pre-iPad or laptop days). His favorite story was about riding the wooden roller coaster at Euclid Beach. He talked about feeling the salt air in his nostrils, his hair flying back and the sensation he was flying. When he told me these stories, he became more animated, he seemed younger and I was happy to know more about him and another era.

In his book *How to Say It to Seniors*, author David Solie writes, "Life review is the dominant psychological event of getting old. The need to be remembered, to uncover their lasting legacy is the other urgent development…senior adults focus on reviewing their lives to find out what it meant for them to have lived."

Give your loved ones the gift of listening. You will learn a lot you may never have known about your family's history and your loved one's thoughts on life. It will, in turn, make you happy to do something so meaningful to them – being interested in their life. You will find you have a deeper relationship which makes both of you happier.

LOST and Found

Support Groups, Professionals, Personal Board of Directors, Friends

In the hit TV series, *LOST*, a group of airline passengers find themselves crashing and surviving on a remote desert island for years (or at least six seasons). They learn to live together, sharing their histories and their daily struggles and they find solace and companionship in their shared survivorship. The concept *no man is an island* first proposed by John Donne, a 17th century poet and contemporary of Shakespeare's, is the same that applies to caregiving. No caregiver can do it alone.

Support groups are a fundamental element of surviving caregiving. Whether you are caring for a loved one with Alzheimer's, coping with the death of a spouse from cancer or parenting a child with autism, support groups are the rescue party in a silent, crazy, lonely world. While many caregivers are not sure if they want to share intimate details with *strangers*, the reality is these strangers can often become your best friends. These fellow caregiving survivors may come to understand you better than your spouse, your sister or your favorite neighbor because they know exactly what you are going through on your caregiving journey (just as Jack, Kate, Sawyer, Hurley and Locke learned to live together and trust each other back on the island in *LOST*).

"Reaching out for help is a sign of strength," says Dr. Leisa Easom, executive director for the Rosalynn Carter Institute for Caregiving. She advises caregivers to not stay quiet about their caregiving situation. "The only way to find the critical support you need is to self-identify as a caregiver."

You can choose from a variety of support groups, both online and in-person to find the one right for you. Some caregivers feel it invades their privacy to share intimate details with an in-person support group and find some of the anonymity of the Internet chat rooms helps them open up. Others need the in-person support where a sympathetic hug after sharing a painful or stressful story can mean everything.

The most important criteria for finding the group that is best for you is to be as specific as possible. When it comes to cancer, there are support groups for spouses of various types of cancer such as lymphoma or breast cancer. For those caring for a veteran, groups such as Vietnam Veterans of America or Wounded Warrior Project or specific conditions such as Disabled American Veterans or Paralyzed Veterans of America can help. There are support groups for young caregivers (teens or college age), for siblings of those with mental health issues and for those LGBT caregivers. Typically, the best place to start is with organizations providing support for the condition impacting your loved one, such as the Alzheimer's Association or Leeza's Place for Alzheimer's disease or Susan G. Komen for the Cure for breast cancer.

Sara Honn Qualls, professor of psychology at the University of Colorado at Colorado Springs says, "Support groups are a major source of comfort for many caregivers who find someone else walking their walk. Caregivers are grateful when someone like the Alzheimer's Association can point to support groups and other resources that speak to the experiences they are going through."

However, Qualls says when a caregiver is simply dealing with an aging parent, sometimes support groups don't offer the specifics needed.

"Sometimes a caregiver is simply taking care of an older parent with no specific illness or disease but finds their parent's mobility is declining," says Qualls. "Well, there is no *diagnostic name* for this issue so caregivers have no identified support group they can turn to in these cases, there is no a support group for low mobility. And while there are support groups for adult children of aging parents, sometimes they cover such a broad spectrum caregivers find them frustrating."

Qualls says this is when caregivers typically turn to informal networks such as friends, other family members and co-workers who they know have been through a caregiving experience and may have some valuable insights.

Circle of Friends

This 1995 movie starring Chris O'Donnell and Minnie Driver was about the strength of friendship. In many ways when a crisis event happens, caregivers are surrounded with well-meaning family and friends who ask, "What can I do to help?" Most caregivers don't have a list in hand to give to someone with exactly the kind of help they need. In addition, coordinating all these requests is beyond the scope of reason for any caregiver at that moment. Until now. Thanks to the digital age, in the last few years several online sites have been created to help caregivers get the support and the break they need and give family and friends a place to create a *circle of support* to give caregivers a break.

Launched in 2008, Lotsa Helping Hands has more than 1 million volunteers who have joined free, private communities performing more than 2.5 million tasks such as delivering meals; doing laundry; providing rides for seniors to the doctor or getting the kids to soccer; finding medical equipment reimbursed by Medicare, etc. Whatever, wherever, whenever the caregiver cannot get to something in her busy life, the circle of care community volunteers fill that gap by performing that task – all from a very detailed online HelpCalendar created with the input of professional nurses and family caregivers.

"When my mother was diagnosed with a brain tumor, our family was devastated," says Wendy Naumann who created a community on Lotsa Helping Hands. "My sister and I live out of state, and even though my brother and other sister live in the same city with my mom, we wanted to be helpful. Volunteers made it much more feasible for us to keep my mom at home during her entire illness; they provided a network for us to tap into when we needed to go beyond the family resources. Some volunteers became an extension of the family."

Lotsa has more than 50 nonprofit organizations using its technology platform as a tool to create online support communities including the Alzheimer's Association, National Family Caregivers Association, Leukemia & Lymphoma Society and the Muscular Dystrophy Association. There are also Open Communities where local community residents can volunteer to help a caregiver and her family even if the volunteer does not personally know the family.

"The power of our communities is caregivers are getting nurturing in body and soul," says Brooks Kenny, chief marketing officer for Lotsa. "The Lotsa communities have become a sacred gathering place for friends and family who want to help a caregiver."

CaringBridge is another online site for caregiver support. This nonprofit organization launched in 1997, was originally established to create an online place where families could send well wishes and post updates on a loved one's condition for concerned family and friends. Entirely funded by donations from families and individuals, more than 43 million people visited the site last year with nearly 400,000 personal pages created over the last 15 years. CaringBridge recently launched a new service called SupportPlanner to help family and friends coordinate tasks and its Amplifier Hub gives volunteers an opportunity to spread the word about CaringBridge and its mission.

We are seeing more people who had a powerful, personal experience using a CaringBridge site to connect family and friends during a health event," says Ronda Maurer, volunteer engagement specialist at CaringBridge. "They in turn realize other people could benefit from the experience and ask us how they can support others in need. We rarely need to recruit volunteers – we have so many people willing to help."

Over the last couple of years and months, other online communities have launched that also offer calendar functions, personal health record information and other caregiver support. Some of these online communities include: CareZone, CareTogether, CarePages, CareFlash, CareTrio and Senior Care Society's Family Portal.

What's Up Doc?

When it comes to caregiving, there are two types of professional experts who can help you:

1. A Geriatric Care Manager (GCM) or a Child Development Specialist (as detailed in the Rehearsals chapter called My Man Godfrey) can help you shoulder the burden of caregiving by giving you peace of mind for the choices you are helping your loved one make or making on their behalf. GCMs are credentialed experts at elder care and understand local resources and how to navigate the health care system. They can help you see the light at the end of the tunnel of caregiving. For those caregivers who are caring for a child with special needs, a child development therapist specializing in the disorder or disease acts in the same way a GCM does for elder care.

2. A Psychiatrist or Psychologist – When friends, family and support groups are not enough, sometimes it is critical to turn to a professional who can lead you through the emotional journey of caregiving. Jill Eikenberry credits her therapist for allowing her to understand her relationship with her mother in a whole different light as she walks her caregiving path. As mentioned in the Misery chapter, a psychiatrist is a health care professional with a medical degree who has studied disorders of the brain. Typically psychiatrists will treat patients with medications. The other type of professional is a psychologist who has studied the pyscho-social behavioral aspects of emotional health. Psychologists are more focused on problem-solving techniques through therapy and counseling. Whichever type of health care professional you choose be certain she or he understands caregiving as this is the foundation for the help you need.

In Good Company

When it comes to starting a new venture, any successful company typically creates a board of directors. Caregiving is really no different. Think of your family members and circle of friends. Is there an attorney in your midst? An accountant, financial planner or perhaps a health insurance executive? How about a nurse or social worker? In life, we all have people around us who we tap for good advice, and we often turn to different people within our circle because they have an expertise in an area where we need help.

Think of caring for your loved one as Caregiving Inc., and you are the Chairman of the Board. Who will be on your personal board of directors? Once you have identified your board, sit with each one and explain where and how you need help. Often, friends and family are eager to lend a helping hand, and if their help happens to be in their wheelhouse of expertise all the better. You will get help, they will feel good about helping you and Caregiving Inc. will be a sustainable, healthy venture.

It's A Wonderful Life

In the great movie, *It's A Wonderful Life*, the angel Clarence tells George Bailey played by the ultimate *every-man* actor, Jimmy Stewart, that, "No man is a failure who has friends."

In your caregiving role, friends are essential. You may count your spouse or a sister as a friend. Maybe it's a neighbor or co-worker. Or it could be someone you meet through a support group or in an online chat room. The important message is friends are essential to your mental wellness.

In a study conducted by Elaine M. Eshbaugh, PhD, at the University of Northern Iowa in Cedar Falls, she wrote in an article for the American Society on Aging newsletter, *Aging Today*, "[I] found that friends living within a 50-mile radius of older adult women were more important in preventing loneliness than was their family who also might live as close."

Her conclusions were five friends seem to be the magic number in combating loneliness among women. And since women tap into more of their *emotional* side while men tap their *physical* side, for male caregivers, taking a jog with a buddy or playing a round of golf with a foursome seems to have the same therapeutic effect to ward off the blues that can arise in caregiving.

Humorist Arnold Glasow said, "A true friend never gets in your way unless you are going down." Caregiving can sometimes make you feel alone and LOST, but seek help and friends and you will be found.

Act III

Coming Attractions

The road to success is always under construction.
— Lily Tomlin

Dialogue Coach – How Do You Start the Conversation?

Motion pictures need dialogue as much as Beethoven symphonies need lyrics.

– *Charlie Chaplin*

Becoming Meryl Streep

On one hand, Charlie Chaplin may have been right – you can entertain without saying a word. Silent films and even the recent Oscar-winning film, *The Artist*, taught us *a picture is worth a thousand words*. When it comes to caregiving it would be nice to rely on images and photos and not have to have those tough conversations with a loved one. However, talking is essential when it comes to caregiving and it is something we do not do enough.

We need to have the conversation with loved ones about a variety of care-related issues. We also need to have the discussions with health care professionals to ensure we are treated as a vital and important member of the care team around a loved one. And we need to share our journey in caregiving with others so we may encourage better understanding of chronic illness, disabilities and disorders, and help others better prepare for a journey most of us will take. The trick is being able to understand how to communicate *effectively* and to understand the conversations swirling around us.

The next chapter is how to have the difficult conversation around caregiving with your older loved one. I call it the C-A-R-E Conversation℠. I focus on conversations with your older parents because those seem to be the toughest to start. One of the techniques in having a conversation with our older parents is to listen. It is difficult because we have our own fears, concerns and ideas about what should happen with their care but it is essential for success that you ask a lot of questions and really *hear* their answers.

In addition to the conversations with older loved ones, you will need to communicate with many health care professionals who throw terminology and insider language around as if we know what they are all about. Caregiving can make you feel like you are a stranger in a foreign land. In the Resources section called Subtitles I have created an alphabetical listing of some of the terminology you may need to know. Consider this a primer on phrases and acronyms you will become familiar with as you take your caregiving journey.

Whether talking to older parents or to health care professionals, listening is critical to your success as a caregiver.

A great example of someone who listens is one of our most celebrated actresses. I am always amazed at how actors can adopt a dialect with such perfection and the consummate artist at this is, of course, Meryl Streep. In her illustrious career, she has played a Polish holocaust survivor, a Danish expatriate in colonial Africa, an Australian mother accused of a heinous crime. She even performed a pitch perfect Julia Child. What makes Meryl so great at these different dialects are two words: She listens. She is like a musical prodigy who can play by ear.

Take a cue from Meryl – stop, focus and pay attention to what others are saying. Only by listening can you learn to speak.

C-A-R-E Conversations^{SM}

Death will be a great relief – no more interviews.

– Katherine Hepburn

Besides managing stress, having the caregiving conversation is one of the toughest tasks a caregiver will encounter. However, we can't avoid these conversations like the plague or shroud them in so much mystery it does us more harm than good to remain silent.

There is a lot of fear and emotion tied up in talking with an older parent about what the future holds. As a caregiver or potential caregiver, it is your responsibility to remove the mystery around the future as much as possible. The *unknown* creates fear, frustration, foolish or costly decisions and conflict that do not need to exist. What is remarkable is how unburdened you will feel once you can have these conversations. It removes a huge obstacle in the roadway of your caregiving journey. Once the conversations are begun you can continue to move on and provide the best care possible for your loved one. And it will spark more dialogue and conversation along the journey that will help both of you.

As you have read in this book, every family is different; every caregiver has a unique situation. There is no script for one conversation. You cannot have one simple conversation and then you are done. One conversation may lead to another and yet another and another. And that is good. As you care for an older parent you will probably have conversations with your spouse, your siblings, your loved one's doctor, etc.

Look Who's Talking

There are two questions I am frequently asked when I talk to caregivers:

1. "When do I have this conversation with my older parent?"
2. "How do I start the conversation with them?"

The first answer is simple: the sooner the better. When it comes to talking to your older parent, HomeInstead, an international organization that provides senior home care, calls it the 40/70 Rule. If you are age 40 or if your parent is age 70, then you should have the conversation.

The second answer is more involved. Every good conversation has to have two sides – you cannot have a one-sided dialogue. In some instances, you want the other person to do more of the talking so you are more of a reporter or investigator – this is a rule of thumb when talking to parents or physicians.

Author David Solie has written a wonderful book called *How to Say It to Seniors* which poignantly reminds caregivers to become empathetic to the person they are talking with – particularly an older parent. He says so often caregivers think they know better – "change is good, I'm the expert on how to manage this, they'll see my way is best."

Solie advises in many ways, our conversations with parents as they age have to follow the same evolution of thinking we took after World War II when child development strategies changed. We became less of a society that said, "Children should be seen but not heard," and became more about listening, explaining and changing our language to provoke less resistance from our kids. Similarly, older parents when approached in the wrong way can become childish. Solie says a two-year old child and an 82-year old parent are not dissimilar at times – they can throw tantrums, want their independence, want to be heard and often feel vulnerable.

Solie says giving unsolicited advice, especially to an older loved one, sets him back on his heels. You are changing the status quo and this creates confusion and conflict. Now you have created a confrontational environment instead of a collaborative one. He advises often we are having conversations about our motivations for doing something (it will save me time, it will save me money) rather than thoughtfully asking our loved one about his motivation.

We have to keep in mind aging and the prospect of death is terrifying for most older Americans. This is the final act in their life's play, which creates fear and a lot of dilemmas for them. Our role as caregivers is to become a partner, a helper, a facilitator not a dictator. We need to create a *safe place* where we can have thoughtful discussions and plan together what is the best course of action. Solie advises to ask a lot of questions to spark dialogue. However, you don't want to sit down with your checklist and fire off questions seeking answers like Mike Wallace on *60 Minutes*. This will make your parent angry, fearful, confused or just answer "yes" or "no" to things. You want *conversation*. You need to ask questions that lead to "explain it to me Mom."

We have to recognize as adult children our lives have changed but so have our parents' lives. We have to match up our situation with the place where our parent may be today. For instance:

You Feel	Your Parent Feels
Fast-paced life	Life slowing down
Forward thinking, looking to future	Backwards reflection
Want to make a difference	Want to leave a legacy
In control	Loss of control
Don't Ask, Just Tell	Need to Decide, Explain
Resignation – let it go	Resolve the conflict
You are losing them	She is losing herself

Older parents may also feel you are violating their privacy or counting your inheritance before it happens when you start the caregiving conversation. Again, fear and panic are taking over in their minds – you are reminding them the end is coming. If you explain to your parents the obstacles, frustration and roadblocks you will encounter if they do not recognize your role as their future caregiver, it may help. Often, they do not want to cause you a world of anxiety and stress. Many parents do not want to burden their children with this information stating instead, "It's all handled honey – don't worry about it."

When you are in a crisis and emotions are running high, it can be an insurmountable task to try to track down information and be able to help make the best decisions for your loved one. Your older parent needs to understand this, the burden is not about having the conversation now, it is about navigating in the dark later. Planning ahead and having the discussion as a family is essential.

Knowing what your loved one wants is another reason the Alzheimer's Association has put so much education around the 10 Warning Signs of the disease. Many people start showing signs of Alzheimer's in their 40s or 50s but these signs go missed or ignored until full-blown dementia makes them unable to contribute to conversations about their future. You will read more about this in the stories of Sylvia Mackey, Jill Eikenberry & Michael Tucker and Joan Lunden.

Studies have shown only one-third of caregivers today have had *the talk* about long-term care with their family member or friend. To ignite the spark of dialogue that needs to happen around caregiving, I have created what I call the C-A-R-E Conversation[SM].

C = Create a conversation about caregiving.

Start with either a personal story or recent news – this can be a story of a friend or a recent news story that touches on caregiving as an important role in our lives. Some recent news stories about high profile people facing care conversations include Catherine Zeta Jones caring for her ill husband Michael Douglas while also caring for their two young children, Glen Campbell and his wife Kim facing his Alzheimer's diagnosis or stories from the high profile people from this book.

This will spark dialogue between you and your loved one on a less personal level and allow her to give opinions. Once the conversation gets going, you can start to ask more pertinent, personal questions relating to her wishes and plans. Again, make sure your loved one is comfortable with the flow of conversation. Don't become over-anxious to have all your answers now. You may need to have this conversation several times over a period of weeks or months. The intent is not to invade her privacy but to have her understand this is a *partnership* for her future care. Explain how anyone who will possibly be acting on her behalf needs to know everything to best help her.

A = Acknowledge first, then Ask.

One word here: Listen. Aging With Dignity has published a great document called *The Five Wishes* which helps older parents and caregivers start the conversation about what they want to have happen as their physical and mental capacities fade. What is important is to ensure your loved one you want to do what is best for her. Having this conversation now, rather than being in a crisis when a sudden illness or other event forces the issue, will make you better equipped to help her when the time comes.

Another important point is not to argue with your loved one if she makes a decision that you don't agree with. You can provide information on why you think an alternative plan is better but in the end, the decisions are hers. You have to let this go. While caregiving is a partnership, these decisions are not yours to make. Keep in mind this is your loved one's final act and it is her monologue to deliver. Your time will come and then you will get to make all the decisions around your future care but for now, this is her show.

Once you have acknowledged your loved one's wishes, you want to continue to ask her and her health care professionals a lot of questions. Only by asking can you get information that will help you in your caregiving role.

R = Review and Reach out.

Now that the caregiving dialogue is rolling, you want to review actuals plans – is there a long-term-care (LTC) policy? Is there legal documentation such as Powers of Attorney or an Advance Directive or a Living Will? Make sure you know what is covered, and more importantly, what may not be covered. This is when you can discover what out-of-pocket expenses may be incurred or you may discover her policy or savings won't cover the cost of her wish to move to that Continuing Care Retirement Community. At this point, you have to be your loved one's guidance counselor and have the discussion about *plan B*. I have seen cases of elders feeling they have taken care of these plans, but very often LTC and other policies do not cover everything and the fall-out is left to the caregiver.

If you don't start the conversation and review the plans already made, it can cause both emotional and sometimes financial challenges for you and your loved one. If your loved one has a legal or estate advisor, you may want to set up a meeting with him and your parent to review your questions regarding the plans in place. Again, make sure your loved one is comfortable with this idea – remember this is a partnership.

Besides reviewing documentation, it is important to reach out for and accept help – through family and friends, through support groups, through professionals, through your workplace HR department or supervisor. Avoiding the *ask* for help or not accepting what others may be offering is what I call the Caregiver's Achilles Heel. Don't let pride or martyrdom take you down. This often happens to the oldest daughter who has taken on the primary caregiver responsibility for a parent.

Dr. Kevin Leman, author of *The Birth Order Book – Why You Are the Way You Are* says, "First borns are programmed to think that 'no one can do it as well as me' and they set very high expectations for themselves – they tell themselves they only count when they do things well." Doing well as a caregiver means reaching out for help.

E = Engage, Educate, Empower.

While you might be the one to take the initiative of starting the caregiving conversation, especially if you feel you will become the primary caregiver, you want to ensure you include any siblings, your other parent, or even your own family (spouse and older children), in the caregiving plan for your loved one. This helps everyone prepare for their role and will help ensure the primary caregiver does not become burned out or bankrupt when taking on caregiving.

Family stress and strife, especially among siblings who do not agree on their parents' care, is common especially as family emotions run high when a caregiving crisis hits. You can hopefully avoid this when the time comes by having these conversations when everyone, including your loved one, can be involved. This ensures all these issues are discussed and decided upon ahead of time. Again, if you are experiencing difficulty getting a sibling to get involved or collaborate with you, Dr. Leman's book offers valuable insights into our relationships with siblings, spouses and even parents.

However, there are going to be times when you just are not able to get all your siblings on the same page. The ongoing stress of these conflicts can create more problems for you as the caregiver. That is when it is time to call in the cavalry – otherwise known as a geriatric care manager (GCM). These professionals are trained to counsel and work with families as an objective, outside expert, and can often bridge the gaps and bring everyone together in tough caregiving situations.

Solie recommends GCMs can become a caregiver's best friend and more importantly, your coach. He says, "In the same way I turn to a golf coach to help me improve my crappy golf swing or you would secure a piano teacher for your child to become the Beethoven you know they are, you need to engage a GCM to help your family navigate the complexities of the caregiving dilemmas you face."

The other role as a caregiver is not just the caring side it is the educational side. You are an advocate for your loved ones – you help ensure health care professionals understand their wishes or needs. You help friends or co-workers understand more about chronic illness such as multiple sclerosis or ALS and what it takes to care for that person. A great example of lightening your caregiving load can be found in Holly Robinson Peete's story about finally telling her friends why R.J. does what he does because of his autism, rather than just telling them he has autism. People will become more engaged in helping you when they truly understand your caregiving situation.

Finally, there is that conversation you need to have with yourself. You need to stop and take the time to acknowledge your wonderful gift as a caregiver. You are allowing an older loved one to live out her last days in dignity and in love. You are reconnecting with loved ones on a different level that brings more meaning to your life. You are educating an ignorant world about illness, disease, disorders and how important it is to be supportive and sympathetic.

You are an ambassador for caregiving and you have empowered yourself. You have added another layer to your life, survived it, and maybe even thrived in it. Celebrate the moments that brought a smile to your face, those times that brought you joy or laughter. And as tough as caregiving can be, you also have rewards along the way. Look in the mirror and say to yourself "thank you."

Reality Show – How Do You Find Time for Yourself?

Love yourself first, and everything else falls into line.

– Lucille Ball

Me Time Monday^{SM}

When you become a caregiver, you often feel like you entered one of today's popular reality TV programs – it is like *Survivor* and *The Amazing Race* all at once. Instead of frantically looking for clues, or worrying about what the tribe will say – I want to change your channel to a *Dancing with the Stars*-type reality show.

Let's call your reality show *Me Time Monday*. If you are asking, "What is *Me Time?*" then we really have to do an extreme makeover on you. Me Time is a concept that has been written about by CNN, *Forbes*, WebMD, BeWell.org and advocated by many of the self-help gurus and health professionals I admire such as Dr. Oz, Louise Hay, Dr. Andrew Weil and Dr. Alice Domar. It is the essence of self-care which is the balance you need when you are caregiving.

You may ask why you need Me Time? If you have read through the chapters on stress, burnout, guilt and depression, you will see why finding Me Time is so critical to your self-care. And self-care is critical to your role as caregiver.

While you may know what Me Time is and why it is important, the bigger question is how do *you* define it and how do you get it? First of all, you need to make a list of all the things you love to do that are just for you – these are probably things you have abandoned or at least don't get to as frequently if you are caregiving. It could be gardening, reading a good book or magazine, painting or sculpting, getting a mani/pedi, going for a drive or bike ride.

Make sure you only list things you love that are just for you – if you wrote down *exercise* but it's something you feel you *have* to do rather than *love* to do, Dr. Domar says do not write it down. In other words, if you feel it is more punishment than passion, it's not Me Time.

Your Me Time activity can take five minutes or five hours – it is yours – no one can give you the list or put restrictions on what you write down. OK. Now you have your list – don't despair when you look at it as you would at Brad Pitt knowing he'll never leave Angelina Jolie to be with you. You will get to the things on the list. Deep breath. Here is how:

Close your eyes and imagine for one minute you have a remote control that could put the entire world on *pause*. Remember – this is your reality show. It is like the game you may have played as a kid – statue maker. Someone twirls you around and tosses you and when you land you have to be as still as a statue. That is what you have just done – tossed your worldly concerns and caregiving responsibilities in the air and they are now in freeze frame (they are not gone they are just on pause).

Now envision yourself doing one of your favorite Me Time activities. Think of how this activity makes you *feel*. Why do you love this so much? Does it bring a smile to your face? When was the last time you engaged in this Me Time activity? Was it more than one week ago?

Next, think of your Me Time activities not as unachievable dreams but as promises. Promises you make to yourself. You are reliable and responsible, you are a maniac multi-tasker, and you probably make a lot of promises to others around you. How many promises do you make to yourself?

A little hint – do not call these promises *resolutions*. Why? Well, that makes it sound too much like the start of the year – we all make New Year's Resolutions but few of us keep them. In fact, according to the University of Scranton researcher John Norcross, one of the authors of *Changing for Good*, 1 in 4 of us make a resolution for the New Year but after six months only 46 percent are still sticking with it.

Richard Wiseman, a psychologist at the University of Hertfordshire in England, author of *:59 Seconds* and creative consultant to the TV show *The Mentalist*, says those who fail to keep their resolution have one common pitfall which is focusing on the downside of the goal. You suppress your cravings, fantasize about being successful, adopt a role model or rely on willpower alone. But these aren't pleasurable experiences, they are torture and you will soon abandon them. He stated in an interview with *The Guardian*, "Failing to achieve your ambitions is often psychologically harmful because it can rob people of a sense of self control."

The way to avoid stress and burn-out is to take control of caregiving and the best way to stay in control is to plan ahead. Which is why the next step is to program yourself to think of or do your Me Time activity every Monday. Just as you plan to watch your favorite reality show every week (or at least DVR it to watch when you can), so too can you plan your weekly Me Time.

Why Monday Matters

In 2010 I met with a nonprofit organization, The Monday Campaigns, which was founded in 2005 in association with Columbia University, Johns Hopkins University and Syracuse University in order to apply marketing best practices to public health challenges. Research conducted by Johns Hopkins indicates the week is a critical unit of time in planning our lives and Monday has special significance as the beginning of the week. People view Monday as a day for a fresh start and a chance to set healthy intentions for the next six days. We are more likely to start diets, exercise regimes, quit smoking and schedule doctor appointments on Monday than any other day. And we're looking for help in setting and carrying out our healthy intentions for the week.

Monday is part of our cultural DNA – for most of us, it is the start of the work week, the school week and we feel renewed energy to start something after a nice weekend break. According to the research, the Monday Campaigns show a projected 74 percent of American adults over age 25 believe giving healthy intentions a Monday start will make them more lasting throughout the week. In 2011, The Monday Campaigns launched Caregivers' Monday, a specific campaign targeted to helping the nation's caregivers take care of themselves and asked my company, Caregiving Club, to participate as a charter partner.

"Day in and day out, millions of caregivers give so much of themselves caring for their loved ones that they often neglect their own health and well-being," says Sid Lerner, founder and chairman, The Monday Campaigns. "Caregivers' Monday encourages them to use that first day of each hectic week as their recharge day, to refocus on their own condition to better serve their dependent parent, child or spouse."

Me Time Monday[SM] became my program, including a weekly video tip, to help caregivers focus on that one day in their week where you check in with yourself. It may not be the day when you actually do your Me Time activity, but it is the day you take your virtual remote control, put the world on *pause* and ask yourself: "What did I do for Me Time last week? What am I going to do this week?"

Now you have your Me Time ideas and you have the rationale for starting and checking in with yourself every Monday, here are the instructions for achieving Me Time Monday success. We are going to take the promises you have made to yourself and follow three simple steps (remember – think of *Dancing with the Stars* – instead of learning a two-step, you are going to learn a three-step).

The Me Time Monday[SM] 3-Step

1. **First of all, you need to have an actual plan for your promises – your Me Time.** If you just have a desire to improve or do something, it is not enough. You will be more successful at achieving your promises if you have steps on how to get there. For instance, one of your promises may be walking for 30 minutes at least three times a week.

    Start by scheduling time and asking someone to watch your loved one or give you a break for whatever length of time you need to walk and recharge your batteries. Maybe you start with buying new walking shoes – this is your Week 1 accomplishment – got the shoes! (For me it is all about the shopping to get me motivated).

    Just do one step in your promise each week – you don't have to start walking 30 minutes three times a week in the first week. Maybe you walk once for 15 minutes. Then the next week, you walk twice for 15 minutes – get the picture? Baby steps are a key part of your plan.

2. **Secondly, you need to track your progress.** This instills a sense of accomplishment. This is why weight loss centers like Weight Watchers or Jenny Craig see high rates of success among their members, because each week they have that sense of accomplishment. And it also helps to talk to someone who is invested in seeing you be successful. Having a

friend or other support person who can be your *cheerleader* – celebrating your milestones toward your promise can help keep you going. Call a friend to join you on your walk or tell your spouse about something you saw while on your walk – celebrate your accomplishments each week to keep you motivated.

3. **Lastly, be committed to your promise.** Keep it simple (one promise at a time is better than two or three) and treat occasional *slips* as temporary setbacks on the path to keeping your promise. You have to commit to change. This is a marathon not a sprint. Be kind to yourself if you have a bad week and did not get to walk at all. Don't be discouraged, just start fresh on the next Monday and evaluate what derailed you last week so you can avoid that in the new week. Now you have learned the steps, every star on *Dancing with the Stars* knows you have to practice.

In the Star Performances section of this book I share with you how these celebrities find their Me Time. They all had great tips because they were all very personal. What I have not told you is how I find my Me Time. This will help you see that practice makes perfect.

As you can probably tell by now, reading even one chapter in this book – I am a movie and TV junkie. If you read the Preface to this book, these seeds were planted in my early childhood sitting in a dark theater in the afternoons escaping into the movies. What still makes me really happy, even giddy, is to go to the movies all by myself in the middle of the afternoon. Not only is the theater mostly empty so you feel like you are at a private screening, but there is delight about escaping into other worlds as the real world carries on outside the theater walls. I get a thrill watching Bruce Willis save the world or Julia Roberts light up the screen with her smile or Tom Hanks enthrall you whether he is playing a World War II soldier or a New York-based publishing executive wooing Meg Ryan via email. And I feel like I am a kid again.

I thought I was all alone in my Me Time delight until I caught an episode of TV's Season 5 of *Mad Men*. There it was – Don Draper, (the anti-hero brilliantly played by Jon Hamm) and Peggy Olson (the heroine played by the wonderful Elisabeth Moss) sneaking out of work during the day to go to the movies. As Peggy says, "Someone told me once, this helps clear the cobwebs."

Indeed it does. Writing is my passion and my work but sometimes I get stuck. When I get writer's block, I take myself to an afternoon matinee. Knowing even the stars (or at least their characters on TV) have the same Me Time pleasure as me makes me feel like I am not alone. By giving myself my Me Time Monday movie, I beat my occasional writer's block and finished this book.

Hopefully, in reading this book about celebrities and hearing from caregiving experts, you see as a caregiver, Me Time is something we all need to keep going. There you have it. You have 52 Mondays in a calendar year and 52 chances to grab some Me Time. Now push *play* on the remote control of your reality show and let your Me Time Monday begin.

That's a Wrap

You as Director of the Caregiving Show

"That's all folks!"

– Bugs Bunny

As a kid, I used to hate seeing this sign-off during my favorite Saturday morning TV cartoons because it meant the show was over. Whether you read this entire book or just a chapter or two I hope you felt it was informative and entertaining. What you should realize is the show is not over for caregivers – it is just beginning.

As you've read, over the next 20-40 years we will have more parents and older people to care for than children. But instead of being caught in an empty theater as the lights go up, you realize every seat around you is filled with other caregivers – and now the light bulb over your head should be on.

When it comes to caregiving, you are the Director (and the star – similar to those director/star examples such as Clint Eastwood, Mel Gibson and Barbra Streisand). You get the final cut on what your caregiving movie will be about. Let's review the Director notes you have learned from this book.

Gather Your Best Crew

It is critical you assemble the best crew around you. You need an expert cameraman – in this caregiving show that is known as a geriatric care manager (GCM) – someone who can see the big picture and help you navigate your caregiving responsibilities. You need experts and their services in specific issues such as Elder Law attorneys, senior housing advisors, home health services, personal care workers, geriatricians, health advocates, CAPs experts, etc. You also need your entourage – those close confidantes who help you out when you need it. Let's face it, as the star Director, you are busy and you need the help. Find your online community, support groups and friends who can *be there for you.*

This is learning to say, "Action!"

In addition, you need to learn how to delegate, to get the expert and volunteer help you need, and you need to learn how to let go of the little things that don't impact the *big picture*. You also need to set realistic expectations for yourself during caregiving. Don't live in absolutes and learn about setting limits.

This is learning how to say, "Cut!"

Review the Script

Understanding the script and the dialogue of your caregiving movie are critical. Health care literacy, care transitions, navigating Medicare and Medicaid and other valuable health care language are part of your Directing duties. You also need to ensure everyone is talking to each other. You are directing this show and your loved one depends on you to help the production stay on track. Because you are the Director, the continuity, consistency and overall outcome of the show depends on you.

Also keep in mind – there are no silent movies anymore (OK – forget the 2012 Oscar winner *The Artist* – that was an anomaly). This is called the C-A-R-E Conversations and you have to speak up and be heard. After all, you are the Director and everyone is looking to you.

Location Scouting

Where to *live for a lifetime* is one of the biggest issues facing Americans as we age. It also affects us as caregivers. As you read, there are experts – in person and online – who can help you scout your locations and come up with the perfect setting for your loved one in this caregiving show. There are also a lot of other things to research – catering and crafts services (known as nutrition and meals), movie insurance (or in this case, health care insurance), understanding where you are filming and how Mother Nature may mess with your production schedule (disaster planning), special effects (known as alternative therapies such as pets or music), traveling, transportation and limo drivers (also known as senior driving issues and alternative transportation), medication management, etc. Many experts and online resources can help you – you just need to know these are all the things you will be Directing.

Production Budget

One of the most critical elements of your Director role is knowing your budget. You can't have flying monkeys in your movie if they cost too much. And if you start filming your caregiving movie without a budget or understand the costs of care – you are sure to blow through your money half way through the film. This is called cost overruns and many films get shut down because of it. Having a budget up-front and understanding the costs over the long haul are critical to ensuring you can finish your movie.

Negotiating Your Perks and Benefits

Every good Director negotiates a contract that includes some significant perks and benefits. Your contract needs to ensure you have scheduled your Me Time Monday – get a break so you don't burn-out. It will help you alleviate the stress that comes with having the entire caregiving show riding on your shoulders. If the Director becomes too ill to finish the caregiving show, what will happen to those depending on her or him?

Applause

In the end, caregiving is like *The Lion King* – it is about the circle of life. Lives begin and end. In between, (sometimes toward the end), there is caregiving. Remember, you are making a moving picture – it is not in freeze frame. One caregiving scene will lead to another until the movie is done. But when it is, I have a feeling you will be hearing those words every star and Director longs to hear,

"And the award goes to…."

Subtitles

Alphabetical List of Caregiving Acronyms, Jargon

Even though the Tower of Babel is an ancient story, the confusion of language still exists today – especially in health care. Every industry has its phrases and acronyms that only those industry insiders know. When I first began working in health care, it was no different. There was a whole new language to learn and there were no Rosetta Stone or Berlitz courses to help me. It took me at least six months to create a list with everything I needed to know to keep up with conversations around me. This list became my little cheat sheet for important insider terminology.

Following is my list for you. I tried to make it as comprehensive as possible. Remember what Larry Minnix of LeadingAge said in the Rehearsals chapter Lost In Translation, some terms today will shift to accommodate a more *age-friendly* attitude tomorrow. Just like Webster's Dictionary, new words will find their way onto this list in the years to come. For today, you may consider this your Cliff's Notes to get you started on the basics.

Health care and the world of caregiving can feel like you are in a foreign film – you cannot understand what anyone is saying. This list is your subtitles so you can focus less on the words and more on what the movie is all about.

AAAs
Area Agencies on Aging. Located in most counties and every state with 629 offices. Collectively these agencies are operated by the federal government under the National Area Agencies on Aging (N4As) to provide local elder care service resources. Most resources are public, government and non-profit organizations. Local offices found through Elder Care Locator.

AAT
Animal-assisted therapy. Also known as pet therapy. Using dogs, cats, rabbits, horses to improve the symptoms and impacts of various diseases including autism, Alzheimer's, Parkinson's and terminal illnesses.

Advance Directive
A written document stating how you want medical decisions to be made if you lose the ability to make them for yourself. It may include a Living Will and a Durable Power of Attorney for health care.

ADLs
Activities of Daily Living. Typically used to identify the intensity of caregiving activities and what a loved one may need help with from their family caregiver. ADLs include: bathing, brushing teeth, dressing, eating, toileting, walking, transferring from bed to bath, wheelchair, etc. See also IADLs.

Adult Day Care
Supervised day care for older adults (typically includes meals). Found in centers in local communities.

Adult Protective Services
Investigates complaints of abuse, neglect or exploitation of older adults and those with disabilities.

AFH
Adult Family Home. Also known as Board-and-Care, these are residential facilities licensed to care for up to six residents at a time.

Aging in Place (AiP)
Phrase used to describe the desire to remain in your home living as independently as long as possible as you grow older and age or health-related issues may make this a challenge.

AIDS
Acquired immune deficiency syndrome. The final stage of HIV disease which causes severe damage to the immune system. The CDC reports there are more than 490,000 living with AIDS in the U.S. with 33 million worldwide living with HIV/AIDS, a number that includes 2.1 million children under age 15.

ALS
Amyotrophic lateral sclerosis. This progressive neurodegenerative disease affects nerve cells in the brain and the spinal cord. Patients in the later stages of the disease may become totally paralyzed and will ultimate die from the disease. More than 30,000 Americans suffer from ALS. Also known as Lou Gehrig's disease.

Alzheimer's disease (AD)
More than 5.4 million Americans and 36 million people worldwide. More than 15 million Americans provide care to someone with Alzheimer's. This progressive disease affects the brain impacting memory, thinking and behavior.

Assisted Living (AL)
Residential housing providing certain level of independence but with supervision of meals, transportation, medication oversight, activities and often minimal nursing care.

ASD
Autism spectrum disorder. A group of complex disorders of brain development that includes difficulties in motor coordination and attention, intellectual disability and physical health issues such as sleep and gastrointestinal disturbances. CDC says 1 in 88 American children are on the ASD. Also known as just autism.

Autism
See ASD above.

Board and Care Facility
(see AFH - Adult Family Home)

BP
Blood Pressure. Normal range is 120/80 and high blood pressure is typically 140/90.

Bradykinesia
Slow movement. Bradykinesia is often associated with an impaired ability to adjust the body's position. It can be a symptom of nervous system disorders such as Parkinson's disease or can be a side effect of medication.

Cancer
Cancer is a group of more than 100 diseases characterized by uncontrolled growth and spread of abnormal cells. If the spread is not controlled, it can result in death. Cancer is caused by both external and internal factors. It is the second most common cause of death in the U.S. after heart disease, accounting for nearly 1 in every 4 deaths annually.

CAPS
Certified Aging in Place Specialist. Expert who advises homebuilders and homeowners on home safety modifications for older Americans and those with disabilities.

Care Manager
See GCM (Geriatric Care Manager).

Case Manager
A professional who handles social aspects of a patient's situation – typically a social worker in an institutional setting such as a hospital.

CCAN
Caregiver Community Action Network. Organized by the National Family Caregiver's Association – a volunteer network of former caregivers found in 68 cities nationwide.

CCRCs
Continuing Care Retirement Communities. Contracted lifelong housing, board and health services provided in residential setting. Typically part of a campus with a variety of senior living/housing options.

Celiac disease (CD)
An autoimmune disease triggered by sensitivity to the food component gluten affecting 1 out of 133 Americans. Contrary to perceptions, celiac disease is not a food allergy. Those with CD can manage the disease but today there is no cure. Left untreated CD can lead to small bowel damage that can be life threatening. CD has been linked to Down syndrome, fibromyalgia and chronic fatigue syndrome.

Cerebral Palsy
A group of disorders that can involve brain and nervous system functions such as movement, learning, hearing, seeing and thinking. There are various types of cerebral palsy including spastic, dyskinetic, ataxic, hypotonic and mixed. The CDC says 1 in 303 children have the disease.

Chosen Family or Family of Choice
Used mostly in LGBT community to define the circle of friends, rather than biological family members, who provide care and can make medical and financial decisions if incapacitated (assuming proper legal documentation is in place).

CMS
Centers for Medicare and Medicaid Services. This is the arm of the federal government that administers all things under Medicare (federal) and Medicaid (federal and state level) programs for those age 65+ or who have disabilities. In addition CMS runs the Children's Health Insurance Programs (CHIP).

CNA
Certified Nurse Assistant
Work under the supervision of the nursing or medical staff typically in an assisted living or nursing home setting. Job duties typically include serving meals, helping patients bathe or dress, transferring them from bed to bath or wheelchair, emptying bedpans, making beds. They do not make independent decisions about your loved one's care.

COPD
Coronary Obstructive Pulmonary Disease. Progressive disease (means it worsens over time) that makes it hard to breathe. Main risk factor is smoking, however in non-smokers COPD can mean a person lacks a protein called alpha-1 antitrypsin which can develop into emphysema. Third leading cause of death in the U.S.

Curb-to-Curb Transportation Service
The most common designation for paratransit services, the transit involves picking up and discharging passengers at the curb or driveway in front of their home or destination. The driver does not assist or escort passengers to the door.

Custodial Care
Non-skilled personal care, such as help with activities of daily living (ADLs). It may also include the kind of health-related care that most people do themselves, like using eye drops.

Cystic Fibrosis (CF)
An inherited chronic illness affecting the lungs and digestive system. More than 30,000 children in the U.S. have CF.

Dementia
Loss of brain function that occurs with certain diseases. It affects memory, thinking, language, judgment and behavior. More than 36 million people worldwide have some form of dementia.

Diabetes
Type 1 diabetes once known as juvenile diabetes or insulin-dependent diabetes is a chronic condition in which the pancreas produces little or no insulin, a hormone needed to allow sugar (glucose) to enter cells to produce energy. Type 2 diabetes is far more common and occurs when the body becomes resistant to the effects of insulin or doesn't make enough insulin. More than 25 million children and adults in the U.S. have diabetes.

DME
Durable Medical Equipment. Items such as a walker, wheelchair, or hospital bed that is ordered by your doctor for use in the home. Costs may be covered under Medicare.

DNR and DNI order
Do Not Resuscitate. Do Not Intubate. Legal documentation for health care professionals to follow your wishes on emergency care and to not perform CPR or life support if the heart or breathing stops.

Door-through-Door Transportation Service
A hands-on service for passengers with significant mobility limitations in which a driver not only escorts the passenger into the apartment, assistance is also given for belongings (e.g., groceries). This service is for those who would otherwise not be able to use regular or even enhanced paratransit services.

Door-to-Door Transportation Service
A form of escorted paratransit service that includes passenger assistance between the vehicle and the door of his or her home or other destination but does not entail the driver going inside the destination.

DS
Down syndrome. A genetic condition that occurs when an individual has 47 chromosomes instead of the typical 46. This additional genetic material alters the course of development and causes both physical and mental problems. One in every 691 babies is born with DS and 400,000 people are living with DS in the U.S.

Dual Eligible
A person who qualifies for both Medicare and Medicaid insurance coverage and benefits through the federal government.

Durable Power of Attorney
You can have a Durable Power of Attorney for medical decisions and for financial decisions. This legal document designates the person you authorize to act on your behalf in the event you become disabled or incapacitated.

EAP
Employee Assistance Program. Administered through the human resources department of employers to provide employee help with services such as child care, elder care, substance abuse counseling, wellness programs, etc.

EHR
Electronic Health Record. EHRs may include a range of data, including medical history, medication and allergies, immunization status, laboratory test results, radiology images, vital signs, personal statistics like age and weight. EHRs are sometimes used interchangeably with EPR (electronic patient record) and EMR (electronic medical record). However, the U.S. Department of Health and Human Services (HHS) says these are distinctly different as EMR and EPRs are used mostly by hospitals and health care providers and EHRs contain holistic health information not just medical information. See also PHR (personal health record).

Elder Law Attorney

An attorney that specializes in trusts, estates, public benefits such as Medicare and Social Security. Elder law differs from state to state so it is critical to find an attorney that operates in the state where you need help.

EMR

See EHR.

EPR

See EHR.

EMT

Emergency Medical Technician. A person trained and certified to appraise and initiate emergency care for victims of trauma or acute illness before and during transportation to a health care facility.

ESRD

End Stage Renal Disease. Permanent kidney failure that requires a regular course of dialysis or a kidney transplant. More than 485,000 Americans are being treated for ESRD.

FMLA

Family & Medical Leave Act. Federal program that provides 12 weeks of unpaid time off in a 12-month work period and 26 weeks for caregivers of military service men and women (exceptions are California, Connecticut, Hawaii, Maine, Minnesota, New Jersey, Oregon, Rhode Island, Vermont, Washington, Wisconsin and the District of Columbia which do provide some pay over that period) with job protection when caring for an ill or injured parent.

Formulary

A list of prescription drugs covered by a prescription drug plan or another insurance plan offering prescription drug benefits.

FQHC

Federally Qualified Health Center. Community-based organizations that provide comprehensive primary care and preventive care and are a reimbursement designation from CMS.

FSA
Flexible Savings Account. Administered by employers through benefit programs where certain medical or health care services can be paid for through pre-tax dollars. FSAs have *use it or lose it* policies where if you don't use all the funds before the end of the plan coverage period, it does not roll over, you lose those unused funds.(see HSA).

FTD
Frontotemporal dementia. Often seen in those who have been in combat, such as veterans, or in professional athletes where severe head trauma is common. Typically diagnosed years after the injury. Affects 50,000-60,000 Americans and represents 10-20% of all dementia cases. One of the most common dementias affecting a younger population.

GCM
Geriatric Care Manager. Also known as Care Manager or PCGM. Health and human services manager who acts as a guide and advocate for families who are caring for older relatives or adults with disabilities. Education and experience typically includes nursing, gerontology, social work, psychology with special training on elder care.

Geriatrician
Physician who specializes in caring for older patients.

Gerontology
Study of the social, psychological and biological aspects of aging.

GLBT
Gay, Lesbian, Bisexual, Transgender (more commonly referred to as LGBT).

HCD
Health Care Directive. Legal documentation that is a set of written instructions that a person gives to specify what actions should be taken for their health if they are no longer able to make decisions due to illness or incapacity.

Heart disease
A condition that develops when plaque builds up in the walls of the arteries. Because the build-up narrows the arteries, it is harder for blood to flow which can cause heart attack or stroke. Leading cause of death in the U.S.

HHA
Home health aide. This is a designation for a registered worker who has trained for in-home care. They may administer medications, check pulse and temperature, provide help transferring from bed to bath or wheelchair, aid in bathing, dressing, feeding, provide personal care services such as light housekeeping or laundering. They do not change catheters, change bandages, give injections or assist with medical equipment such as breathing devices.

HIPAA
Health Insurance Portability and Accountability Act. Instituted in 1996, this is a privacy and security rule that protects an individual's health information. Health care providers, insurers and others must adhere to this national standard for the security and confidentiality of electronic protected health information.

HIV
Human Immunodeficiency Virus. HIV infection gradually destroys the immune system which makes it harder for the body to fight infection. Worldwide 33 million people are living with HIV.

Hospice
A facility or program provided in the home where a multi-disciplinary team provides *comfort care* (rather than curative care) for the physical and emotional needs of someone with a terminal illness and their family.

Hospitalists
Doctors who are trained in critical care, who only see patients in hospital settings and are available all hours of day and night. Typically directs the health care needs within the hospital setting but does not create an ongoing health care relationship with the patient (as opposed to a Primary Care Physician).

HRA
Health Risk Assessment. Health questionnaire evaluating health risks and quality of life.

HSA
Health Savings Account. Administered by employers through benefit programs where certain medical and health care services can be paid for through pre-tax dollars. HSA funds can be held until retirement if you choose – there is no *use it or lose it* such as with an FSA (see FSA).

IADLs
Instrumental Activities of Daily Living. Typically used to identify the intensity of caregiving activities and what a loved one may need help with from their family caregiver. IADLs include: cooking, driving, keeping track of finances, managing medications, shopping, using the telephone or computer. See also ADLs.

Independent Living
Any housing arrangement designed exclusively for seniors, generally those aged 55 and over.

IU
International Unit. Used in pharmacology as a unit of measurement of a substance based on biology activity or effect.

LEP
Limited English Proficient. Relates to health care literacy and the risk of non-computer savvy, some minority or non-English speaking individuals and low-income persons who struggle with English – spoken conversations and/or reading comprehension.

Lewy Body
A pattern of cognitive decline that can be similar to Alzheimer's disease. Involves memory impairment, poor judgment, confusion and excessive sleepiness. Fifty percent of patients experience rapid eye movement (REM) sleep behavior disorder.

LGBT
Lesbian, Gay, Bisexual, Transgender. Also GLBT or LGBTQ.

Living Will
A legal document also known as a medical directive or advance directive. It states your wishes regarding life-support or other medical treatment in certain circumstances, usually when death is imminent.

LPN
Licensed Practical Nurse. Can give injections, operate a feeding pump, administer oxygen, clean wounds, prepare and administer medications. Cannot set-up and operate IVs.

LTC
Long Term Care. Insurance plans that cover some costs for nursing home, community-based care or in-home care services.

MCI

Mild Cognitive Impairment. This is a diagnosis that falls in between the severe (Alzheimer's disease) or the normal (typical forgetfulness that is a natural part of aging) ranges for memory and brain health. MCI patients can remain independent and manage daily functions but have more memory loss or recall issues than normal older persons.

Medicaid

A joint Federal and state program that helps with medical costs for some people with limited income and resources. Medicaid programs vary from state to state.

Medical Home

A cultivated partnership between the patient, the family and primary provider in cooperation with specialists and support from the community. Built around care coordination, medical homes sometimes include additional resources such as health information technology, and appropriately trained staff. In the medical home, the patient has open access to see whatever physician they choose. No referral or permission is required.

Medicare

The Federal health insurance program for people who are age 65 or older, certain younger people with disabilities, and people with End-Stage Renal Disease (permanent kidney failure requiring dialysis or a transplant, sometimes called ESRD). Original Medicare is fee-for-service coverage under which the government pays your health care providers directly for your Part A and/or Part B benefits.

Medicare – Part A

Part A which is coverage for inpatient hospital stays, care in a skilled nursing facility, hospice care, and some home health care.

Medicare – Part B

Part B which covers certain doctors' services, outpatient care, medical supplies, and preventive services.

Medicare Advantage (Part C)

A type of Medicare health plan offered by a private company that contracts with Medicare to provide you with all your Part A and Part B benefits.

Medicare – Part D
Part D is optional benefits for prescription drugs available to all people with Medicare for an additional charge. This coverage is offered by insurance companies and other private companies approved by Medicare.

Mental illness
Any of various psychiatric conditions, usually characterized by impairment of an individual's normal cognitive, emotional or behavioral functioning and caused by psychological or psychosocial factors. One in 17 people in the U.S. suffer from a serious mental illness.

mHealth
Known as mobile health this is a subset of telehealth. It is the delivery of health-related services and information via mobile communication devices such as cell phones and smartphones.

MPERS
Mobile Personal Emergency Response Systems. Technology devices, typically including a cellular or texting service that alerts a caregiver their loved one has fallen. Devices range from watches to belt clips to lavaliers to cell phones with special services. See also PERS.

MS
Multiple Sclerosis. Auto-immune disease, currently with no cure, that attacks the central nervous system and can result in paralysis and loss of physical functions such as eyesight, pain in chest or limbs, etc. Impacts 2.1 million people worldwide and 400,000 Americans, most diagnosed between ages of 20-50 years old.

Muscular Dystrophy (MD)
Muscular dystrophy is a group of inherited disorders that involve muscle weakness and loss of muscle tissue, which get worse over time. The term that encompasses more than 40 neuromuscular diseases that affect more than 1 million Americans and can occur in childhood or adulthood.

NORCs
Naturally Occurring Retirement Communities. NORC Aging in Place Initiative is a program of The Jewish Federations of North America (JFNA). The 157 Federations comprise a community-based network of 1,300 health and social services providers that provide humanitarian assistance to millions of people nationally who want to age in place.

NP
Nurse Practitioner. NPs are advanced registered nurses (RNs) who provide preventive and acute health care services. They can perform exams, diagnosis conditions, provide immunizations, order lab tests and prescribe medication.

OT
Occupational Therapy. This type of treatment helps you return to your usual activities (like bathing, preparing meals, and housekeeping) after an illness.

OTC
Over-the-Counter. Refers to any medication that does not require a prescription from a doctor.

PACE
Programs of All-inclusive Care for the Elderly. A special type of health plan that provides all the care and services covered by Medicare and Medicaid as well as additional medically-necessary care and services based on your needs as determined by an interdisciplinary team. PACE serves frail older adults who need nursing home services but are capable of living in the community. PACE combines medical, social, and long-term care services and prescription drug coverage.

Palliative Care
This is comfort care provided at any stage to someone who has a terminal illness. The care relieves symptoms of disease or illness but does not provide curative measures.

Paratransit
The word *paratransit* can mean several different alternative modes of flexible passenger transportation that do not follow fixed routes or schedules. Depending on your particular need and the population density of your area, you may request a door-to-door pickup for your doctor's appointment, or you may be picked up in front of your home as part of a group heading to a fixed location such as a grocery store.

Parkinson's disease (PD)
A chronic degenerative brain disorder that affects one in 100 people over age 60 although people can be diagnosed as early as age 18. Loss of cells in the brain affects control of bodily movements. One million people in the U.S. and 5 million people worldwide are diagnosed with PD.

Patient Navigator
Also known as Health Navigators or Health Advocates. Professionals who help caregivers and patients with care coordination and interfacing with insurance companies on claims or provider billing departments on the family's behalf.

PCP
Primary Care Physician. A physician/medical doctor who provides first contact for a person with undiagnosed condition and continuing care for various medical conditions.

PERS
Personal Emergency Response Systems. Technology devices such as sensors in the home or mobile devices such as cell phones with special services, watches, belt clips, lavaliers that have a special GPS chip or alert/alarm in case a loved one has fallen. See also MPERS.

Personal Care Aide (PCA)
Also called a personal care attendant. An in-home care worker who performs tasks such as light housekeeping, meal preparation and in some cases help feeding, bathing, dressing, toileting or transferring a loved one. Not as credentialed as a home health aide who can also help administer medications, take blood pressure and temperature readings.

PGCM
Professional Geriatric Care Manager. See GCM.

PHR
Personal Health Record. See EHR.

PMR
Progressive Muscle Relaxation. Used in stress reduction techniques.

Power of Attorney
A medical power of attorney is a document that lets you appoint someone you trust to make decisions about your medical care. This type of advance directive also may be called a health care proxy, appointment of health care agent, or a durable power of attorney for health care.

Preventive Services
Health care to prevent illness or detect illness at an early stage, when treatment is likely to work best (for example, preventive services include Pap tests, flu shots, and screening mammograms).

PT
Physical Therapy. Treatment of an injury or a disease by mechanical means, like exercise, massage, heat, and light treatment.

PTSD
Post Traumatic Stress Disorder. A mental health problem that can occur after someone goes through a traumatic event such as war, assault or disaster.

Respite
Also known as companionship services. Respite is provided to give the family caregiver a break from day-to-day care activities and responsibilities for a loved one. Respite care can be delivered in the home or via outside services. Respite workers or volunteers do not perform the functions of a personal care aide or home health aide.

RFG
Registered Financial Gerontologist. A special credential provided to financial planners and CPAs who have completed a course in aging issues.

RN
Registered Nurse. Provide and coordinate care, educate patients and the public about various health conditions and provide advice and emotional support to patients and family members. They can specialize in various fields including ER medicine, podiatry, obstetrics and gynecology, geriatrics, surgery, etc.

SAD
Seasonal affective disorder. A type of depression associated with winter months or geographic locations which lack sunshine for many months of the year. Affects more women than men.

SCU
Special care unit. Also called memory care facilities. A designation for assisted living facilities that care for dementia residents.

Senior Centers
More than 11,000 senior centers are located in cities across the country. They provide information, education, socialization, outings and events for adults age 60+.

Shelter-in-Place
In the case of an emergency or disaster situation, this does not mean to go to a shelter. Rather this means to find a small, interior room with no or few windows and take refuge there.

SHIP
State Health Insurance Assistance Program. A state program that gets money from the Federal government to give free local health insurance counseling to people with Medicare.

SNF
Skilled Nursing Facility. A nursing facility with the staff and equipment to give skilled nursing care and, in most cases, skilled rehabilitative services and other related health services.

SPAP
State Pharmacy Assistance Program. A state program that provides help paying for drug coverage based on financial need, age, or medical condition.

SSI
Supplemental Security Income. A monthly benefit paid by Social Security to people with limited income and resources who are disabled, blind, or age 65 or older. SSI benefits are not the same as Social Security retirement or disability benefits.

SSRI
Selective Serotonin Reuptake Inhibitors. Create effect on brain's chemistry by increasing the serotonin levels to improve mood. Also known as an anti-depressant typically used to treat anxiety disorders and depression.

Sundowning or Sundowners
A symptom of those suffering from dementia and Alzheimer's where paranoia and irrational behavior occur at dusk or sundown.

TBI
Traumatic Brain Injury. A form of acquired brain injury that occurs when a sudden trauma causes damage to the brain. TBI can result when the head suddenly and violently hits an object, or when an object pierces the skull and enters the brain tissue.

Telehealth
Clinical and non-clinical health information, administrative services and research information typically delivered via online through email or video chat.

Telemedicine
Medical or other health services provided to a patient using a communications system (like a computer, telephone, or television) by a practitioner in a location different than the patient's. Includes a consult, possibly diagnostics and prescriptions if needed.

Telephone Reassurance
A program that promotes the security of *at risk* senior citizens by providing daily telephone reassurance calls. Typically managed by volunteer organizations.

Transportation Services
Services for older citizens include: Paratransit, Door-to-Door, Door-Through-Door, Curb-to-Curb (CTC). See separate listings for definitions.

Tricare
A health care program for active-duty and retired uniformed services members and their families.

Visitation Services
Home visitation/socialization programs for homebound older adults and those with disabilities.

VSOs
Veterans service organizations. There are many different organizations, typically associated with a particular war (Vietnam Veterans of America, National Military Family Association) or a veteran's condition (Wounded Warrior Project, Disabled American Veterans). These organizations are affiliated with but not part of the Departments of Veteran's Affairs (VA) operated by the federal government.

Work-Life Benefit
Provided by employers as part of overall employee benefit package to promote preventive care and improved health and wellness. Varies by employer but can include: flex time, telecommuting, paid FMLA, etc.

Resources – You Are Not Alone

Knowledge is power.

—*Sir Francis Bacon*

Caregiving Advocacy and Service Organizations

AARP aarp.org	
Administration on Aging aoa.gov	American Society on Aging asaging.org
Association for Conflict Resolution (professional) acrnet.org	Aging with Dignity agingwithdignity.org
American Association of Caregiving Youth aacy.org	ARCH National Respite Network and Resource Center archrespite.org
BenefitsCheckUp benefitscheckup.org	Caring caring.com
Caring Connection - part of National Hospice and Palliative Care Organization caringinfo.org	Caring From a Distance cfad.org

Caregivers' Monday part of the Healthy Monday Campaigns mondaycampaigns.org/ caregivers-Monday	Center for Medicare and Medicaid Services (CMS) – Caregiver Information medicare.gov/caregivers/
Easter Seals easterseals.com	Family Caregiver Alliance caregiver.org
Family Caregiving 101 familycaregiving101.org	Family Doctor (American Academy of Family Physicians) familydoctor.org
Health Care Advocates healthcareadvocates.com	Healthcare and You Coalition healthcareandyou.org
Kaiser Family Foundation kff.org	Leading Age leadingage.org
Long-Term Care Ombudsman Program theconsumervoice.org/ombudsman	National Alliance for Caregiving caregiving.org
National Asian Pacific Center On Aging napca.org	National Association of Professional Geriatric Care Managers caremanager.org
National Council on Aging (NCOA) ncoa.org	NCOA Benefits Check-up benefitscheckup.org
National Council on Patient Information and Education talkaboutrx.org	National Family Caregivers Association nfcacares.org
National Hispanic Council on Aging nhcoa.org	National Hospice and Palliative Care Organization and Caring Connections nhpco.org
National Patient Safety Foundation npsf.org	National Resource Center on LGBT Aging lgbtagingcenter.org
Next Step in Care – United Hospital Fund nextstepincare.org	Patient Advocate Foundation patientadvocate.org

Rosalynn Carter Institute for Caregiving (RCI) at Georgia Southwestern University rosalynncarter.org	Services and Advocacy for GLBT Elders (SAGE) sageusa.org
The Veneration Project venerationproject.org	WellSpouse Foundation wellspouse.org

Caregiving Products and Technology

Active Forever activeforever.com	ADT Security Services adt.com
AgeTek Alliance agetek.org	Aging in Place Technology Watch ageinplacetech.com
BeClose beclose.com	The CareGiver Partnership caregiverpartnership.com
Ceiva ceiva.com	ComfortZone by the Alzheimer's Association alz.org/comfortzone/
EasyConnect earlybirdalert.com	firstStreet for Boomers and Beyond firststreetonline.com
Home Health Tech Store homehealthtechstore.com	Independa independa.com
Intel GE Care Innovations careinnovations.com	iPad apple.com
GlowCaps from Vitality vitality.net	Grandcare Systems grandcare.com
Great Call, Jitterbug phone greatcall.com	Kindle amazon.com
Kinect xbox.com/KINECT	Lifecomm lifecomm.com
Lifestation lifestation.com	Medic Alert medicalert.org
Paro Robots parorobots.com	Philips Lifeline lifelinesys.com

Posit Science – DriveSharp software positscience.com	Presto presto.com
SecuraTrac securatrac.com	Skype skype.com
Smart Silvers Alliance smartsilvers.com	Tabsafe tabsafe.com
Telikin telikin.com	USC Center for the Digital Future digitalcenter.org
VibrantNation vibrantnation.com	WiiFit wiifit.com

Celebrity Web Sites

David Osmond davidosmond.com	TheFamily (Alan Osmond) thefamily.com
Farrah Fawcett Foundation (Alana Stewart) thefarrahfawcettfoundation.org	HollyRod Foundation (Holly Robinson Peete) hollyrod.org
Joan Lunden joanlunden.com	

Disease Organizations and Support Groups

AIDS Healthcare Foundation aidshealth.org	ALS Association alsa.org
Alzheimer's Association alz.org	American Cancer Society cancer.org
American Diabetes Association diabetes.org	American Heart Association heart.org
American Psychological Association apa.org	Association of Frontotemporal Degeneration theaftd.org

Autism Speaks autismspeaks.org	BringChange2Mind bringchange2mind.org
Cancer Support Community and Gilda's Club cancersupportcommunity.org	Center for Autism and Related Disorders (CARD) centerforautism.com
Cystic Fibrosis Foundation cff.org	Dream Foundation dreamfoundation.org
Eva's Heroes evasheroes.org	Farrah Fawcett Foundation thefarrahfawcettfoundation.org
HollyRod Foundation hollyrod.org	Michael J. Fox Foundation for Parkinson's Research michaeljfox.org
Nancy Davis Foundation for Multiple Sclerosis and the Race to Erase MS erasems.org	National Down Syndrome Association (NDSA) ndss.org
National Alliance on Mental Illness (NAMI) nami.org	National Institute for Mental Health (NIMH) nimh.nih.gov
National Kidney Foundation kidney.org	National Multiple Sclerosis Society nationalmssociety.org
National Parkinson Foundation parkinson.org	Susan G. Komen for the Cure ww5.komen.org
United Cerebral Palsy ucp.org	

Driving

AARP – Driver Safety Course aarpdriversafety.org	Alzheimer's Association (online instructional videos) alz.org

American Occupational Therapy Association aota.org	Automobile Club of America "Roadwise Review" seniordriving.aaa.com
Car Fit car-fit.org	Posit Science – DriveSharp software positscience.com
The Hartford – Safety for a Lifetime Program on Senior Driving thehartford.com/Advance50	ITNAmerica itnamerica.org
National Center for Senior Transportation (NCST) seniortransportation.easterseals.com	National Mobility Equipment Dealers Association nmeda.com
SilverRide silverride.com	

Employers

Family and Medical Leave Act (FMLA) dol.gov/whd/fmla	ReACT (Respect a Caregiver's Time) reactconnection.com
Society of Human Resources Management (SHRM) shrm.org	

Financial - Costs of Caregiving

American Institute of Financial Gerontology aifg.org	Genworth Cost of Care Study genworth.com
Women's Institute for a Secure Retirement (WISER) wiserwomen.org	

Government Services

Administration on Aging – National Family Caregiver Support Program aoa.gov	Administration on Aging – National Clearinghouse for Long Term Care Information longtermcare.gov
Alzheimer's alzheimers.gov	Ask Medicare (see CMS below)
Centers for Disease Control and Prevention (CDC) cdc.gov/aging/caregiving	Centers for Medicare and Medicaid Services "Ask Medicare" for Caregivers medicare.gov/caregivers
Elder Care Locator (also see National Association of Area Agencies on Aging below) eldercare.gov	Medline Plus (National Institutes of Health) nlm.nih.gov/medlineplus
National Adult Protective Services apsnetwork.org	National Association of Area Agencies on Aging and the Eldercare Locator n4a.org eldercare.gov
National Clearinghouse for Long Term Care Information longtermcare.gov	National Institute for Mental Health (NIMH) nimh.nih.gov
National Resource Directory nationalresourcedirectory.gov	Questions are the Answer ahrq.gov/ questionsaretheanswer
State Health Insurance Assistance Program (SHIP) shiptalk.org	U.S. Department of Veteran's Affairs (VA) – Caregiver caregiver.va.gov
U.S. Department of Veterans's Affairs - My HealthE Vet myhealth.va.gov	

Healthy Caregiver

Alzheimer's Association – Caregiver Stress Test alz.org	American Medical Association Caregiver Self Assessment ama-assoc.org
AmeriDoc ameridoc.com	Be Well bewell.org
Caregivers' Monday mondaycampaigns.org/ caregivers-monday	Getnumune getnumune.net
Health Finder healthfinder.gov	Healthy Monday Campaigns mondaycampaigns.org
MD Live Care mdlivecare.com	Medline Plus medlineplus.gov
My Consult – Cleveland Clinic eclevelandclinic.org/ myConsultHome	National Institutes of Health nih.gov
National Sleep Foundation sleepfoundation.org	Real Age realage.com
RingADoc ringadoc.com	

Home, Housing and Caregiving Hotels

AARP Caregiving Help and Advice from Genworth genworth.com/caregiving	Aging in Place Institute louistenenbaum.com/ the-aging-in-place-institute
American Cancer Society Hope Lodges cancer.org/Treatment/ SupportProgramsServices/ HopeLodge	A Place for Mom aplaceformom.com
Care care.com	CarePlanners careplanners.com
CareLinx carelinx.com	CareScout, a Genworth company carescout.com

Eden Alternative edenalt.org	Fall Prevention Center for Excellence stopfalls.org
Fall Stop Move Strong fallstop.net	The Fisher House Program fisherhouse.org
Green House Project thegreenhouseproject.org	The Hartford "Home for a Lifetime" thehartford.com/Advance50
HelpGuide helpguide.org	Home Instead homeinstead.com
Leeza's Place leezasplace.org	Martha Stewart Center for Living (MSCL) The Mt. Sinai Hospital mountsinai.org
Med Cottage medcottage.com	National Association of Homebuilders – Certified Aging in Place Specialists (CAPS) nahb.org
National Association of Professional Geriatric Care Managers caremanager.org	National Center for Assisted Living ahcancal.org
Naturally Occuring Retirement Communities – An Aging in Place Initiative norcs.org	Next Door Garage Apartments nextdoorgarageapartments.com
Practical Assisted Living Solutions (PALS) palsbuilt.com	Rebuilding Together rebuildingtogether.org
Right At Home rightathome.net	Senior Bridge seniorbridge.com
Senior Helpers seniorhelpers.com	Silverado Senior Living silveradosenior.com
Snapfor Seniors snapforseniors.com	Village Movement - Beacon Hill Village beaconhillvillage.org
Village to Village (VtV) Network vtvnetwork.org	Visiting Nurses Association of America vnaa.org

Legal

Medicare Rights Center medicarerights.org	National Academy of Elder Law Attorneys (NAELA) naela.org

Meals and Nutrition

Dinewise dinewise.com	Meals on Wheels Association of America mowaa.org
Mom's Meals momsmeals.com	National Institute on Aging – Healthy Eating After Age 50

Membership Groups

AARP aarp.org	Motion Picture and Television Fund mptvfund.org
The Transition Network (TTN) thetransitionnetwork.org/connect/ connect-caring-collaborative/	WomanSage womansage.org

Specialized Caregiving Help

American Music Therapy Association (AMTA) musictherapy.org	Pet Partners deltasociety.org
Pets for the Elderly Foundation petsfortheelderly.org	Pet Therapy pet-therapy.org
Powerful Tools for Caregivers powerfultoolsforcaregivers.org	Therapy Dogs Inc. therapydogs.com

Travel

Angel Flight Angelflight.com	Automobile Association of America aaa.com
MedJet Assist medjetassist.com	NetJet netjets.com
Society for Accessible Travel and Hospitality sath.org	

Veterans Caregiver

Help Our Wounded helpourwounded.org	Joining Forces whitehouse.gov/joiningforces
National Military Family Association militaryfamily.org	National Resource Directory nationalresourcedirectory.gov
Project Sanctuary projectsanctuary.us	ReMIND – Bob Woodruff Foundation remind.org
U.S. Department of Veteran's Affairs (VA) - Caregiver Support caregiver.va.gov	Wounded Warrior Project woundedwarriorproject.org

Volunteer to Help Caregivers

(For specific diseases or disorders, see Disease Organizations above)

Care2 care2.com	CaringBridge caringbridge.org
Center for Volunteer Caregiving volunteercaregiving.org	Lotsa Helping Hands lotsahelpinghands.com
National Family Caregivers Association – Caregiver Community Action Network (CCANers) nfcacares.org	National Volunteer Caregiving Network (formerly known as Faith in Action Network) fianationalnetwork.org
Volunteer Match volunteermatch.org	

Acknowledgements

To the following people – thank you for sharing and caring.

My Personal Board of Directors, Producers, Critics, Fans and Dear Friends

Vicki Guttridge, Alex Witt, Molly Ballantine, Laurie Mahoney, Debbie Cifone, Gretchen Benes, Michelle Hudspeth, Merritt Meade Loughran, James Grant, David Palmer, Michael Duffett, Brent Parkhouse.

My Three Fairy Godmothers

Everybody needs great mentors in your life – I've been blessed with three of the best. Mary Furlong whose belief in me gave me the gumption to go for it; Joni Evans, who gave me my first writing job and encouragement in writing this book; and Myrna Blyth, who gave my writing a place to flourish and reach millions of readers.

Behind the Scenes

I am grateful to Mary Ellen Hurrell who edited parts of this book and helped in this entire endeavor. The one person I trust to understand my vision and create something memorable is my book designer, Jennifer Jacquez, a friend and colleague (who started her career creating movie posters). And to my wonderful research assistant, Val Gilmore, who was exceptionally thorough and quick to respond to my every request and I had many. Also thanks to my team at Balboa Press especially Madison Lux, Heather Perry and Andrea Geasey who kept the book on track with their weekly check-ins.

Walk of Fame

This book would not exist if it were not for the gracious and generous celebrities who agreed to be interviewed. Each one shared so many intimate moments of their caregiving story. They talked about emotions that were real and raw and in the end their goal was to help you in your caregiving journey – I am just the messenger. I am eternally grateful and indebted to them: Jill Eikenberry and Michael Tucker, Marg Helgenberger, Joan Lunden, Sylvia Mackey, Alan and David Osmond, Holly Robinson Peete and Alana Stewart. Also a big thanks to their hard working publicists and assistants, Lori Glass Berk, Lianne Cashin, Andy Gelb, Judy Katz, Zuzana Korda, Elaine Silvestri.

Best In Show

There are too many to list here but I am grateful to all the wonderful experts I interviewed and who are quoted or contributed valuable information for this book. I am happy to call all of them colleagues and many of them friends. They are all stars in the caregiving constellation. Special shout outs to: Lisa Blaney-Koen, Lori Bitter, Andy Cohen, Jeff Cole, Nancy Cullen, Dr. Neal Cutler, Judy Diaz, Eric Dishman, Cherry Duhamel, Gary Drevitch, Rich Eisenberg, Jane Farrell, John Feather, Erin Heintz, Gail Hunt, Cindy Hounsel, Nicole Kaplan, Brooks Kenny, Sid Lerner, Carol Levine, Nancy Lewin, Jeff Maltz, Larry Minnix, Lea Pipes, Peter Radsliff, Ken Scherer, Paula Serios, Bob Stein, Susan Ayers Walker.

All In the Family

Of course, none of this would have been possible without family, especially my parents: Sally and Don Phelps, and Jim and Debbie Snelling.

References and Notes

Throughout this book are cited sources for various data. Following is a listing of these sources. Unless otherwise noted, all studies, surveys and research was conducted with U.S. population or groups.

Studies and Surveys

AARP – *Beyond Happiness - Thriving* (June, 2012)
AARP - *Healthy@Home 2.0* (April, 2011)
AARP Foundation – *Food Insecurity Among Older Adults* (August, 2011)
AARP Policy Institute in collaboration with Harris Interactive Survey – *We Can Do Better: Lessons Learned for Protecting Older Persons in Disasters* (May, 2006)
AARP Public Policy Institute – *Valuing the Invaluable: 2011 Update The Growing Contributions and Costs of Family Caregiving* (2011)
Administration on Aging – *A Profile of Older Americans 2011* (2012)
Alzheimer's Association – *2012 Alzheimer's Disease Facts and Figures* (March, 2012)
Alzheimer's Association *Generation Alzheimer's – The Defining Disease of the Baby Boomers* (2011)
Alzheimer's Association and First Lady of California Maria Shriver - *The Shriver Report™ – A Woman's Nation Takes on Alzheimer's* (October, 2010)
Alzheimer's Association – *Younger-Onset Alzheimer's – I'm Too Young to Have Alzheimer's disease* (2011)
American Academy of Family Physicians – *Seniors and Caregivers Online Survey* (April, 2012)
American Association of Geriatric Psychiatry (AAGP) – *Dating and Remarriage Over the First Two Years of Widowhood* by D. Schneider, P. Sledge, S. Shuchter and S. Zisook (1996), published in Annals of Clinical Psychiatry
American Cancer Society – *2012 Facts and Figures*

American College of Rheumatology - *Conflict Resolution Quarterly*, Volume 29 (2001)
American Psychological Association – *2012 Stress In America™ Survey*
American Society on Aging, in collaboration with MetLife Mature Market Institute - *Still Out, Still Aging – The MetLife Study of Lesbian, Gay, Bisexual and Transgender Baby Boomers* (March, 2010)
Berg Insights – *mHealth and Home Monitoring Report* (December, 2010)
Bill and Melinda Gates Foundation, in collaboration with Civic Ventures – *The Silent Epidemic – Perspectives of High School Dropouts* (2005)
Bowling Green State University, Ohio – *Negative and Positive Caregiving Experiences: A Closer Look at the Intersection of Gender and Relationship* by I-Fen Lin, Holly R. Fee, Hsueh-Sheng Wu (April, 2012)
Bowling Green State University, Ohio – *Does Informal Care Attenuate the Cycle of ADL/IADL Disability and Depressive Symptoms in Late Life?* By I-Fen Lin and Hsueh-Sheng Wu (July, 2011)
Bureau of Labor Statistics – *Labor Force Projections to 2020* (February, 2012)
Caring.com and National Safety Council – *Mature Drivers Survey* (2008)
Caring.com – *Caregiving and Depression Online Survey* (April, 2011)
Center for American Progress – *Protecting Workers and Their Families with Paid Leave and Caregiving Credits* (April, 2012)
Center for Public Integrity – iWatchNews *Report on Top 10 FEMA Disaster Designations* (2011)
Centers for Disease Control and Prevention – *Prevalence of Autism Spectrum Disorders* (Monitoring Network 2008 data, Surveillance Summaries 2012)
Centers for Disease Control and Prevention – *Wireless Substitution Early Release of 2012 National Health Interview Survey* by Stephen J. BlumbergPhD, Julian V. Luke – National Center for Health Statistics (2011)
Centers for Disease Control and Prevention – *2009-2010 National Survey of Children with Special Health Care Needs* (2011)
Centers for Disease Control and Prevention, National Center for Injury Prevention and Control - Web–based Injury Statistics Query and Reporting System (WISQARS) (November 30, 2010)
Centers for Disease Control and Prevention, National Center for Injury Prevention and Control - Web-based Injury Statistics Query and Reporting System for Seniors, Depression and Suicide Rates (WISQARS) (January, 2007)
Centers for Disease Control and Prevention – *Adults and Older Adult Adverse Drug Events* (web site data)
Centers for Disease Control and Prevention - *National vital statistics reports; vol 56 no 10 - National Center for Health Statistics.* By Kung HC, Hoyert DL, Xu JQ, Murphy SL. Deaths: Final data for 2005. Hyattsville, MD: National Center for Health Statistics. 2008.; Heron MP, Hoyert DL, Murphy SL, Xu JQ, Kochanek KD, Tejada-Deaths: Final data for 2006.. (2009)
Centers for Disease Control and Prevention - *National Health Interview Survey – Complementary and Alternative Medicine (CAM)* (July, 2009)
Centers for Disease Control and Prevention – *Lumbar Spine and Proximal Femur Bone Mineral Density, Bone Mineral Content and Bone Area – U.S. 205-2008* (March, 2012)
Center for Health Care Strategies – *Health Strategies Fact Sheet*
Center for Poverty Research - *Senior Hunger in the United States: Differences Across States and Rural and Urban Areas* by James P. Ziliak & Craig Gunderson, U. Ky. (September, 2009)
Commonwealth Fund - *A Look at Working-Age Caregivers Roles, Health Concerns and Need for Support* (2005)
Families and Work Institute, in collaboration with Alfred P. Sloan Foundation – *2008 National Study of Employers* (May, 2008)
FGI Research Survey – *The Cultural Significance of Monday* by JP Fry and RA Neff (December, 2008)
Genworth – *Genworth 2012 Cost of Care Survey*
Genworth – *Beyond Dollars – The True Impact of Long Term Caring* (2010)
Georgetown University - Center on an Aging Society – *Low Health Literary Skills Survey Increase Costs Survey* (1999)

Harris Interactive, in collaboration with Amedysis – *Annual Home Care Matters Initiative on Caregiver Costs* (2011)
The Hartford – Your Road Ahead – A Guide to Comprehensive Driving Evaluations and We Need to Talk – Family Conversations with Older Drivers
The Hartford – Boomers in Transition – Where Will They Live Next? Survey Findings (June, 2011)
Harvard University Press – Social Trends in the United States by A.J. Cherlin (1992)
Harvard University - Harvard Law School and Harvard Medical School "Medical Cost Bankruptcy" (February, 2005)
HomeInstead Senior Care Network – *2012 Poll on Seniors and Volunteering* (2012) Institute of Medicine Health Roundtable on Health Literacy – *How Can Health Care Organizations Become More Health Literate?* (July, 2012)
Institute of Medicine – *Dietary Reference Intakes – Water, Potassium, Sodium, Chloride, and Sulfate* (February, 2004)
JMed Internet Research – *Periodic Prompts and Reminders in Health Promotion and Health Behavior Interventions* by JP Fry and RA Neff (2009)
Kaiser Family Foundation – *Talking About Medicare – Your Guide to Understanding the Program* (2012)
Kaiser Family Foundation – *Kaiser Commission on Medicaid Facts* (February, 2009)
Kelton Research in collaboration with eHealthInsurance – *Health Insurance IQ Survey* (November, 2011)
Mayo Clinic – *Optimism-Pessimism Assessed in the 1960s and Self-reported Health Status 30 Years Later Study*, T. Maruta, RC Colligan, M. Malinchoc, KP Offord (2009)
MetLife Mature Market Institute in collaboration with Louis Tenenbaum – *The MetLife Report on Aging in Place 2.0 – Rethinking Solutions to the Home Care Challenge* (September, 2010)
Microsoft Corporation – *The Convergence of the Aging Workforce and Accessible Technology* (2003)
Minnesota Department of Human Services – *Tranform 2010 Project*, in collaboration with Minnesota Board on Aging and Minnesota Department of Health – Policy Brief Examining Issues Critical to the Agewave, What Will Keep Family Caregivers Caring? (March, 2009)
MIT AgeLab in collaboration with The Hartford – *Who Drives Older Driving Decisions? Study* (June, 2004)
National Academy on an Aging Society - *Caregiving: Helping the Elderly with Activity Limitations. Challenges for the 21st century: Chronic and Disabling Conditions* (2000)
National Academy on an Aging Society – *Low Health Literacy Increase Annual Health Care Expenditures* (2000)
National Alliance for Caregiving in collaboration with AARP and funded by MetLife Foundation – *Caregiving in the U.S.* (2009)
- A Focused Look at Those Caring for Someone 50 or Older
- A Focused Look at the Ethnicity of Those Caring for Someone
- A Focused Look at Those Caring for a Child with Special Needs Under the Age 18
- A Focused Look at Those Caring for Someone Age 18-49

National Alliance for Caregiving in collaboration with Easter Seals –*Caregiving in Rural America* (2006)
National Alliance for Caregiving, in collaboration with Evercare – *The Evercare Survey of the Economic Downturn and Its Impact on Family Caregiving* (2009)
National Alliance for Caregiving in collaboration with Evercare – *The Evercare Study of Hispanic Family Caregiving in the U.S.* (2008)
National Alliance for Caregiving in collaboration with Evercare – *The Evercare Study of Family Caregivers – What They Spend, What They Sacrifice* (2007)
National Alliance for Caregiving in collaboration with Evercare – *The Evercare Study of Caregivers in Decline – A Close-up Look at the Health Risks of Caring for a Loved One* (September, 2006)
National Alliance for Caregiving in collaboration with MetLife Mature Market Institute and University of Pittsburgh - *MetLife Study of Working Caregivers and Employer Health Care Costs* (2010)
National Alliance for Caregiving in collaboration with the MetLife Mature Market Institute – *The MetLife Study of Caregiving Costs to Working Caregivers – Double Jeopardy for Baby Boomers Caring for Their Parents* (June, 2011)

National Alliance for Caregiving in collaboration with Towson University and MetLife Mature Market Institute – *The MetLife Study of Sons at Work – Balancing Employment and Elder Care* (2003)

National Alliance for Caregiving in collaboration with the National Multiple Sclerosis Society and Southeastern Institute of Research funded by Sanofi U.S. – *Multiple Sclerosis Caregivers* (March, 2012)

National Alliance for Caregiving in collaboration ReACT with funding by Pfizer and Janssen – *Best Practices in Workplace Elder Care* (March 2012)

National Alliance for Caregiving in collaboration with Richard Schulz PhD, Thomas Cook PhD, University Center for Social and Urban Research, Department of Psychiatry at University of Pittsburgh, Alzheimer's Immunotherapy Program – Pfizer, Janssen – *Caregiving Costs Declining Health in the Alzheimer's Caregiver as Dementia Increases in the Care Recipient* (November, 2011)

National Alliance for Caregiving in collaboration with UnitedHealthcare – *The eConnected Family Caregiver – Bringing Caregiving Into the 21st Century* (2010)

National Alliance for Caregiving in collaboration with UnitedHealth Foundation – *Caregivers of Veterans – Serving on the Homefront* (November, 2010)

National Alliance for Caregiving in collaboration with United Hospital Fund – *Young Caregivers in the U.S.* (September, 2005)

National Association of Female Executives – *Top 50 Companies for Executive Women* (2012)

National Cancer Institute – *Overweight and Obesity Associated With Increased Risk* (2010)

National Center on Elder Abuse at the American Public Human Services Association in collaboration with Westat, Inc. prepared for the Administration on Aging – U. S. Department of Health and Human Services – *National Elder Abuse Incidence Study* (September, 1998)

National Citizens' Coalition for Nursing Home Reform - *Emergency Preparedness: Questions Consumers Should Ask* (2008)

National Institute on Aging Center, National Institute of Health, U.S. Department of Health and Human Services – *Healthy Eating After 50* (June, 2008)

National Institute of Mental Health – Older Adults - Depression and Suicide Fact Sheet (April, 2007)

Northwest Institute for Children and Families – *African American Kinship Caregivers Principles for Developing Supportive Programs* (2002)

Norwegian University of Science and Technology Department of Public Health – *Article on Insomnia and Heart Attack Risk* by Lars J. Vatten, M.D., PhD; Carl Platou, M.D. and Imre Janszky, M.D., PhD, Trondheim (2011)

Northwestern Mutual – *The State of Planning in America Study* (2012)

Partners Healthcare Center for Connected Health – *Clinical trial study of technology usage in medication adherence* (2006)

Pets Are Wonderful Support (PAWS) in collaboration with Banfield Charitable Trust – *The Health Benefits of Companion Animals* (2007)

Pew Research Center – *The Return of the Multigenerational Family Household* (March, 2010)

Pew Research Center – *Family Caregivers Online* (July, 2012)

Pew Research Center – *Generations and Their Gadgets* (February, 2011)

Pfizer/ReACT in collaboration with Gallup – *Working Caregivers Poll* (July, 2011)

Points of Light Institute – *Facts on Volunteering in the Points of Light Era* (2009)

Resource Renewal Institute – *Extreme Weather and Community Resilience Field Notes* (2012)

Services and Advocacy for Gay, Lesbian, Bisexual and Transgender Elders (SAGE), National Academy on an Aging Society – *Public Policy and Aging Report* (Summer 2011)

Services and Advocacy for Gay, Lesbian, Bisexual and Transgender Elders (SAGE) – *Caregiving in the LGBT Community* (July, 2012)

Services and Advocacy for Gay, Lesbian, Bisexual and Transgender Elders (SAGE), in collaboration with United Hospital Fund – *Next Step in Care – Family Caregivers and Health Care Professionals Working Together* (2011)
Society for Human Resource Management (SHRM) – *2011 Employee Benefits – Examining Employee Benefits Admidst Uncertainty* (2011)
Working Mother Research Institute – *Women and Alzheimer's Disease The Caregivers' Crisis* (January, 2012)
UCLA Longevity Center - *Aging Forecast* by S.Y. Woo and G.W. Small, UCLA Center on Aging (2003)
UCLA Center for Health Policy Research - *Stressed and Strapped: Caregivers in California*, by G. Hoffman (2011)
University of California at San Francisco Center for AIDS Prevention Studies at the AIDS Research Institute – *Stress and Coping in Gay Male Caregivers of Men with AIDS* (June, 2000)
UnitedHealthcare, in collaboration with Volunteer Match – *Volunteering and and Your Health – How Giving Back Benefits Everyone* (March, 2010)
University of Southern California, Andrus Gerontology Center – *A Sociocultural Stress and Coping Model for Mental Health Outcomes Among African American Caregivers in Southern California* by Bob G. Knight (1999)
United Nations – *The Demography of Population Ageing* by Barry Mirkin and Mary Beth Weinberger (2005)
University of Virginia – James Coan PhD – *Toward the Neuroscience of the Social Regulation of Emotion* (2012)
University of Washington at St. Louis School of Medicine - *Study on Alzheimer's and Sleep Deprivation Links* by Yo-El Ju, MD, assistant professor of neurology, presentation at American Academy of Neurology, New Orleans (April 21-28, 2012)
U.S. Bureau of Labor Statistics – *Volunteering in the United States 2010 Report* (2010)
U.S. Census Bureau – *Remarriage in the United States* (2006)
U.S. Census Bureau - *Projections of the Population by Age and Sex for the United States: 2010 to 2050* (August, 2008)
U.S. Census Bureau – *The Older Population 2010 Census Brief* (2010)
U.S. Census Bureau – *American Fact Finder 2010 data from American Community Survey* (2010)
U.S. Department of Health and Human Services – Office of the Inspector General – *Gaps in Nursing Home Emergency Preparedness and Response During Disasters 2007-2010 Report* (April, 2012)
U.S. Department of Education – *The Health Literacy of America's Adults Report* (September, 2006)
U.S. Department of Transportation National Highway Traffic Safety Administration – *Traffic Safety Facts 2009 Data* (2009)
U.S. Equal Employment Opportunity Commission (EEOC) - Unlawful Disparate Treatment of Workers with Caregiving Responsibilities (May, 2007)
U.S. Preventive Services Task Force – *Primary Care – Relevant Interventions to Prevent Falling in Older Adults* (December, 2010)
Virginia Commonwealth University – *Factors Affecting Elder Caregiving in Multigenerational Asian American Families* by Suzi S. Weng and Peter V. Nguyen (January, 2010)

Articles and Journals

Aging Today – newsletter of the American Society on Aging - *Friends Play a Key Role in the Lives of an Increasing Demographic of Women Living Solo* (July, August, 2012)
Aging Today – newsletter of the American Society on Aging – *At Now! OAA Reauthorization Must Include Services for LGBT Elders* (July-August, 2012)
American Journal of Clinical Nutrition – *Differential Effects of Coffee on the Risk of Type 2 Diabetes According to Meal Consumption in a French Cohort of Women* (February, 2010)
American Journal of Epidemiology - *Caregiving Intensity and Change in Physical Functioning Over a 2-Year Period: Results of the Caregiver-Study of Osteoporotic Fractures,* Lisa Fredman PhD, Jane A. Cauley, Dr. Ph., Marc Hochberg MD, MPH, Kristine E. Ensrud MD, MPH (April, 2009)

Archives of Internal Medicine – *Prospective Study on Occupational Stress and Risk of Stroke* by Akizumi Tsutsumi, MD; Kazunori Kayaba, MD; Kazuomi Kario, MD; Shizukiyo Ishikawa, MD (2009)

Everyday Health – *Pets for the Elderly – A Therapeutic Match* (August 1, 2009)

Forbes – *Stressed Out? Find Some Me Time* (January 23, 2009)

The Guardian – *New Year's Resolutions Doomed to Failure, Say Psychologists* (December, 2009)

Harvard Health Letter – *Senior Citizens Do Shrink – Just One of the Body Changes of Aging* (November, 2005)

Health Affairs - *Informal Caregiving By and For Older Adults*, by D. Wagner and E. Takagi (February 2010)

International Journal of Geriatric Psychiatry – *UCLA pilot study of yoga meditation for family dementia caregivers with depressive symptoms*, H. Lavretsky, E.S. Epel, P. Siddarth, N. Nazarian, N. St. Cyr, D.S. Khalsa, J. Lin, E. Blackburn, M.R. Irwin (March, 2012)

Japan Journal of Nursing Science – *Foot Bath Effect on Cardiac Parasympathetic* (2011)

Journal of American Geriatrics Society – *Mortality Associated with Caregiving, General Stress and Caregiving – Related Stress in Elderly Women*, Lisa Fredman PhD, Jane A. Cauley, Dr. Ph., Marc Hochberg MD, MPH, Kristine E. Ensrud MD, MPH (March, 2010)

Journal of Aging and Health - *Caregiving and Cognitive Function in Older Women: Evidence for the Healthy Caregiver Hypothesis* - Rosanna M. Bertrand, PhD, *Health Policy, Abt Associates Inc., Cambridge, MA, USA,* Jane S. Saczynski, PhD *Domestic Health Division, Health Policy, Abt Associates Inc., Cambridge, MA, USA,* Catherine Mezzacappa *Boston University School of Public Health, Boston, MA, USA,* Mallorie Hulse, MPH *Boston University School of Public Health, Boston, MA, USA,* Kristine Ensrud, MD, MPH, FACP *Center for Chronic Disease Outcomes Research, Minneapolis, MN, USA; University of Minnesota School of Medicine, Minneapolis, MN, USA,* Lisa Fredman, PhD *Boston University School of Public Health, Boston, MA, USA*

Journal of the American Medical Association (JAMA) - *Caregiving as a Risk Factor for Mortality* published by Richard Schulz, PhD and Scott Beach, PhD, University of Pittsburgh (1999)

Journal of the American Medical Association - *Incidence of Adverse Drug Reactions in Hospitalized Patients* by Jason Lazarou, MSc; Bruce H. Pomeranz, MD, PhD; Paul N. Corey, PhD (April, 1998)

The Journal of Gerontology - *Caregiving and Volunteering: Are Private and Public Helping Behaviors Linked?* by *Jeffrey A. Burr, Namkee G. Choi, Jan E. Mutchler, Francis G. Caro (2005)*

Journal of Marriage and Family – *Late life widowhood* (66)4 1051-1068 by D. Carr (2004)

Journal of Nursing Scholarship – *A Conceptual Framework of Nursing in Native American Culture* by John Lowe, R.N. PhD and Roxanne Struthers, R.N. PhD (2001)

Journal of the Transportation Research Board – *Effects of Age on Spinal Rotation During a Driving Task*, Bryan Reimer, Lisa A. D'Ambrosio, Joseph F. Coughlin, Rozanne M. Puleo, Jaclyn E. Cichon, John Daniel Griffith – MIT AgeLab (January, 2009)

Mintz Levin – Employment, Labor and Benefits Newsletter - U.S. Equal Employment Opportunity Commission (EEOC) - *Unlawful Discrimination Against Pregnant Workers and Workers with Caregiving Responsibilities* presentation topic at EEOC February 15, 2012 meeting reported by Martha Zackin

New England Journal of Medicine – *Care for the Dying Falls Mostly on Family Members* by Ezekiel J. Emanuel, M.D., Ph.D., chair of the department of bioethics at the National Institutes of Health, Linda L. Emanuel, M.D., PhD., vice president of the Institute of Ethics, American Medical Association (1999)

New England Journal of Medicine - *Emergency Hospitalizations for Adverse Drug Events in Older Americans* by Daniel S. Budnitz, M.D., M.P.H., Maribeth C. Lovegrove, M.P.H., Nadine Shehab, Pharm.D., M.P.H., and Chesley L. Richards, M.D., M.P.H. (November, 2011)

Science Daily – Article stating divorce rate no higher among parents of autistic children vs. non-autistic children from 2010 Kennedy Krieger Institute research by Brian Freedman, PhD, lead author of the study and clinical director of the Center for Autism and Related Disorders (May 19, 2010)

Sleep – SE Goldman SE, et al. *Association between nighttime sleep and napping in older adults* (2008)

Stroke – The Journal of the American Heart Association and American Stroke Association - *Caregiving Strain and Estimated Risk for Stroke and Coronary Heart Disease Among Spouse Caregivers Differential Effects by Race and Sex* by William E. Haley, PhD; David L. Roth, PhD; George Howard, DrPH; Monika M. Safford, MD - University of South Florida in Tampa (2010)

United Features Syndicate – *Ways to Make Your Home More Senior-Accessible* (January 30, 2011)

WebMD.com – *Why Men and Women Handle Stress Differently*

WebMD.com – *Sleep and Weight Gain*

Working Mother – *2011 Best Companies* by Working Mother Research Institute (2011)

Books/DVDs

Benson, Dr. Herbet, M.D. – *The Relaxation Response* (HarperTorch, 1976)

Brody, Elaine M. – *Women in the Middle: Their Parent Care Years* (Springer Publishing, 1990)

Buettner, Dan – *The Blue Zone – Lessons of Living Longer From the People Who've Lived the Longest* (National Geographic Society, 2008)

Burning Hay Wagon Productions, Mike Bernhagen and Terry Kaldhusdal executive producers – *Consider the Conversation™ – A Documentary Film About a Taboo Subject* (DVD or purchase, also seen on PBS affiliates, 2011)

Caregiving Club Productions – Sherri Snelling executive producer, Kyle Burke, producer – *Handle With Care* (original broadcast on RLTV cable channel, 2011)

Carter, Rosalynn – *Helping Yourself Help Others – A Book for Caregivers* (Three Rivers Press, 1995)

Denholm, Dr. Diane – *The Caregiving Wife's Handbook – Caring for Your Seriously Ill Husband, Caring for Yourself* (Hunter House, 2012)

Furlong, Dr. Mary S. – *Turning Silver Into Gold – How to Profit in the Boomer Marketplace* (Financial Times Press, 2007)

Gandolfini, James and Sheila Nevins, executive producers – *Wartorn 1861-2010* (HBO Documentary Films and Attaboy Films)

Hawn, Goldie – *Ten Mindful Minutes* (Perigee Trade, 2011)

Hay, Louise L. – *The Power Is Within You* (Hay House Inc., 1991)

Keaton, Diane – *Then Again* (Random House, 2011)

Kübler-Ross, Elisabeth and Kessler, David – *On Grief and Grieving – Finding the Meaning of Grief Through the Five Stages of Loss* (Scribner, 2007)

Leman, Dr. Kevin – *The New Birth Order Book – Why You Are the Way You Are* (Revell, a division of Baker Publishing Group, 2009)

Love, Susan M., M.D. and Domar, Alice, PhD – *Live a Little!* (Crown Publishers, division of Random House, 2009)

Louv, Richard – *Last Child in the Woods – Saving our Children from Nature-Deficit Disorder* (Algonquin Books, 2008)

Lunden, Joan and Amy Newmark – *Chicken Soup for the Soul – Family Caregivers* (Chicken Soup for the Soul Publishing, Inc., 2012)

Lyubomirsky, Sonja, PhD – *The How of Happiness – Getting the Life You Want* (Penguin Books, 2008)

McClellan, Stephanie, M.D. and Hamilton, Beth, M.D. – *So Stressed – The Ultimate Stress Relief Plan for Women* (Free Press, 2010)

Norcross, John, PhD, Prochaska, James O., PhD, DiClemente, Carl, PhD – *Changing for Good – A Revolutionary Six-Stage Program for Overcoming Bad Habits and Moving Your Life Positively Forward* (William Morrow Paperbacks, 1995)

Peete, Holly Robinson and Peete, Ryan Elizabeth – *My Brother Charlie* (Scholastic, 2010)

Peete, Rodney – *Not My Boy! A Father, A Son and One Family's Journey With Autism* (Hyperion, 2010)

Perricone, Nicholas, M.D. – *Dr. Perricone's Seven Secrets to Beauty, Health and Longevity – The Miracle of Cellular Rejuvenation* (Ballatine Books, 2007)

Pomerantz, Celia – *Alzheimer's - A Mother-Daughter Journey* (CreateSpace, 2011)

RLTV, Elliott Jacobson, executive producer – *Taking Care with Joan Lunden* (RLTV cable channel original 4-part series, 2010)

Roizen, Michael F., M.D. and Oz, Mehmet C., M.D. – *You – The Owner's Manual* (Harper Resource, division of Harper Collins, 2005)

Russo, Francine – *They're Your Parents, Too! How Siblings Can Survive Their Parents' Aging Without Driving Each Other Crazy* (Bantam Books, 2010)

Sapolsky, Robert M. – *Why Zebras Don't Get Ulcers – The Acclaimed Guide to Stress, Stress-Related Diseases and Coping* (Holt Paperbacks, 2004)

Saunders, Dr. Charmaine – *Women & Stress* (Harper Collins, 2010)

Shook, Loren and Winner, Stephen – *The Silverado Story – A Memory Care Culture Where Love Is Greater Than Fear* (AJC Press, 2010)

Shriver, Maria and Sheila Nevins, executive producers - *Hopeless – The Alzheimer's Project* (HBO 4-part documentary series in collaboration with The National Institute on Aging (2009)

Solie, David – *How to Say It© to Seniors – Closing the Communication Gap with Our Elders* (Prentice Hall Press, 2004)

Small, Dr. Gary – *Alzheimer's Prevention Program* (Workman Publishing, 2011)

Smith, Dr. Ian K. – *Happy – Simple Steps to Get the Most Out of Life* (St. Martin's Press, 2010)

Stewart, Alana – *My Journey With Farrah – A Story of Life, Love and Friendship* (Harper Collins, 2009)

Stewart, Alana, Fawcett, Farrah, O'Neal, Ryan – *Farrah's Story* (Windmill Productions, NBC News, May 15, 2009)

Tucker, Michael – *Family Meals – Coming Together to Care for an Aging Parent* (Atlantic Monthly Press, 2009)

Weil, Andrew, M.D. – *Spontaneous Happiness* (Little Brown and Company, 2011)

Wiseman, Richard - *:59 Seconds – Think a Little, Change a Lot* (Knopf, 2009)

Zucker, Gary – *Spiritual Partnership – The Journey to Authentic Power* (Harper One, imprint of Harper Collins, 2010)

About the Author

Sherri Snelling, CEO and founder of the Caregiving Club, is a nationally recognized expert on America's 65 million family caregivers with special emphasis on how to help caregivers balance *self-care* while caring for a loved one. She is the former Chairman of the National Alliance for Caregiving based in Washington, D.C. and directed caregiving initiatives at a leading health and wellness company. In 2012, Sherri was named #4 on the Top 10 Influencers on Alzheimer's disease list by Sharecare, the online site created by Dr. Mehmet Oz and Jeff Arnold for content contributors that represent the world's foremost medical, health and wellness expertise.

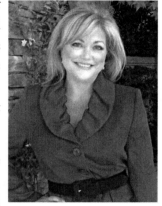

As contributing editor and blogger on caregiving for Next Avenue (the PBS web site for baby boomers), ThirdAge, Huffington Post, Alzheimer's Association and others, Sherri has also been interviewed on CBS Evening News, ABC World Evening News, MSNBC, Fox Business Network, CNN, and in the *New York Times, USA Today, PARADE, Prevention, AARP Bulletin* and WebMD. She is creator, executive producer and host of a caregiver self-help reality cable TV program, *Handle With Care*, and the Me Time Monday[SM] weekly videos in support of Caregivers' Monday. She also interviews celebrities about caregiving at red carpet events in Hollywood and New York City.

Sherri has participated on various caregiving advisory councils: White House Middle Class Task Force, Centers for Medicare and Medicaid Services (CMS), Centers for Disease Control and Prevention (CDC), and Alzheimer's Association. She is a frequent speaker on caregiving and boomer women self-care topics and is represented by the internationally prestigious American Program Bureau. She has received numerous awards throughout her career and for her programs including the U.S. Department of Justice and National Center for Missing & Exploited Children Award, American Society on Aging – Aging & Business Award and a National Women in Communications Award. Sherri holds a B.A. in journalism and political science from the University of Southern California and resides in Newport Beach, California.

Index

Symbols

9/11 9, 75, 122, 175, 337, 417
40/70 Rule 454

A

AARP xxi, 123, 235, 237, 245–247, 250, 253, 281, 286, 310, 322, 328, 380, 434, 493, 496, 498
Accenture 305
acceptance 150, 374, 375, 423, 426
ActiveForever 334
activities of daily living (ADLs) 26, 199, 391, 476
Ad Council 123, 340
Administration on Aging 229, 249, 260, 261, 276, 281, 283, 489, 495
ADT 491
Adult day care 133, 156, 236, 261, 316, 320, 472
Adult Family Homes (AFH) 270
adult orphan 373
Advanced Driving Dynamics 247
Advance Directive 29, 144, 225, 366, 457, 472
Agency for Healthcare Research and Quality (AHRQ) 295
AgeTek Alliance 305, 323, 334, 491
Aging and Disability Resource Center (ADRC) 281
Aging in Place Institute (AiP) 256, 496
aging in place or age in place 238, 254–258, 278, 324, 472, 474, 483, 491, 496, 497
Aging In Place Technology Watch 324
Aging With Dignity 366, 489
AIDS 86, 93, 403, 406, 409
airlines 80, 82
airports 77, 96, 348

alkaline diet 47, 312
Alley, Kirstie 78
ALS 79, 80, 144, 204, 262, 286, 459, 473, 492
alternative therapies 91, 355, 469
Alzheimer's 26–35, 57, 73–75, 77–82, 203–207, 250, 271–272, 282, 491–493
   10 Warning Signs 204, 456
   Association 26, 27, 35, 57, 60, 77, 79, 199, 204, 205, 213, 250, 271, 276, 282, 325, 347, 351, 390, 428, 456, 491–493, 496
   Comfort Zone 282
   Lewy Body 481
   National Alzheimer's Plan 205, 282
   Navigator 282, 283
   Safe Return 282
   Sundowning, sundowners 26, 27, 31, 206, 357
Alzheimer's Prevention Program 74, 398, 405
American Association of Caregiving Youths (AACY) 48, 186, 489
American Association of Geriatric Psychiatry (AAGP) 131
American Cancer Society 106, 107, 110, 350, 358, 492, 496
   Bark for Life 358
   Hope Lodges 350, 496
American Diabetes Association 25, 492
American Heart Association 330, 402, 439, 492
American Institute of Financial Gerontology (AIFG) 237
American Medical Association 288, 300, 303, 389–391, 496
   Caregiver Self-Assessment 390
American Music Therapy Association (AMTA) 361
American Occupational Therapy Association 245, 246, 380

American Psychological Association (APA) 318, 393, 422
　Caregiver Briefcase 282, 393
　Stress in America Survey 318
American Society on Aging 192, 194, 245, 448, 489
American Speech and Hearing Association 357
AmeriDoc 290, 496
Angel Flight 350, 499
anger 13, 66, 131, 145, 146, 276, 413, 415, 416, 418, 439
Animal Assisted Therapy (AAT) 355, 472
A Place for Mom 31, 32, 285, 496
Apple 332, 334, 491
　iPad 322, 332, 333, 402, 439, 442, 491
ARCH National Respite Network and Resource Center 212
Area Agencies on Aging (AAA) 212, 259, 283, 293, 312, 379, 380, 472, 495
Argon, Dianne 187
aromatherapy 92, 93, 401, 409
Assisted Living Facility (AL) 27, 35, 56, 58, 80, 99, 138, 236, 253, 262, 271, 331, 349
Association of Frontotemporal Degeneration (AFTD) 74, 81
ataxia 151
AT&T 329
autism and autism spectrum disorder (ASD) 3, 7, 10–17, 19, 20, 122, 149, 151, 152, 163, 204, 212, 213, 272, 284, 311, 312, 314, 326, 332, 345, 346, 349, 355–357, 360, 368, 377, 443, 459, 472, 473, 493
Autism Speaks 19, 213, 284, 493
Automobile Club of America and AAA Foundation for Traffic Safety 244, 246, 380

B

baby boom, baby boomers xxii, 38, 39, 128, 138, 151, 186, 192, 244, 256, 270, 299, 376, 377, 403, 418
Baldwin, Alec 125
Baldwin, Candace 220, 257
Bates, Doug 223, 363, 371
BeClose 491
Benefits Check-up 236, 490
Benson, Herbert 389, 393, 394
Bensussan, Gale 403
BeWell 461

Bill and Melinda Gates Foundation 187
bisexual 191, 193, 284, 479, 481
blame 33, 105, 150, 414
Blaustein, Alan 291
BMI (body mass index) 205, 377, 404, 405
board-and-care 270, 472
Borden, Enid 310
Brazeal, Michael 409
breathing techniques 395
BringChange2Mind 163, 493
Brosnan, Pierce 157
Bua, Robert 287
Buettner, Dan 397
burn-out xxii, 383, 384

C

Cameron, David – British Prime Minister 437
Campbell, Glenn 203, 456
Camp Reveille 38, 351
cancer 103–116, 424
　anal cancer 106, 107
　breast cancer 4, 42, 43, 49, 50, 69, 90, 99, 125, 157, 181, 405, 406, 426, 444
　cervical cancer 107, 110
　chemotherapy 42, 44, 92, 103, 107, 113, 114, 223, 350, 371, 374, 411
　City of Hope 110
　Leonardis Clinic in Bavaria 110
　radiation 42, 107, 113
C-A-R-E Conversations xxii, 36, 48, 132, 144, 169, 293, 453–459, 469
Care Cottage 269, 496
CareFlash 446
Caregiver Partnership 491
Caregiver's Achilles Heel 458
Caregivers' Monday 463, 464, 490, 496
Caregiver's Touch 333
Caregiver Walkabout xxiv
Caregiving Club 463
caregiving matchmakers 280, 285–287
Caregiving Movement xxii
Caregiving Wife's Handbook, The 145
Care Innovations 328, 491. *See also* Intel/GE
CareLike 283
CareLinx 259, 260, 286, 496

care manager 30, 31, 132, 145, 168, 211, 217, 255, 278, 280, 281, 301, 343, 458, 468
CarePages 446
CarePlanners 291
CareScout 276, 286, 287, 293, 496
CareTogether 446
care transitions 30, 32, 219–224, 274, 275, 282, 284, 304, 468
CareTrio 446
CareZone 446
CarFit 245, 252, 380
CaringBridge 378, 446, 499
Caring.com 249, 276, 421
   Alzheimer's Steps and Stages 282
   Caring Advisor 283
Caring Connections 367, 490
Caring From a Distance (CFDA) 29, 57, 293, 489
Carlucci, Celeste 263
Carter, Dixie 157
Carter, Rosalynn 123, 180, 400, 414, 424, 444, 491
casein-free diet 312
case manager 298
Cash & Counseling 240
Ceiva 331, 491
celiac disease 474
Center for Autism and Related Disorders (CARD) 14
Center for Volunteer Caregiving 378, 499
Centers for Disease Control and Prevention (CDC) 12, 56, 89, 256, 262, 283, 303, 324, 340, 341, 421, 473, 475, 495
Centers for Medicare and Medicaid Services (CMS) 276, 282, 298, 304, 339
   Ask Medicare 282, 495
cerebral palsy 262, 349, 475, 493
certified aging in place specialist (CAPS) xxi, 255, 256, 265, 278, 474, 497
Certified Nurse Assistant (CNA) xxi, 259, 475
Challenge Aspen 351
Chapman, Sandra 388
childhood x, 12, 38, 68, 129, 131, 151, 187, 415, 439, 442, 465, 483
childish 67, 410, 454
chosen family 193, 475
Churchill, Winston 429, 438
circadian rhythms 403, 427, 438
Cleveland Clinic 289, 496
   My Consult 289, 496

Close, Glenn 163
Cohen, Richard 143
Cole, Jeff 128, 321, 327, 332, 334
comfort care 223, 370, 480, 484. *See also* hospice and palliative care
Commonwealth Fund 384, 437
compassion fatigue 399
concierge 257, 258, 279, 280, 300
Consider the Conversation: A Documentary Film About a Taboo Subject DVD 367
Consumer Electronics Show (CES) 334
Continuing Care Retirement Communities (CCRCs) 272, 457, 474
Cooper, Martin 323, 331, 334
COPD (chronic obstructive pulmonary disease) 180, 223, 475
coping, cope 11, 15, 19, 60, 88, 92, 96, 97, 100, 132, 180, 187, 193, 307, 308, 338, 360, 388, 393, 418, 425, 428, 441, 442, 443
Corporation for National and Community Service 376
cortisol 46, 313, 356, 388, 390, 407
Couric, Katie 146
Cranston, Bryan 155
Creagan, Edward 356
Cutler, Neal 237, 238
cystic fibrosis 151, 476, 493

D

dance, dancing xxiii, 20, 59, 83, 86, 97, 209, 263, 359, 361, 408
Darwin, Charles 423
Davis, Nancy 43, 47, 49, 50, 85, 91, 95, 99, 434, 493
daydream 439
death, dying 363–381
dementia 23–35, 55–57, 77–82, 204–207
   vascular 57, 205
Denholm, Dr, Diane 145
denial 10–12, 25, 27, 39, 48, 58, 63–65, 75, 78, 89, 106, 122, 131, 216, 299, 374
Department of Transportation (DOT) 249
depression xxii, 25, 38, 60, 129, 138, 145, 149, 193, 221, 262, 264, 272, 307, 311, 317, 356, 359, 360, 374, 377, 383, 384, 397, 403, 404, 406, 421–429, 437, 442, 461, 486, 487
diabetes 23–25, 77, 79, 99, 162, 163, 173, 198, 205, 262, 305, 313, 345, 404, 406, 407, 439, 476, 492

Dinewise 312, 498
disability xi, 47, 60, 66, 94, 98, 99, 104, 121, 145, 161, 239, 281, 418, 433, 473, 487
Disabled American Veterans 444, 488
disaster planning 282, 337–344, 469
Dishman, Eric 322, 323, 326, 331, 334
divorce 8, 11, 15, 28, 89, 94, 105, 132, 137, 145, 146, 150, 162, 180, 227, 238, 351
DMV 251
DNA 463
doctors, physicians 220–224, 296–301, 303–308
Domar, Alice 387, 392, 461, 462
Do Not Resuscitate (DNR) xxi, 225, 366, 476
Douglas, Michael 424, 456
Down syndrome (DS) 13, 121, 149, 151, 157, 162, 204, 205, 272, 346, 368, 474, 477, 493
DRA (deficit reduction act) 228
Dream Foundation 368, 493
Driver Seat Game app by Liberty Mutual 251
DriveSharp 246, 332, 492, 494
driving 132, 145, 221, 238, 243–252, 257, 260, 277, 281, 282, 310, 322, 323, 332, 349, 350, 380, 417, 434, 469, 481, 493, 494
   alternative transportation 221, 243, 246, 248, 251, 252, 342, 469
   assessment 244–246
   retirement 221, 243, 249, 251, 252
Dr. Oz 394, 438, 440, 461
Dr. Seuss (Theodor Geisel) 156, 157
drug interactions 306
durable medical equipment (DME) 318, 476
Durable Power of Attorney 225, 230, 232, 366, 472, 477, 485
Dworkin-Bell, Sharon 256

E

EAP (employee assistance program) 293, 294, 316, 320, 477
Easom, Leisa 123, 444
Easter Seals 13, 249, 351, 380, 490
EasyConnect from Early Bird Alert 333, 491
Eden Alternative 273, 274, 497
Eikenberry, Jill 4, 54–69, 131, 143, 155, 212, 225, 259, 274, 275, 346, 395, 447, 456
Elder 411, Elder 911 333
elder abuse 260, 287

Elder Care Locator 212, 259, 283, 379, 472, 495
Elder Law attorney 28, 60, 225, 227, 228, 232, 237, 240, 242, 283, 468, 478
elder neglect 287
electronic health record (EHR) 299, 301, 306, 477, 478, 485
electronic medical record (EMR) 299, 477, 478
electronic patient record (EPR) 299, 477, 478
Ellis, Terri 16
emergency preparedness 337–344
emphysema 180, 475
employee 121, 285, 293, 315–320, 393, 436, 477, 488
employer 197, 236, 289, 291, 293, 294, 315–320, 477, 479, 480, 488, 494
end-of-life 46, 51, 59, 112, 122–124, 144, 194, 222, 223, 363–381, 416
Ephron, Nora xix, 130, 143, 431
Epstein, Lawrence J. 402
Eshbaugh, Elaine M. 448
Espinoza, Robert 194
ESRD (end stage renal failure) 228, 478, 482
Eva's Heroes 163, 493

F

faith 5, 42, 43, 50, 86, 89, 91, 92, 95–98, 100, 105, 112, 113, 203, 249, 262, 370, 372, 378, 392, 416, 418, 441, 499
faith-based organizations 262, 378, 441
Falls Free Program 264
falls risk 92, 256, 263, 266
Fall Stop Move Strong 263, 497
Family and Medical Leave Act (FMLA) 319, 320, 478, 488, 494
Family Caregiver Alliance 284, 490
Family Caregiving 101 283, 490
Family Care Navigator 283
Farrah Fawcett Foundation 113, 114, 117, 350, 492, 493
Farrah's Story documentary 108
Fawcett, Farrah xi, 5, 102–117, 192, 350, 375, 492, 493
FDA 47, 91, 114, 303
fear 13, 14, 48, 50, 60, 65, 67, 75, 131, 276, 370, 410, 413–415, 424, 431, 433, 434, 452, 453, 455
Feather, John 192
fee-for-service 222, 229, 482
FEMA (Federal Emergency Management Agency) 338–340

financial planning 237, 238
firstStreetOnline 334, 491
Fisher House Program 350, 497
Five Wishes document 366, 457
flex time 316, 318, 319, 488
forgiveness 370, 413, 415, 418, 419, 441
Fox, Michael J. 8, 9, 19, 145, 210, 437, 493
Foxx, Jamie 157
French, Steve 376
friends, friendship 14–16, 37–39, 102–113, 191–193, 356–358, 374–376, 445–448
frontotemporal degeneration (FTD) 74, 81, 479
FSA (flexible spending account) 236, 479, 480
Fun Theory from Volkswagen 440
Furlong, Dr. Mary xxii

G

Gallagher, Peter 155
Gallup/ReACT survey 315
Garber, Victor 155
gay xxii, 191–194, 284, 319, 479, 481
GE 325, 328, 491. *See also* Care Innovations
Genworth 228, 236, 281, 286, 287, 293, 349, 494, 496
Gen X 138
geofence 325
geriatric care manager xxi, 30, 31, 132, 145, 169, 211, 217, 255, 276, 278, 280, 281, 301, 343, 446, 458, 459, 468, 474, 479, 485
Girl Scouts 435
GlowCap 304, 305, 323, 491
gluten-free 12, 47, 92, 311, 312
Goldberg, Whoopi 78
Goldilocks Syndrome 30, 31, 274, 278
Google xxi, 9, 19, 280, 285, 290, 299, 325, 334
GoogleHealth 290, 299
Government Health Insurance Counselors 231, 292
GPS 304, 322, 325, 330, 347, 485
GPS Shoe 322
Grandcare Systems 329, 491
gray market 260, 287
Great Call 305, 330, 491
Great Grabz 267
Green House Project 273, 274, 497
grief 67, 112, 131, 146, 150, 216, 363, 374, 375, 390, 410, 416, 421, 422, 423

guilt xi, xxii, 3, 10, 18, 19, 33, 34, 36, 37, 45, 46, 56, 66, 67, 110–112, 114, 129, 133, 138, 145, 363, 367, 383, 384, 413–419, 422, 461

H

Habitat for Humanity 269
HAL (Hybrid Assisted Limb) 327
Hamilton, Beth 389, 410
Hamlin, Harry 78
Handle With Care TV program 333
Hands On Network 377
happiness ix, 34, 110, 200, 355, 419, 422, 431–442
Harden, Don 403
Harris, Arlene 323, 331
Harris Poll 338
Hartford, The 244, 249, 250, 256, 494, 497
Hawn, Goldie 435
Hay, Louise H. 438, 461
health advocates 231, 291, 299, 424, 468
Health Care Directive 194, 222, 479
health care insurance 225–232, 291, 295, 299, 318, 469
health care IQ 297
health care literacy 222, 295–298, 301, 468, 481
health care proxy or agent 230, 485
Health First Aging Institute 30, 104, 151, 205, 210, 275, 379
health savings account (HSA) 236, 295, 479, 480
Healthy Monday 490, 496
heart disease 25, 144, 173, 204, 205, 389, 396, 404, 406, 407, 439, 474, 479
Helgenberger, Marg 4, 40–52, 124, 129, 179, 187, 210, 212, 395
HelpGuide 275, 497
Help Our Wounded 381, 499
Heston, Charlton 71, 203
HIPAA (Health Insurance Portability and Accountability Act) 226, 289, 296, 480
hippotherapy 357
HIV 223, 473, 480
Holbrook, Hal 157
Hole In the Wall Gang 351
HollyRod Foundation 16–19, 332, 377, 492, 493
home care 25, 31, 32, 80, 169, 209, 228, 235, 236, 237, 253–278, 285, 286, 287, 293, 294, 377, 454, 480, 481, 485. *See also* in-home care
Home for Life Solutions 329

home health aide xxi, 61–63, 169, 236, 238, 259, 267, 269, 287, 316, 326, 480, 485, 486
Home Health Tech Store 491
HomeInstead 249, 259, 269, 377, 454, 497
homeopathic medicine 150
home safety 236, 239, 253–278, 324, 328, 474
hope xx, 10, 12, 15, 18, 45, 79, 95, 98, 99, 110, 111, 112, 203, 243, 258, 296, 298, 334, 350, 431, 433, 441, 467, 496
hospice 32, 219–242, 271, 274, 357, 358, 363–372, 376, 378, 411, 480, 482, 489, 490
hospitalist 221, 222, 224, 298, 480
hospitals, hospitalization 219–224, 297–308, 303–306
Hounsel, Cindy 234, 235, 238
HPV (human papilloma virus) 107
hugs, hugging 411, 431, 444
Human-Animal Interactions 356
Human resource departments (HR Departments) 236, 289, 293, 316, 318, 436, 458
humor 6, 7, 39, 61, 68, 87, 96, 115, 116, 216, 371, 431, 433, 436
Hunt, Gail 316
Hurricane Katrina 122, 316, 337–340, 342, 343
hydrated, hydration 349, 401, 407
hydrotherapy, hydro-exercise 93, 409
hygge 435

I

iClouds app 439
identity theft 260
incontinence 77–79, 82, 239, 271
Independa 305, 330, 491
Independent Transportation Network (ITN) 248, 249
in-home care 25, 32, 235–237, 258, 258–260, 278, 285–287, 294, 480, 481, 485
inner child 38, 410, 435, 438
insomnia 138, 307, 394, 396, 400–402, 409, 422
Institute of Medicine (IOM) 297, 407
Intel 322, 323, 325, 328, 491
  Intel/GE Care Innovations 328, 491
Internet xxii, 10, 19, 169, 213, 280, 288, 293, 297, 331, 333, 361, 417, 444
isolation 132, 193, 194, 198, 221, 262, 264, 273, 278, 311, 321, 332, 377, 422, 427, 428, 431, 442

J

Jaycees 47, 262
Jefferson, Thomas 439
Jenkens, Robert 274
Jewish Federations of North America (JFNA) 258, 483
Jitterbug 305, 323, 330, 331, 491
Johnson, Dwayne (the Rock) 156
Joining Forces 380, 499
journaling 425
joy 38, 179, 361, 375, 433–435, 459
Junior League 262

K

Kaiser Family Foundation 228, 258, 490
Kallmyer, Beth 27, 35, 60, 77, 79, 276
Kataria, Madan 436
Keaton, Diane 130, 139
Kennedy, John F. 376, 438
Kenny, Brooks 446
Kessler, David 131, 150, 374, 375, 416, 421, 425
kidney failure 223, 228, 478, 482. *See also* ESRD
Kindle 332, 491
kinship caregiving 198, 199
Kübler-Ross, Elisabeth 131, 150, 374, 375, 416, 421, 425

L

Laird, Rosemary 30, 35, 104, 112, 151, 205, 210, 275, 379
Lantern Festival 419
laughter, laughing 6, 14, 20, 50, 68, 69, 96, 101, 103, 115, 116, 303, 307, 397, 435–437, 441, 459
Leading Age 490
Leeza's Place 444, 497
Lehrer, Paul 307
Leiner Health Products 403
Leman, Dr. Kevin 130, 458
LEP (low English proficiency) 297, 481
Lerner, Sid 464
lesbian 191–194, 284, 319, 479, 481
Levine, Carol 61, 220–222, 226, 298, 304, 306
Levin, Nora Jean 29, 30, 45, 57, 167, 168, 169, 293

LGBT (lesbian, gay, bisexual, transgender) 191–195, 284, 319, 475, 479, 481, 490
Licensed Practical Nurse (LPN) 481
Lifecomm 325, 491
LifeStation 329, 491
Lin, I-Fen 11, 388
LivHome 259
Living Will 59, 144, 194, 222, 225, 232, 366, 367, 457, 472, 481
long-distance caregiving 57, 167–171
Longoria, Eva 162
long-term care xxi, 48, 51, 58, 59, 67, 121, 122, 125, 194, 216, 226, 227, 229, 233, 235, 237, 257, 274, 276, 277, 281, 284, 316, 318, 370, 456, 484, 490
Long Term Care Ombudsman 276, 490
look back period 228
Lotsa Helping Hands 378, 445, 499
Louv, Richard 426
Love, Susan 387, 392
Lowe, John 200
Lunden, Joan xi, 4, 22–39, 139, 167, 206, 225, 231, 274, 275, 285, 298, 351, 438, 456, 492
Lynn, Christine E. 200
Lyubomirsky, Sonja 433, 434, 437

M

Mackey, John 71–83
Mackey, Sylvia 4, 70–83, 205, 216, 272, 345, 348, 456
Macular Degeneration Partnership 244
Maltz, Jeff 248
Mandel, Debbie 387
Martha Stewart Center for Living at Mt. Sinai Hospital 263, 264, 497
Martin, Kathleen 240
massage therapy 355, 393, 397, 486
Matsunga, Judd 227, 228
Maurer, Ronda 446
Mayo Clinic 47, 107, 311, 347, 356, 390, 396, 397, 437
Mazmanian, Vic 112, 372, 416, 441
McCartney, Linda 157
McCartney, Paul 157
McClellan, Stephanie 389, 410
M.D. Anderson Cancer Center – University of Texas, Houston 92, 409
MDLiveCare 289, 290, 496
meal delivery 199, 236, 238, 311, 312, 314, 316, 378

Meals on Wheels Association of America 309–312, 378, 498
MedCottage 269, 497
Medicaid xxi, 28, 46, 59, 156, 221, 225–233, 237, 240, 242, 257, 276, 279, 281, 282, 292, 294, 298, 304, 305, 312, 339, 342, 468, 475, 477, 482, 484, 490, 495
MedicAlert 282, 329, 491
Medicare 28, 46, 156, 221–223, 225–233, 235, 237, 242, 260, 276, 279, 281, 282, 289, 291, 292, 294, 298, 304, 339, 342, 346, 371, 445, 468, 475–478, 482–484, 487, 490, 495, 498
Medicare Rights Center 230, 498
medications 296–308, 303–308, 330–332
meditation 50, 69, 117, 318, 389, 393, 394, 396, 439
MedJet Assist 347, 499
Medline Plus 288, 495, 496
Mehl-Madrona, Lewis 200
memory care facilities 59, 271, 338, 356, 486
mental health, mental illness 163, 421–429
  bi-polar disorder 163, 175, 422, 423, 424
  schizophrenia 175, 422, 424
Me Time xxiii, 3, 5, 11, 21, 38, 39, 52, 69, 83, 101, 117, 261, 379, 414, 438, 454, 461–466, 469
Me Time Monday xxiii, 414, 461–470
MetLife Mature Market Institute, Metlife Foundation 192, 194, 262, 317
Michael J. Fox Foundation for Parkinson's Research 19, 493
Microsoft 290, 299, 329
  Esoma Exercise System 329
  Health Vault 290, 299
  Kinect 329, 491
  Xbox 329
Minnix, Larry 270, 293, 299, 327, 338, 340, 341, 343, 471
MIT AgeLab 244, 245, 256, 333
Mom's Meals 312, 498
Monday Campaigns 463, 464, 490, 496
Moore, Demi 139
Motion Picture and Television Fund (MPTF) 223, 258, 277, 332, 363, 369, 371, 374, 379, 426
Multicultural 197–201
multigenerational housing 268

multiple sclerosis (MS) 4, 5, 43, 44, 46, 47, 49, 50, 77, 85, 87–99, 101, 122, 143, 144, 187, 204, 210, 213, 256, 262, 284, 286, 311, 312, 314, 355, 357, 396, 397, 404, 409, 434, 439, 459, 483, 493
multiple support declaration 239
muscular dystrophy 92, 149, 151, 394, 445, 483, 496
music therapy 12, 150, 355–361, 498

N

Nancy Davis Foundation and Race to Erase MS 43, 47, 49, 85, 91, 99, 434, 493
naps 438
NASA 288
National Alliance for Caregiving (NAC) 7, 46, 47, 59, 90, 95, 104, 124, 127, 144, 149, 161, 163, 169, 173, 174, 179, 185, 192, 197, 198, 219, 235, 239, 240, 247, 262, 268, 283, 307, 312, 315–317, 327, 384, 393, 422, 425, 440, 490
National Alliance on Mental Illness (NAMI) 264, 493
National Association of Area Agencies on Aging (N4As) 212, 283, 472
National Association of Elder Law Attorneys (NAELA) 227, 498
National Association of Family Caregivers (NFCA) 283, 379, 445, 490, 499
   Caregiving Community Action Network (CCAN) 379, 474, 499
National Association of Homebuilders (NAHB) 255, 497
National Association of Professional Geriatric Care Managers (NAPGCM) 293
National Cancer Institute 405
National Center for Health Statistics 408
National Center for Senior Transportation (NCST) 249, 380, 494
National Clearinghouse for Long-Term Care 229, 284, 495
National Council on Aging (NCOA) 229, 236, 264, 490
National Elder Abuse Incidence Study 260
National Family Caregiver Support Program 249, 260, 261
National Family Caregiving Month (November) 379, 419
National Football League (NFL) 4, 9, 11, 32, 71, 71–73, 76, 78–82, 272

National Highway Traffic Safety Administration (NHTSA) 244, 250, 401
National Hospice and Palliative Care Organization (NHPCO) 367, 371, 378, 489
National Institute of Health (NIH) 356, 423
National Institute of Mental Health (NIMH) 433, 493, 495
National Mobility Equipment Dealers Association 248, 494
National Multiple Sclerosis Society 88, 213, 493
National Parkinson Foundation 19, 493
National Patient Safety Foundation 297, 490
National Resource Center for Patient-Directed Services (NRCPDS) 240, 260
National Resource Center on LGBT Aging 193, 284, 490
National Resource Directory 176, 284, 495, 499
National Safety Council 249
National Volunteer Caregiving Network 378
Natural Marketing Institute 376, 403
nature deficit disorder 426, 427
Naumann, Wendy 445
NCB Capital Impact 257, 274
Network of Care 285
Next Door Garage Apartments 269, 497
Next Step in Care 221, 224, 284, 301, 304, 490
Nguyen, Peter 199
Nintendo WiiFit 329, 492
Norcross, John 462
NORCs (naturally recurring retirement communities) 258, 483
Northwestern Mutual 235
Nursebot 326
nursing home 63, 80, 129, 206, 228, 236, 237, 253–278, 285, 327, 337–341, 355–358, 361, 370, 378, 475, 481, 484
nutrition 138, 205, 221, 257, 309–314, 353, 393, 401, 403, 407, 411, 469, 498
nutritional supplements xxii, 334, 401, 403

O

O'Connor, Sandra Day 206
O'Doherty, Jim 371
O'Neal Ryan 104, 105, 106
optimism, pessimism 145, 437, 439
Orlov, Laurie 324, 334
Osborn, Jim "Oz" 333

Osmond, Alan 5, 84–101, 143, 144, 357, 404, 409, 436, 492
Osmond, David 5, 84–101, 436, 492
Osmond, Suzanne 94, 143
Osmond, Valerie 85, 91, 143
over-the-counter (OTC) 306, 403, 484
OXO Good Grips 325
oxytocin 388, 440

P

palliative care 219–224, 363–372, 378, 484, 489, 490
PALS (Practical Assisted Living Solutions) 269, 497
Paralyzed Veterans of America 444
Parker Jewish Institute for Health Care and Rehabilitation 379
Parkinson's disease (PD) xi, 3, 7–21, 74, 80, 145, 204, 205, 210, 256, 262, 327, 331, 349, 355, 377, 437, 472, 474, 484, 493
   Bradykinesia 8, 474
Paro the robot 326, 491
Partner Healthcare's Center for Connected Health 305
patient advocate 290, 291, 299, 490
Patient Advocate Foundation 291, 490
Patient Directed Services Program 240
PBS 8, 117, 367
Peace Corps 376
Peete, Holly Robinson xi, 3, 6–21, 122, 139, 143, 150, 152, 163, 179, 212, 216, 312, 360, 377, 426, 459, 492
Peete, Rodney 9–12, 14, 16, 20, 143, 150, 212, 216
Perricone, Nicholas 407
personal emergency response systems (PERS) xxi, 263, 325, 483, 485
personal health record (PHR) 175, 290, 333, 446, 477, 485
Pet Partners 356, 358, 498
Pets for the Elderly Foundation 358, 498
pet therapy 355–358, 362, 472, 498
Pew Research Center 198
pharmacists, pharmacies 231, 249, 257, 290, 305, 306, 334, 346, 487
Philips Lifeline 329, 491
physical touch 410, 411
Pierce, David Hyde 377
Pipes, Lea 277
Points of Light Institute 377

Pollan, Tracy 145, 210
Pomerantz, Celia 361
Posit Science 246, 332, 492, 494
Post Traumatic Stress Disorder (PTSD) 124, 146, 162, 174, 175, 204, 212, 346, 422, 486
Powerful Tools for Caregivers 316, 498
Power of Attorney 59, 225, 226, 230, 232, 366, 472, 477, 485
prescriptions 249, 296–308, 330–333
Presto 305, 323, 331–334, 492
professional therapist 65, 66, 282, 375, 415
Project Sanctuary 351, 499
psychiatrist 200, 425, 428, 447
psychologist 186, 296, 359, 392, 393, 428, 447, 463

Q

Qualls, Sara Honn 296, 413, 423, 428, 444, 445

R

Radner, Gilda 371
Radsliff, Peter 305, 323, 334
RAND Corporation 405
raw food movement 92
Reagan, Nancy 34, 206, 262
Reagan, Ronald 34, 84, 191, 203, 204, 206, 438
RealAge Calculator 440
Rebuilding Together 255, 497
Red Cross 248, 339, 341, 342
Registered Financial Gerontologist (RFG) 237, 238, 242, 486
regrets 9, 36, 37, 415, 416
Relaxation Response 389, 393
ReMIND 381, 499
remote monitoring 293, 327, 328, 329, 330
respitality 262, 349
respite 38, 63, 83, 117, 169, 175, 212, 214, 253, 261, 262, 286, 316, 320, 349, 351, 353, 378–380, 411, 424, 486, 489
Richards, Denise 139
Right At Home 249, 259, 497
RingaDoc 290, 496
Rinna, Lisa 78
RLTV 23, 333
RN (registered nurse) 259, 347, 484, 486
Robertson, Pat 146

Robert Wood Johnson Foundation 274
Robinson, Matthew T. 8
Robots 322, 326, 327, 333, 491
Rogen, Seth 156
Roizen, Michael 438, 440
Romney, Ann 95, 357
Rosalynn Carter Institute for Caregiving at Georgia Southwestern State University 123, 424, 491
Rosenberg, Rabbi Arthur 369, 370, 374, 426
Rowe, Tim 323
Rubin, Gretchen 434
Russo, Francine 130

S

Sacks, Oliver 359
SAD (seasonal affective disorder) 404, 486
Safe Return® 282
SAGE (Services and Advocacy for LGBT Elders) 192–194, 284, 491
Sandwich Generation 3, 7, 8, 24, 137–139, 174, 198
Sapolsky, Robert 388, 389
SATH (Society for Accessible Travel & Hospitality) 345
Saunders, Charmaine 392
Schiavo, Terri 144, 366
Schlossberg, Caroline Kennedy 139
SecuraTrac 325, 347, 492
self-care xx, xxii, 126, 138, 319, 383–385, 424, 461
Seligman, Martin 435
SeniorBridge 293, 497
SeniorCare Society's Family Portal 446
Senior Helpers 497
setting limits 399, 401, 468
sex 107, 157, 192, 367, 390, 399, 401, 402, 410
Seymour, Jane 167
shabaz 273, 274
Sheik, Sherwin 286
shelter in place 340
Shields, Brooke 139
shingles 375
SHIP (State Health Insurance Assistance Program) 292, 487, 495
Shook, Loren 32, 271
Shriver, Maria 139
Shriver Report: A Woman's Nation Takes on Alzheimer's, The 26, 317
Shriver, Sargent 376

siblings ix, 13, 46, 57, 58, 88, 94, 124, 129, 130, 131, 151, 156, 161–163, 179, 181, 185, 187, 212, 215–217, 227, 230, 235, 236, 239, 311, 360, 363, 400, 417, 444, 453, 458
Silverado Senior Living 32, 112, 271, 356, 357, 372, 416, 441, 497
SilverRide 248, 494
Silvers & Fit 263
Silver Sneakers 263
SilversSummit Conference 334
Siskowski, Connie 48, 186, 187, 188
skilled nursing facility (SNF) 220, 229, 273, 339, 482, 487
Skype 289, 331, 492
sleep 27, 46, 69, 79, 117, 175, 205, 307, 340, 360, 392, 393, 399–403, 427, 438, 440, 473, 481, 496
Small, Dr. Gary 74, 398, 405
SmartSlippers 329
SmartStart 12
smile, smiling 34, 116, 130, 331, 358, 414, 418, 434, 437, 441, 459, 462, 465
Smith, Ian K. 441, 442
Snap for Seniors 276, 497
Snelling, Jim 247
Snyderman, Nancy 291
Social Security 28, 128, 225, 227, 232, 234, 235, 239, 317, 478, 487
social worker 31, 213, 220, 223, 224, 285, 298, 300, 363, 371, 447, 474
Society for Human Resources Management (SHRM) 316, 494
Society of Actuaries (SOA) 234
Solie, David 293, 415, 442, 454, 455, 458
Sorensen, Caroline 311
Special Care Unit (SCU) 271, 486
special needs child 8, 11, 13–15, 149–152, 216, 280, 283, 361, 368, 410, 422
spirituality 50, 104, 113, 198–200, 369, 441
spousal refusal 237, 242
SSRI (selective serotonin reuptake inhibitor) 428, 487
SSR (special service request) 348
Stern, Charlotte 291
Stewart, Alana xi, 5, 102–117, 146, 192, 298, 350, 375, 395, 436, 492
Stewart, Martha 263, 264, 497
Stowe, Madeleine 187

stress xxii, 66, 76, 112, 124, 125, 129, 132, 133, 138, 145, 146, 162, 163, 174, 186, 193, 200, 212, 223, 259, 282, 307, 308, 313, 316–318, 326, 346, 356, 358, 360, 375–377, 383, 384, 387–393, 396, 400, 403–405, 407–410, 422, 425, 435–438, 440, 441, 453, 455, 458, 461, 463, 469, 485, 486, 496
stretching 408
Summitt, Pat 203
sunshine 92, 263, 399, 401, 403, 404, 421, 427, 439, 486
super foods 313, 406
support groups 81, 186, 211–214, 282, 285, 316, 318, 352, 376, 378, 379, 397, 415, 428, 441, 443, 444, 447, 458, 468, 492
survivor guilt 417
Susan G. Komen for the Cure 42, 49, 444, 493
Swayze, Lisa Niemi 146

T

Tabsafe 305, 492
Tai chi 257, 263, 395, 396
taxes, caregiver tax credits 122, 239, 242
technology xxi, xxii, 122, 128, 175, 244, 246, 263, 267, 273, 288, 304, 305, 308, 321–336, 367, 379, 445, 483, 485, 491
telehealth 289, 328, 483, 487
telemedicine 279, 280, 288–290, 294, 488
Telikin 331, 333, 492
Tenebaum, Louis 256, 265–268
Texas Instruments 329
Thomas, William 274
Thomson, Andy 425
Thoreau, Henry David 426, 427
Thurston, Catherine 192–194
transgender 191, 193, 284, 319, 479, 481
Transition Network, The 379, 498
traumatic brain injury (TBI) 124, 146, 162, 174, 175, 381, 487
travel 37, 56, 76, 77, 79, 82, 96, 114, 176, 225, 244, 325, 342, 345–351, 353, 499
treated and streeted 304
TSA (Transportation Security Administration) 75–77, 82, 346
Tucker, Michael 4, 54–69, 143, 155, 212, 225, 259, 274, 275, 346, 436, 456

U

United Cerebral Palsy of America 262, 349, 493
UnitedHealthcare 293, 327, 377
United Hospital Fund 61, 194, 220, 221, 226, 284, 298, 304, 306, 490
universal design 255, 256, 265–268, 324, 325, 330
USC Center for the Digital Future 128, 321, 492
U.S. Census Bureau 121, 127, 131, 186, 268
U.S. Department of Education 297
U.S. Department of Health and Human Services 229, 282, 284, 299, 339, 477
U.S. Department of Homeland Security 340
U.S. Department of Labor 235
U.S. Equal Employment Opportunity Commission 318

V

vacations 56, 228, 261, 345, 349, 353, 379
VA (Department of Veteran's Affairs) 175, 350, 380, 381, 488, 495, 499
Van Cauter, Eve 402
veterans 59, 124, 146, 156, 157, 162, 173–176, 212, 213, 225, 255, 258, 284, 350, 351, 380, 381, 444, 479, 488, 495, 499
VibrantNation.com 333, 492
video chat 288, 289, 328, 331, 487
Vieira, Meredith 122, 143, 144
Vietnam Veterans of America 284, 444, 488
Village Movement 168, 257, 258, 279, 497
Visiting Nurses Association 259, 497
visualization 394
Vitality 304, 323, 491
Vitamin D *(also Vit D)* 92, 263, 404, 406, 427, 439
volunteer 168, 248, 249, 255, 257, 258, 262, 269, 276, 292, 310, 311, 320, 332, 350, 358, 366, 371, 376–381, 411, 426, 441, 445, 446, 468, 474, 486, 488, 499
Volunteer Match 499
VSOs (veterans service organizations) 284, 380, 488

W

Walker, Susan Ayers 323, 324, 325
walking x, 8, 31, 52, 69, 72, 79, 90, 96, 115, 280, 322, 325, 338, 346, 356, 391, 394, 408, 417, 439, 441, 444, 464, 472

Wartorn documentary 174
WebMD 288, 388, 401, 406, 461
weight management (gain, loss) 312, 404, 408
Weil, Andrew 200, 422, 427, 461
well spouse 237
Well Spouse Foundation 491
Weng, Suzy 199
West Nile virus 88, 89
Willing Hearts, Helpful Hands 379
Wilson, Lynn 77, 78
Winner, Steve 271, 357
Wiseman, Richard 463
WomanSage 351, 379, 498
Women for a Secure Retirement (WISER) 234, 235, 238, 494
Wounded Warrior Project 284, 352, 380, 444, 488, 499

Y

yoga 52, 69, 93, 117, 393, 395, 396, 397, 436
Young@Heart documentary 360

Z

Zarfarlotfi, Susan 401
Zeer, Darrin 397
Zeta-Jones, Catherine 423, 424, 456
Zukav, Gary 434